Essentials of Pediatric Cataract Surgery

Sudarshan Kumar Khokhar
Chirakshi Dhull
Editors

Essentials of Pediatric Cataract Surgery

Springer

Editors
Sudarshan Kumar Khokhar
Professor Ophthalmology
Dr. RP Centre for Ophthalmic Sciences
All India Institute of Medical Sciences
New Delhi
India

Chirakshi Dhull
Eye Q Hospital
Rohtak
Haryana
India

ISBN 978-981-16-0211-5 ISBN 978-981-16-0212-2 (eBook)
https://doi.org/10.1007/978-981-16-0212-2

This Springer imprint is published by the registered company Springer Nature Singapore Pte Ltd.
The registered company address is: 152 Beach Road, #21-01/04 Gateway East, Singapore 189721, Singapore

Contents

About the Editors

Sudarshan Kumar Khokhar is currently working as Professor and Head at Dr. Rajendra Prasad Centre for Ophthalmic Sciences, All India Institute of Medical Sciences (AIIMS), New Delhi, India. He has more than 20 years of clinical, teaching, and research experience at AIIMS, with particular expertise in pediatric cataracts and complicated adult cataracts. He is a well-published author with over 80 publications in peer-reviewed journals and numerous book chapters. Over the last decade Professor Khokhar has offered instruction courses on pediatric cataracts at various national and international conferences, e.g., for the American Academy of Ophthalmology (AAO), European Society of Cataract and Refractive Surgeons (ESCRS), Asia-Pacific Academy of Ophthalmology (APAO), World Ophthalmology Congress (WOC), and American Association for Pediatric Ophthalmology and Strabismus (AAPOS). Professor Khokhar has designed a special cannula—Khokhar's capsular painting cannula—for phacoemulsification in white cataracts and was a pioneer in using the plasma blade in persistent fetal vasculature (PFV) eyes. He has received many achievement awards from international bodies, including the APAO and AAO.

Chirakshi Dhull is currently working as a Consultant for Eye Q India. She has previously worked as Senior Resident in cataract and refractive surgery at Dr. Rajendra Prasad Centre for Ophthalmic Sciences, All India Institute of Medical Sciences (AIIMS), New Delhi. A postgraduate from AIIMS, she has over 50 publications in peer-reviewed journals and book chapters to her credit. She has previously served as an editor for two textbooks in ophthalmology. She was awarded the prestigious G Venkataswamy Gold Medal in Ophthalmology in 2017. She received ET SELVAM Award from All India Ophthalmological Society in 2020. She has presented papers at both national and international conferences, including the American Academy of Ophthalmology (AAO), World Society of Pediatric Ophthalmology and Strabismus (WSPOS), European Society of Cataract and Refractive Surgeons (ESCRS), Asia-Pacific Academy of Ophthalmology (APAO), and Asia-Pacific Glaucoma Congress (APGC).

List of Videos

Part I

Management of Pediatric Cataract

Preoperative Evaluation and Investigative Modalities in Pediatric Cataract

1

Amber Bhayana, Chirakshi Dhull, and Sudarshan Kumar Khokhar

1.1 Introduction

There are no substitutes to thorough history and careful clinical examination while planning for any surgery and pediatric cataract is no different. Preoperative evaluation should be performed keeping the differential diagnoses in mind. Questions like cause of the cataract, whether to operate, when to operate, and how to operate should be answered by the preoperative examination. Preoperative biometry and deciding the postoperative target refraction are challenging in children but essential to decide details of intraocular lens implantation.

Pediatric cataract is a major preventable cause of childhood blindness across the world with prevalence being more common in developing countries [1]. The adjusted annual age-specific incidence of new diagnosis of congenital and infantile cataract has been reported to be 2.49 per 10,000 children in first year of age, around 3.18 per 10,000 in cumulative 5 years, and increasing to 3.46 per 10,000 by 15 years. Incidence of bilateral cataract was noted to be higher than that of unilateral [2]. Most common causes in Indian setting are developmental and posttraumatic, other being cataracts with retinal detachment, persistent fetal vasculature, subluxated/dislocated lens, uveitic cataracts, spherophakia, etc. Developmental cataract was seen in 45.6% and posttraumatic cataract in 29.7% of pediatric patients less than 14 years of age in Indian population [3]. Pediatric cataracts need to be timely treated surgically in order to prevent amblyopia and blindness.

1.2 History

A pediatric eye preoperative evaluation requires specialized techniques of history taking and examination as many of the times the child himself is not very cooperative nor can express him/herself. Communication with children is an art in which the examiner has to be patient, friendly, and in synchrony with the child's psychology which will vary according to the age. The toddlers are the sort difficult to examine. One should create a warm and friendly atmosphere for the child to be comfortable in.

A detailed medical history should include his basic information—name, age, gender, date of birth, height, weight, and if required head circumference, arm span, upper segment, lower segment ratio significance of which will be described later. Major symptoms as noticed by the parents

A. Bhayana · S. K. Khokhar (✉)
Professor Ophthalmology, Dr. RP Centre for Ophthalmic Sciences, All India Institute of Medical Sciences, New Delhi, India

C. Dhull
Eye Q Hospital, Rohtak, Haryana, India

S. K. Khokhar, C. Dhull (eds.), *Essentials of Pediatric Cataract Surgery*,
https://doi.org/10.1007/978-981-16-0212-2_1

include leukocoria or more commonly what they call as white spots in the black part of eye, strabismus, abnormal ocular movements, or delayed visual milestones. Parents often notice the child falling frequently and getting hurt, keeping objects too close to face, reading at a very short distance, sitting too close to the television, rubbing eyes too frequently, or photophobia. Diminution of vision might be reported by the child himself mature enough to notice or pointed out by teachers regarding poor vision in school going children. The child may also be referred by some primary physician who might have noticed cataract in the first place or as a part of routine eye examination following eye trauma. History of present illness includes when first the present complaint was noticed, other coexisting ocular anomalies, how it has progressed, and associated systemic symptoms.

Past medical history includes records of previous ocular examinations, any medical or surgical treatment history (like any surgery for glaucoma or retinopathy of prematurity), any history of laser intervention, and any drug allergies. All treatment history including oral, topical ophthalmic, and topical dermatological medications should be documented to rule out drug induced cataracts.

Antenatal history is as important and includes the age of mother at the time of conception, nature of conception whether it was spontaneous or assisted, history of any gestation-related disorders like gestational diabetes, or pregnancy-induced hypertension group of diseases, any history of maternal infections like TORCH (toxoplasma, cytomegalovirus, rubella, herpes), history of exposure to X-ray, CT scan or any other ionizing radiations, history of exposure to any teratogenic drugs, or other risk factors like smoking, alcohol, etc. Mother should be inquired about infections or exanthematous fever episodes during her antenatal period as first trimester rubella infection is a common cause of congenital cataracts in developing nations. These children require a detailed systemic evaluation to rule out other systemic involvements (Table 1.1).

Table 1.1 Suggested workup for an infant with suspected Rubella syndrome

Maternal history	Exanthemotous fever during antenatal period
Common clinical features in child	Microphthalmos
	Iris atrophy, iritis, iris hypoplasia
	Posterior synechiae
	Congenital cataract
	Pigmentary retinopathy
Investigations	IgM and IgG titers
	Detection of virus
	Polymerase chain reaction
	Cardiology opinion and echocardiography to rule out cardiac anomalies
	Brainstem evoked response audiometry to rule out sensorineural hearing loss

Perinatal history includes period of gestation at birth, route of delivery whether normal vaginal, Cesarean section or forceps assisted, history of delayed cry or asphyxia, and any history of hospital admission.

About one-third of children with congenital cataracts have positive family history. Siblings and parents should always be screened in cases of non-traumatic congenital or developmental cataracts and pedigree chart for at least three generations documented. Genetic workup is warranted in presence of positive family history. Even in sporadic cases, genetic mutations might be involved, most common of which are five nucleotide variations: CRYBA4:p.Y67N, CRYBB1:p.D85N, CRYBB1:p.E75K, CRYBB1:p.E155K, and GJA3:p.M1V [4]. Some of the inheritance patterns of the diseases are as shown in Table 1.2.

In cases of trauma, the history is usually obvious. Details about the mechanism will point toward whether it was an open or a closed globe injury. In open globe, a primary repair becomes essential. A rupture of the anterior or posterior lens capsule may alter the surgical plan as discussed later. In closed globe injury, subluxation of lens, angle recession, sphincter, or retinal tears are possible (Table 1.3).

Table 1.2 Inheritance patterns of cataracts [5]

Autosomal dominant	Autosomal recessive	X-linked recessive	X-linked dominant
Hyperferritenemia cataract syndrome	Congenital cataract fascial dysmorphism and neuropathy	Norrie disease	Hunnerman-Conradi syndrome
Coppock like cataract	Warburg micro syndrome	Nance–Horan syndrome	
Posterior polar cataract	Martsolf syndrome		
Zonular pulverulent cataract	Hallerman streiff syndrome		
Anterior polar cataract	Smith–Lemli–Opitz syndrome		
Cerulean type cataract			
Volkmann type congenital cataract			

Table 1.3 Approach to a child with leukocoria

1. Opacity anterior to lens	Peter's anomaly
	Corneal opacity
2. Lenticular opacity	Isolated cataract
	Complicated cataract
3. Opacity posterior to lens	Retinopathy of prematurity
	Retinal detachment
	Persistent fetal vasculature
	Vitreous hemorrhage
	Coat's disease
	Toxocariasis

Other positive systemic history may point toward a syndromic disorder. A thumb rule to keep in mind is that in cases of unilateral cataracts suspect something wrong in the eye itself, whereas in cases of bilateral cataracts some systemic or genetic disorder might be the culprit. It should also be remembered that many seemingly unilateral cataracts are actually asymmetrically bilateral. It would be useful here to go through the etiology of cataract in children in Table 1.4.

Table 1.4 Etiology of cataract in children

Bilateral cataracts	Unilateral cataracts
Idiopathic	Idiopathic
Hereditary cataracts (Autosomal dominant inheritance is commonest)	Ocular anomalies—persistent fetal vasculature, anterior segment dysgenesis, posterior lenticonus, posterior pole tumors
Genetic and metabolic diseases—Down syndrome, Lowe syndrome, galactosemia, Marfan's syndrome, trisomy 13–15, hypoglycemia, Alport syndrome, myotonic dystrophy, Fabry disease, hypoparathyroidism	Traumatic
Maternal infection—rubella, cytomegalovirus, varicella, syphilis, toxoplasmosis	Rubella
Ocular anomalies—aniridia, anterior segment dysgenesis	Asymmetric bilateral cataract
Corticosteroid induced	

1.3 Examination

Babies who have not yet developed neck holding can be examined in mother's lap. Those with neck holding are most comfortable in shoulder hold as shown in the Fig. 1.1 [6]. This position increases the area of contact with the mother and the child is at ease. Children older than 3–4 years can be assessed on slit lamp. Children with age less than 1 year can still be tried for an examination under slit lamp using assistance from parents where they hold the baby under the armpits with head leaning forward over the examining strap of the slit lamp biomicroscope [7].

1.3.1 Vision Assessment in Children

Children can verbalize what they understand from what they see. That makes vision assess-

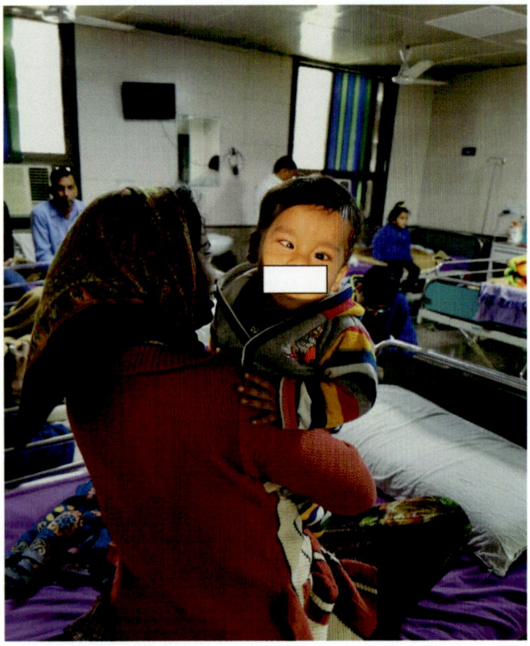

Fig. 1.1 Shoulder hold position to examine the child

ment in them equally tactful. Child's willingness to cooperate and his intelligence and visual function vary significantly with age and accordingly the methods to assess them have to be tailor made.

The most basic form of vision assessment is seen by analyzing "fixation" of the child. The child is asked to look at a visually catchy object placed at a distance of 25–30 cm which can be a pen, a torchlight, or a colorful toy. It is observed if the child can visually fix on the object and follow it in all directions. Test should be done both monocularly and binocularly. A normal response should be that the child is able to "fix" and "follow" the object. Alternatively he can be described to have a central, steady, and maintained fixation that is the child should be able to look at a fixating target without any involuntary or wandering eye movements and should be able to follow it in all directions without any squint or nystagmus [8]. Another examining technique is to cover alternate eyes and look for change in response. The child will stay cooperative as long as the uncovered eye has well fixating vision and will defy occlusion of his only normal seeing eye.

For preverbal children the following tests can be used: (1) Catford drum test [9] uses a motor driven drum with black dots of different sizes on a white background projected through a central aperture measuring 4 × 6 cm. The drum can be rotated right to left or vice versa. The patient is seated at 60 cm and asked to fixate on the moving dot. The visual acuity is indicated by the smallest dot which doesn't produce optokinetic nystagmus in the patient [10]. (2) Teller acuity cards are based on preferential looking. It is a semi-quantitative assessment of visual acuity. It measures the spatial contrast sensitivity. It has alternating black and white stripes against a blank background. A couple of the black and white stripes comprise a cycle and the maximum detectable cycles per degree of visual angle gives the measure of visual acuity. Preference of the child to look at gratings (indicated by the child's head position and reaction) of alternating black and white stripes of maximum detectable frequency rather than a plain background forms the basis of the test. The child is first presented with thickest stripes followed by thin stripes successively. (3) Electrophysiological tests for vision assessment include visual evoked response (VER), electroretinogram (ERG), and electro-oculogram (EOG) which have the advantage of being non-contact, noninvasive, and objective. These tests are not a function of media clarity and are dependent solely on the retina, nerve, and cerebral function. Visual evoked response detects potential generated in the cerebral cortex in response to light stimulation. They are good predictors of vision gain postsurgery. (4) Pupillary response is another indirect method to detect vision where an equal and brisk response grossly suggests normal visual pathway. A normal direct response indicates a normal afferent pathway (optic nerve) and a normal efferent pathway (oculomotor nerve parasympathetic) of the same eye. A normal consensual response means a normal afferent pathway of the other eye and a normal efferent pathway of the same eye. Any absolute or relative defect as compared to the other eye should be documented and is the simplest way to quantify nerve function. This test is

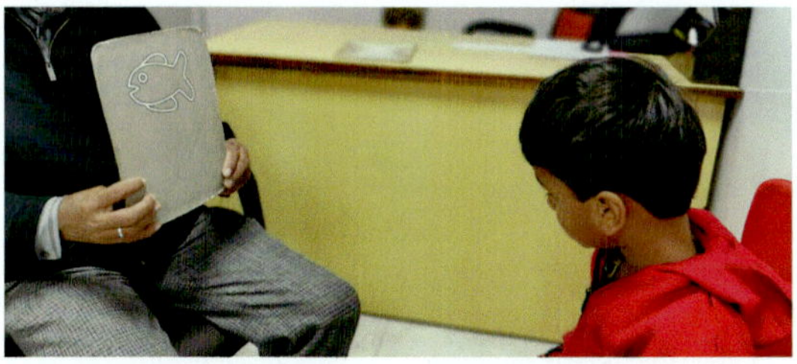

Fig. 1.2 Vision assessment using Cardiff acuity cards

independent of media opacity and solely depends on retina and nerve function.

For preschool children (about 2 years of age) following can be used: (1) Cardiff acuity cards (Fig. 1.2) based on the principle of vanishing optotypes where pictures are drawn of the same size but are drawn with black lines with white space of varying width so that they disappear at particular distance. It is performed at a distance of 50 cm for 0–12 months and at a distance of 100 cm for 12–24 months. The visual acuity corresponding to the thinnest detectable optotype is assigned. (2) Boeck candy test, where the child is offered candies of different sizes and guided to his/her mouth; smallest detectable candy being a measure of visual acuity. (3) Worth's ivory ball test, where balls of different sizes are rolled across the floor; the smallest ball which the child can retrieve is a measure of visual acuity. (4) Similarly, in Sheridan's ball test fixation on rolling balls is assessed. (5) In STYCAR (screening tests for young children and retards), child is asked to name the shown toy or pick up its miniature form from the stock.

For ages more than 5 years Tumbling E, Landolt's C charts can be used and Snellen's thereafter [11, 12].

Table 1.5 summarizes different methods to assess visual acuity in different ages.

Table 1.5 Different methods to assess visual acuity in different ages

Preverbal children	Pupillary reflexes
	Visual evoked response
	Optokinetic nystagmus
	Teller's acuity
	Pattern of fixation
1–2 years of age	Worth's ivory ball test
	Boeck's candy test
	Screening test for the young children and retards
	Cardiff's acuity test
2–3 years of age	Miniature toy test
	Coin test
	LEA Symbols
3–5 years of age	Allen's picture card
	Lippman's HOTV test, letter test
>5 years of age	Tumbling E
	Landolt's broken ring
	Snellen's chart
	LogMAR chart

1.3.2 Ocular Movements

Nystagmus usually develops in children with visually significant cataracts with onset before 3 months of age because the media opacity prevents the fixation reflex from developing which is likely to persist even after media clarity is restored. Best corrected vision in such patients is seldom better than 20/100 posttreatment. Similarly wandering eye movements and ocular deviation are generally associated with poor prognosis. Presence of strabismus indicates chronicity in cataracts [8]. Tendency of the eye to go into esodeviation or exodeviation depends on the tone of medial recti and refractive status of the other eye. Assessment of squint/nystagmus can be done by torch light examination visualizing the corneal reflex and cover uncover tests. A video recording can be done preoperatively to document ocular movements and compared postoperatively. Nystagmus sometimes may improve post-surgery however parents should be explained about the guarded prognosis [8, 13, 14].

1.3.3 Oculo-Digital Phenomenon

Infants with gross visual deprivation as in dense cataracts are seen to poke their fingers in the groove between their brow and eyeball which

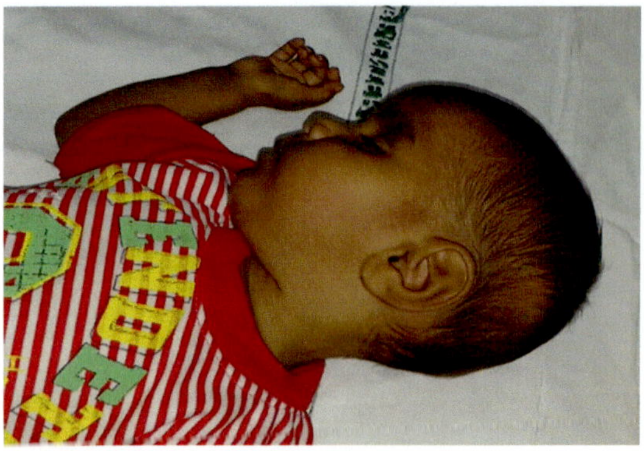

Fig. 1.3 Child with orbital fat atrophy secondary to excessive oculo-digital phenomenon

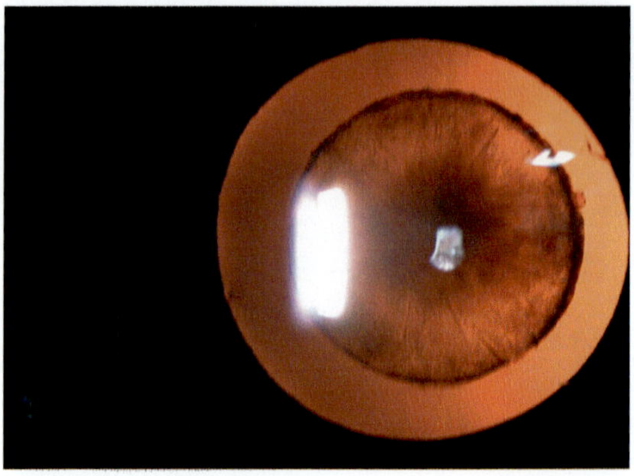

Fig. 1.4 Bruckner test showing OD esotropia with cataractous lens, OS clear lens

is hypothesized to stimulate their retinal photoreceptors so as to have some perception of light in the form of flashes. Such children are seen to have loss of orbital fat with deep set globes with poor fixation, wandering eye movements, all indicating poor visual prognosis (Fig. 1.3) [15].

1.3.4 Pupils

Pupils should be examined before dilation. Size, shape, interocular symmetry should be documented. Signs of blunt trauma like sphincter tears, iridodialysis should be looked for in respective cases. Direct and consensual responses should be checked and any relative afferent pupillary defect should be carefully looked for; if present indicates neuronal damage.

1.3.5 Red Reflex Test

Distant direct ophthalmoscopy enables assessment of the red glow of the eye which is sensitive for detection of visual-axis opacities, refractive errors, anisometropia, and strabismus (Bruckner's test) (Fig. 1.4). It is a handy and useful test which can be used in the most uncooperative of children [16–19]. It may be done after mydriasis or prior to it in a dark room.

1.3.6 Anterior Segment Examination

Evaluation of anterior segment can be done on slit lamp biomicroscope if the child allows or with torch light. Any doubt should warrant an examination under sedation or anesthesia. Lid and adnexa should be thoroughly checked for any discharge, nasolacrimal duct obstruction, blepharitis, or any other foci of active infection. Corneal opacities, abnormalities of anterior chamber, iris, and pupil should be documented. Micro-ophthalmos and typical colobomas are frequently associated. The form of cataract or rather any abnormality can be documented using slit lamp photography which can be repeated to see real-time progression, can serve as a teaching tool and also be used to council the parents regarding the disease.

1.3.6.1 Lens Examination

Location and type of the opacity in the crystalline lens may help in morphological classification and etiology (Table 1.6 and Figs. 1.5, 1.6, 1.7, 1.8, and 1.9) [20]. On the basis of etiology, cataracts can be classified as shown in Table 1.2 [21].

Bilateral zonular ones are most commonly sporadic/developmental. Unilateral cataracts may be post trauma, iatrogenic post-surgery

Table 1.6 Morphological classification of pediatric cataract based on location of the opacity

Whole lens	Central	Anterior	Posterior	Miscellaneous
Total	Lamellar/ zonular	Anterior polar: (a) dot like (b) plaque like (c) pyramidal	Posterior polar	Oil droplet
Congenital morgagnian	Nuclear	Anterior subcapsular	Posterior subcapsular	Wedge shaped
Membranous/partially absorbed	Central pulverulent	Anterior lenticonus	Posterior lenticonus	Coralliform
	Ant egg			Floriform
	Cerulean cataract			Dandelion like
	Cortical			Starry Sky cataract
	Sutural			Stud button
				Reduplicated cataract
				Linear opacities
				Crystalline
				Nodular
				Stem of cactus
				Barbed fence-like cataract

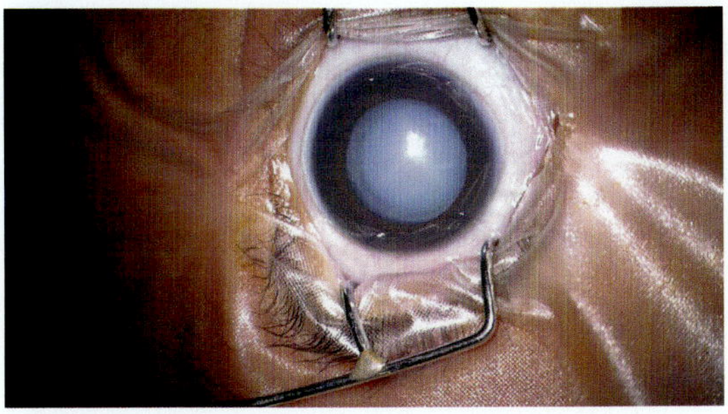

Fig. 1.5 Zonular cataract

(such as after trabeculectomy [22] and retinopathy of prematurity (ROP) [23] surgeries), post injection in ROP; most commonly posterior subcapsular variants. Traumatic cataracts can be post closed globe injury or more commonly post open globe injuries (Fig. 1.10) [24]. Total cataracts may be present in chromosomal anomalies or metabolic disorders. Bilateral posterior subcapsular cataract (PSCs) may indicate chronic steroid intake. Poorly dilating pupils with partially absorbed cataract and posterior synechiae in a microphthalmic eye may indicate rubella.

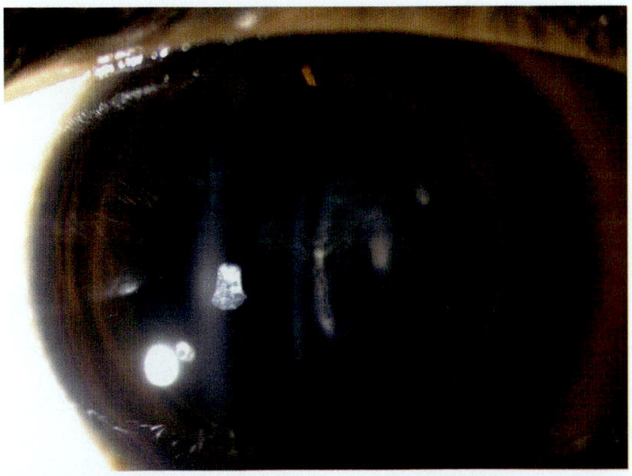

Fig. 1.6 Total white cataract

Children with complicated cataract secondary to uveitis may be have active cells in anterior chamber, band shaped keratopathy, posterior synechiae. Flattening of anterior curvature of the lens may indicate loss of volume of the lens due to posterior capsular rupture which may be picked up on slit lamp biomicroscopy as "fish-tail" sign or on ultrasound B-scan and ultrasound biomicroscopy.

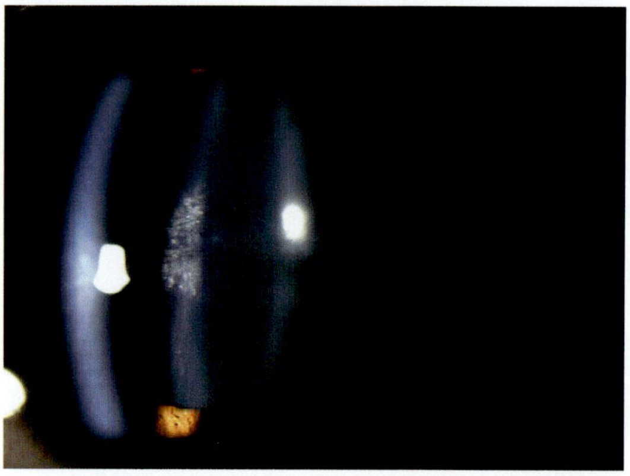

Fig. 1.7 Sutural cataract

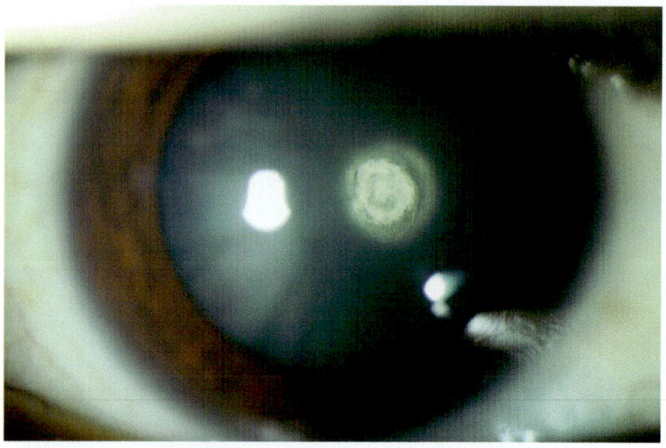

Fig. 1.8 Anterior capsular cataract

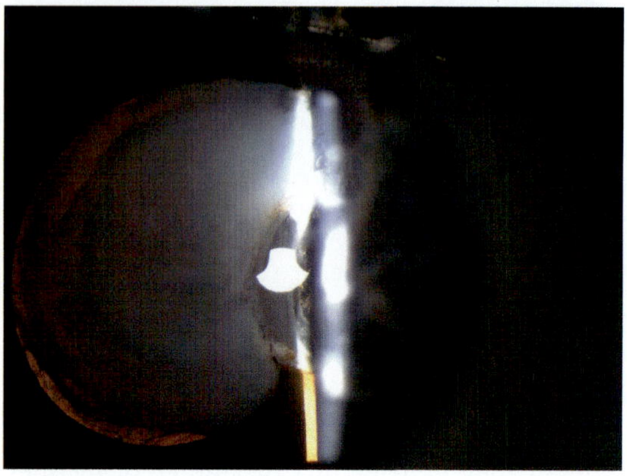

Fig. 1.9 Posterior polar cataract

Cataracts which cause significant obstruction to fundal glow and opacities greater than 3 mm in the visual axis need to be operated. Lenticular

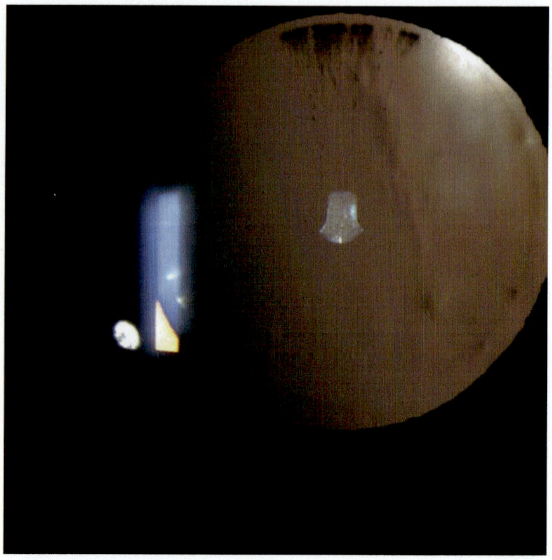

Fig. 1.10 Cataract post corneal perforation

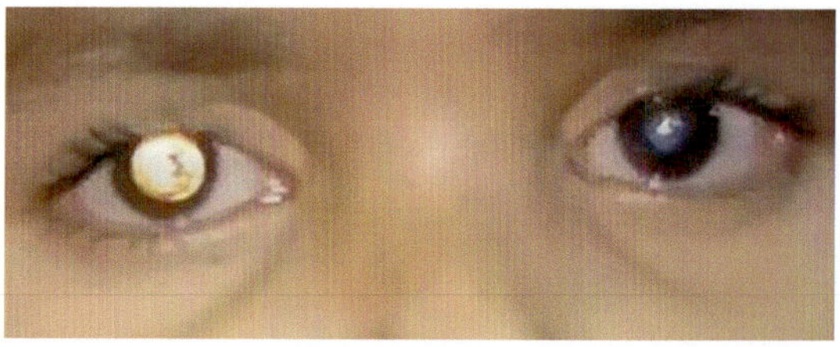

Fig. 1.11 Visually insignificant cataract

opacities in the periphery not causing hindrance to visual axis can simply be observed over time (Fig. 1.11).

Persistent pupillary membrane might be a coexisting finding which is indicative of remnant fetal lenticular vasculature found attached at the collarette.

1.3.7 Intraocular Pressure Measurements

Pediatric cataract eyes with cataract may be associated with preoperative or postoperative pseudophakic glaucoma. Rubella cataracts, post-traumatic, and uveitic cataracts may also be associated with raised IOP. Intraocular pressure documentation before surgery is of paramount importance both in terms of preoperative control of glaucoma and also for prognosticating the outcome, depending on the optic nerve status. In this regard, preoperatively, Perkins tonometer may be used during examination under general anesthesia. It can also be done with non-contact tonometer or tonopen which is useful in cases of corneal opacity.

1.3.8 Posterior Segment Examination

Fundus examination with indirect ophthalmoscope is essential to rule out any posterior segment anomaly that may prevent the child from gaining vision even after a successful cataract surgery. Indirect ophthalmoscopy with scleral indentation is the gold standard if the child and media clarity allow. If view of the retina is not possible, ultrasound B-scan should be done to rule out vitreous hemorrhage/exudates, retinal detachment persistent fetal vasculature or any intraocular mass in posterior segment.

1.3.9 Examination Under Anesthesia

Anesthesia is warranted in children uncoopearative enough to not allow any examination. It starts with examining the child under operating microscope for complete anterior segment starting from cornea upto the back of lens and if media permits the fundus as well using indirect ophthalmoscopy. Any corneal scar needs to be noted with special attention to pupillary membranes which may indicate a form of persistent vasculature. A snapshot can be taken during video recording of the examination to maintain a documentation of the same. White to white corneal diameter is measured using manual or digital callipers. A small white to white is an indirect indicator of small lens bag size and will be a contraindication to IOL implantation. Keratometry is measured using a portable autorefractor-keratometer. Axial length of the eye is measured using A-scan ultrasonography. Posterior segment can be assessed in cases of significant media opacity using ultrasound B-scan to rule out retinal detachment, retinoblastoma, or any other pathology. Ultrasound biomicroscopy of the anterior segment with water bath can be done to get a status of lens such as size and shape of the lens, any subluxation, any plaque on the anterior and posterior capsule, any specs of calcification, any evidence of lens volume loss as in partially absorbed cataract, any evidence of opening of the anterior or posterior capsule or presence of anterior or posterior capsular plaque.

1.4 Investigations

1. Majority of the cataracts are idiopathic in nature and don't require any investigation as such, but it is always better to keep this as a diagnosis of exclusion. A child having cataract with hepatomegaly with jaundice should be suspected for galactosemia and investigated for urinary reducing substance and enzyme levels for galactokinase, galactose1-phosphate uridyl transferase. For suspected infectious etiology like rubella, immunoglobulin levels are warranted along with polymerase chain reaction targeted toward other viruses in TORCH spectrum. Echocardiography is required to rule out cardiac anomalies in rubella which might also be present in cases of Marfan's syndrome. The common anomalies encountered are atrial septal defects, patent ductus arteriosus, aortic root dilatation. In suspected cases of hypothyroidism, serum calcium and phosphorus levels need to be looked into. In patients with juvenile idiopathic arthritis-related cataracts, detailed rheumatology workup is warranted. Genetic testing is warranted in cases of hereditary cataracts.
2. Imaging:
   (a) Ultrasound B-scan
   Ultrasound B-scan is warranted in cases of significant media opacities where fun-

dus evaluation on indirect ophthalmoscopy is not possible as in cases with total cataracts or poorly dilating pupils to at least get an idea of what the posterior segment beholds. Retinal detachments (Fig. 1.12a), fundal colobomas (Fig. 1.12b), persistent fetal vasculature (Fig. 1.12c), or any mass in posterior segment like retinoblastoma or melanoma (Fig. 1.12d) can be easily picked up [25]. It is also used in very small children who are uncooperative.

(b) Ultrasound A on B-scan (axial length)
A vector modality over B-scan is used to take ocular measurements mainly of the axial length or can be used to measure intraocular dimension of any mass.

(c) **Ultrasound biomicroscopy** Ultrasound biomicroscopy (UBM) is used to image the anterior segment of an eye using higher frequencies of 35 MHz, and 50 MHz as compared to conventional USG. UBM can be used for ocular biometry including anterior chamber depth (ACD), lens thickness (LT), angle to angle (ATA), sulcus to sulcus (STS), and bag diameter (BD). With the increase in frequency, ocular penetration decreases. UBM can also be used preoperatively to assess the sulcus and assessment of anterior capsule for secondary intraocular lens (IOL). It is also used in evaluation of morphology of lens and detection of abnormalities like capsular plaque, posterior lenticonus, persistent fetal vasculature (PFV), bupthalmic eyes, etc. which helps in better planning and management. UBM may also help evaluate for subluxation, iridodialysis, cyclodialysis, foreign body localization in anterior segment, lens evaluation in corneal opacity, posterior capsular dehiscence and postoperative IOL centration and tilt.

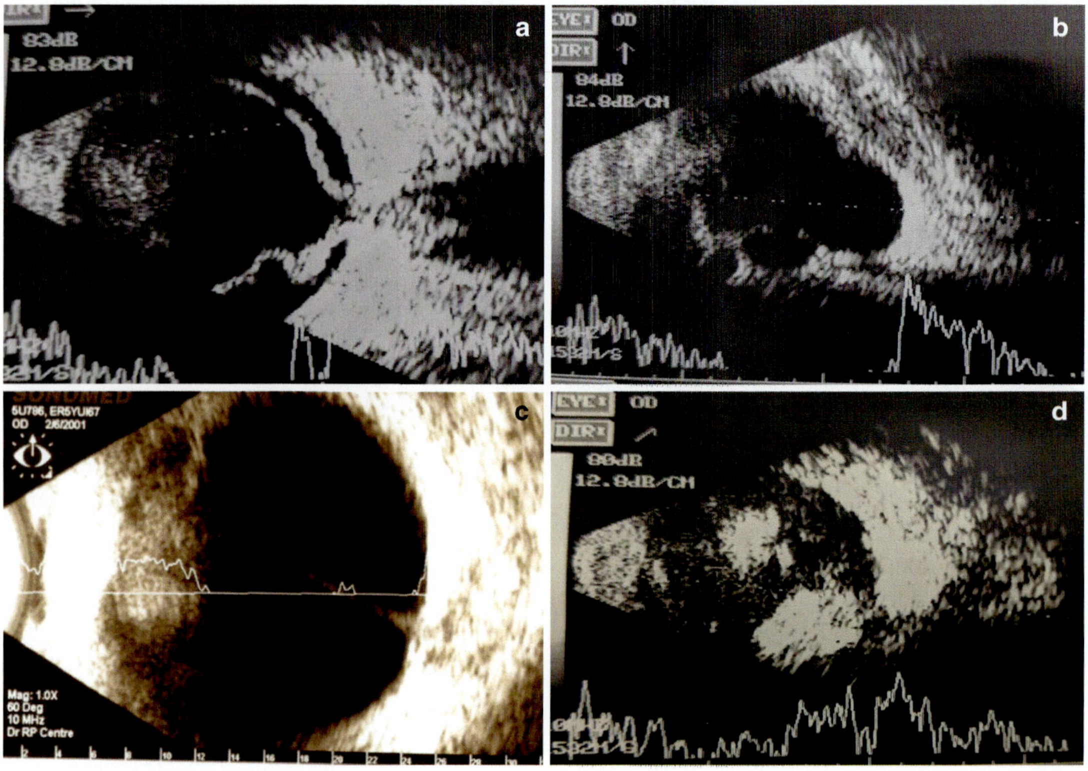

Fig. 1.12 Posterior segment ultrasound B-scan images showing: (**a**) Retinal detachment; (**b**) Fundal coloboma; (**c**) Persistent fetal vasculature; (**d**) Retinoblastoma. (Courtesy—Sudarshan Khokhar, Chirakshi Dhull, Springer Ltd.)

3. For anesthesia
   Complete blood counts with electrolytes are required as planning for any surgery under anesthesia. For too small children, hemoglobin, bleeding and clotting times with urine routine microscopy, and culture sensitivity can be a viable alternative. Targeted investigations like chest X-ray, ECG, and echocardiogram should be done in patients with diagnosed respective systemic disorders for preanesthetic fitness. A consultation from the respective specialist should be sought. A child with seizure will require antiepileptic dose modification for the perioperative and intraoperative period which has to be sought after by the treating neurologist. Final clearance is given by the anesthetist after complete systemic evaluation.

1.5 Surgical Planning

1. Biometry/IOL formulae/target post op refraction/considering aphakia in small eyes, younger age
   Axial length of the eye can be measured by ultrasound A-scan. When the probe is placed perpendicular to the eyeball parallel to its axis, the retina is picked up as a sharply rising echo spike. This is the contact method in which the probe may indent the cornea and may give falsely lower value of axial length. Another method is the immersion method in which a coupling fluid is used between the probe and the cornea.
   On the other hand, axial length measurement optically using partial coherence interferometry (as using IOLMaster, Carl Zeiss) is a non-contact, observer independent, reproducible, and more accurate method. But again, it can be used only for cooperative grown up kids making ultrasound under anesthesia just prior to surgery the only option in small and uncooperative kids.
   Keratometry can be measured using autorefractor-keratometers and portable ones for examination under anesthesia. Partial coherence interferometry utilizing machines (like IOLMaster, Carl Zeiss Meditec; and LenStar, Haag Streit) can be used wherever possible.
   Pediatric eyes are supposed to grow until their pre-programmed adult sizes are reached. If emmetropia is planned for the current surgery, every 1 mm growth will make the eye nearly 3 D more myopic. So an undercorrrection is performed while routinely planning for pediatric IOL power so as to make the eye closest to emmetropic after its growth has stabilized. But again there are conflicting reports in literature regarding which IOL formulae to use for calculation. Dahan et al. [26] proposed 20% reduction for children less than 2 years of age and 10% reduction for children between 2 and 8 years of age and emmetropic power thereafter. On the basis of axial length he proposed 22 D for 21 mm, 24 D for 20 mm, 26 D for 19 mm, 27 D for 18 mm, and 28 D for 17 mm. Enyedi et al. [27] proposed age (years) + post of refractive error (diopters) should be equal to 7.
   What we follow for our patients is 20% undercorrection for less than 6 months age, 15% for 6 months to 1 year, 10% for 1–2 years, 5% for 2–5 years, and emmetropic power thereafter. The less undercorrection in Indian pediatric eyes is justified by a study done by the authors in which growth rate in Indian eyes was found to be less than the western data [28]. We prefer not to put an implant if the axial length is less than 17 mm or white to white corneal diameter is less than 9 mm [21]. Secondary IOL implantation can be planned later on in these cases.
2. Delayed sequential/Simultaneous sequential
   The main advantage of simultaneous bilateral cataract surgeries include medical benefits like preoperative care and medications, hospitalization and undergoing anesthesia only once; and social benefits like requiring lesser time from parents or relatives as it will require lesser follow ups saving costs. Risks include bilateral endophthalmitis and inability to evaluate refractive outcome after first eye surgery which can be later used to modify IOL power for the second eye [29]. At our center for the same rea-

son we routinely prefer second eye surgery after a gap of 3 days or later. Simultaneous surgeries can be planned for small infants where an intraocular implant is not planned for because here we don't have any IOL power to modify after evaluating refractive results of the first eye, plus it will give added advantage to children being exposed to anesthesia only once with systemic issues.

3. Preoperative regimen of oral/topical medication
   Preoperatively the children are started on 0.5% moxifloxacin eye drops in both eyes for perioperative antibiotic coverage 2 days prior to surgery. 2% homatropine hydrobromide are also instilled 1 day prior to surgery to keep pupil dilated. Non dilating pupils may require 1% atropine.
4. When to consider additional procedures like primary posterior capsulectomy, etc.
   One of the very common complications post pediatric cataract surgery is visual-axis opacification which occurs due to proliferation of remnant lens epithelial cells over the posterior capsule and/or vitreous scaffold. It occurs more commonly in children due to more proliferative tendencies on account of younger age. In such cases all our efforts to give a clear medium to the child to prevent amblyopia go in drain. Cooperative adults can easily undergo a laser capsulotomy to encounter the same. But a child will always require a second surgery under anesthesia. Thence came the importance of primary posterior capsulorhexis which we recommend in children upto 8 years of age; with limited anterior vitrectomy which we recommend in children upto 6 years of age. Size of the opening should be 4–4.5 mm about 1 mm smaller than anterior opening [21].

Options of IOLs (in brief)

Single piece lens are meant for single site: in the bag only. Multipiece IOL can be used at multiple sites: in the bag, sulcus with or without capture or scleral fixated. In the bag hydrophobic acrylic white lenses is one of the most common implantations done in cases of pediatric cataracts with/without posterior rhexis with good bag size. In cases of small bag size, complicated cases with extension of rhexis, inadvertent large posterior capsular opening, cases post trauma with good sulcus support a multipiece lens can be implanted in the sulcus whose optic can be captured behind the posterior capsular opening to enhance its stability. Cases with subluxation greater than 8 clock hours that can't be managed by capsular tension ring or cionni bag fixation, are usually planned for scleral fixation of a multipiece lens in cases not having connective tissue disorders with normal sclera or anterior chamber IOL and iris claw lens otherwise. The same options hold true for secondary IOL placement in cases left primarily aphakic with an additional choice of multipiece IOL placement in the sulcus in cases of good sulcus support.

1.6 Syndromic Associations

Down's syndrome (trisomy 21) is one of the most common genetic disorders having a wide range of ocular manifestations like mongoloid slant, esotropia, nystagmus, refractive errors and astigmatism, lacrimal duct obstruction, brushfield's spots on iris, keratoconus. Prevalence of cataracts in such patients varies from 4% to 37% [30].

Lowe's syndrome (oculocerebrorenal disorder) involves congenital cataracts (lenticonus—Fig. 1.13 or other forms) in children with mental retardation and renal dysfunction [31].

Congenital rubella syndrome involves microcephaly, sensorineural deafness, patent ductus arteriosus and ocular involvements some of

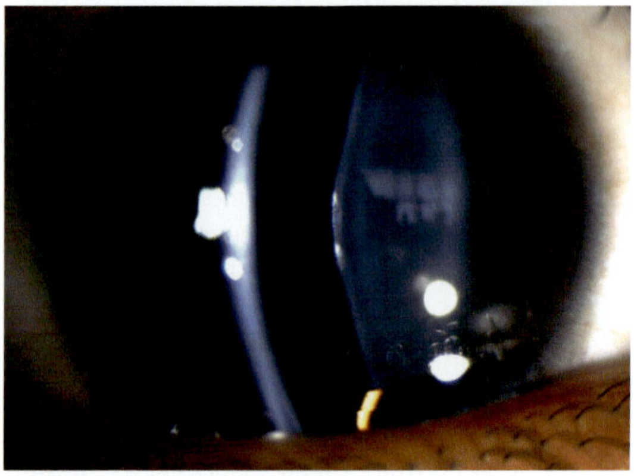

Fig. 1.13 Anterior lenticonus

which include membranous cataract with poorly dilating pupil, posterior synechiae, microphthalmos and salt and pepper retinopathy [32]. IgM and IgG titers should be sent for if suspected.

Cataract in an infant with hepatomegaly, failure to thrive and jaundice should raise suspicion for galactosemia and accordingly investigated (Tables 1.7 and 1.8) [35].

Table 1.7 Syndromic associations of cataract [33]

Syndrome	Genetic loci	Inheritance pattern	Phenotypic features
Autosomal recessive congenital infection-like syndrome (pseudo-TORCH syndrome)	USP18—22q11.21	AR	Microcephaly, intracranial calcification, congenital cataracts, clinical course resembles congenital TORCH infection
Cerebro-oculo-facio-skeletal syndrome (COFS)	ERCC6—10q11.23	AR	Microcephaly, congenital cataracts, microphthalmia, arthrogryposis (congenital joint contractures), rocker-bottom feet, severe developmental delay, growth failure, dysmorphism with prominent nasal root and overhanging upper lip
Rhizomelic chondrodysplasia punctata type 1	PEX7, 6q23.3	AR	Systemic shortening of proximal limb bones (i.e., rhizomelia), seizures, recurrent respiratory tract infections, congenital cataracts
Conradi–Hünermann–Happle syndrome (X-linked dominant chondrodysplasia punctata type 2)	Emopamil-binding protein (EBP) gene—Xp11.23-p11.22	XLD	Chondrodysplasia (rhizomelic type), growth retardation, frontal bossing, flat nasal bridge, down-slanting space between eyelids, cataracts (mostly sectoral), antimongoloid slant, asymmetrically short limbs, macrocephaly, patchy alopecia, scaly/flaky skin, ichthyosis, flexion deformities or spasms of interphalangeal joint, kyphosis or scoliosis, calcaneus valgus
Craniosynostosis-cataract syndrome	–	–	Severe craniosynostosis, bilateral nuclear cataracts, bifid nose-tip in the female offspring of nonconsanguineous parents
Cri-du-chat (cat cry) syndrome [13]	5p deletion most commonly	Sporadic, isolated cases	High shrill cry (cat cry), microcephaly, cataract, hypertelorism, round face, mental retardation, antimongoloid slant of palpebral fissures, epicanthic folds, anteverted pinnae, preauricular skin tags, prominent nasal bridge, micrognathia, muscular hypotony, congenital heart, and genitourinary defects
Czeizel Lowry syndrome CAMFAK (congenital cataracts, microcephaly, failure to thrive, and kyphoscoliosis)/CAMAK (cataract, microcephaly, arthrogryposis, and kyphosis) syndrome	–	AR	Microcephaly (with changes seen on CT scan of head), bilateral infantile cataracts, mental retardation and Perthes disease-like hip deformities, kyphoscoliosis, bird-like face

(continued)

Table 1.7 (continued)

Syndrome	Genetic loci	Inheritance pattern	Phenotypic features
Down's syndrome	21q22.3	Isolated cases	Flat occiput, flat facies, brachycephaly, epicanthal fold, flat nasal bridge, upslanting palpebral fissure, Brushfield spots, protruding tongue, small nose and mouth, diastasis recti, generous nuchal skin, short fifth finger with clinodactyly, single transverse palmar crease, sandal gap (wide space between first two toes), short, broad hands, short fifth middle phalanx, joint hyperflexibility, hypotonia, premature aging, dry skin, congenital heart defects, congenital or infantile cataracts (particularly cerulean blue dot cataract)
Early onset Cockayne syndrome	ERCC8 gene, 5q12.1	AR	Early cataracts, microcephaly, joint contractures, kyphosis, mental retardation, large ears, enophthalmos, prominent nasal
Edwards syndrome	Trisomy 18	Isolated cases	Aniridia, cataracts, microcephaly, microphthalmos, choanal atresia, small jaw, bullous nose
HEC syndrome [18] (Hydrocephalus, endocardial fibroelastosis, and cataract)	–	–	Communicating hydrocephalus, endocardial fibroelastosis and congenital cataracts
Hyperferritinemia-cataract syndrome	19q13.33, FTL gene	AD	Congenital nuclear cataract [19] (autosomal dominant inheritance), elevated serum ferritin levels
Hallermann–Streiff–Francois (oculomandibulofacial or Aubrey syndrome or Francois dyscephalic syndrome)	6q22.31, GJA1 gene	Autosomal recessive	Essential seven features: Craniofacial malformations and bird-like facies, abnormal dentition, hypotrichosis, skin atrophy (esp. on nose), microphthalmia, congenital cataract, proportionate dwarfism
Lowes/oculo-cerebro-renal syndrome	OCRL gene, Xq26.1	XLR	Triad of: congenital cataracts (can be posterior or anterior lenticonus or even other morphologies), neonatal/infantile hypotonia with mental retardation and renal tubular dysfunction. Other features: ocular keloid, rickets, osteopenia, osteomalacia, glaucoma, joint swelling, arthritis, tenosynovitis, growth parameters like weight and length fall below third percentile by 1–3 year age, delayed teeth eruption, teeth crowding, hypoplastic enamel, constricted palate. Carrier females may have snowflake-like opacities

Table 1.7 (continued)

Syndrome	Genetic loci	Inheritance pattern	Phenotypic features
Majewski syndrome (short rib polydactyly syndrome)	NEK1 gene, 4q23	AR	Lethal syndrome includes neonatal dwarfism, short ribs, polydactyly, cleft lip, epiglottic anomalies, oval-shaped tibia, ambiguous genitalia, cataracts, hypertelorism, colobomata, microphthalmos
Marinesco–Sjogren syndrome	5q31.2, SIL1 gene	AR	Cerebellar ataxia, mental retardation, short stature, congenital cataracts, muscle weakness, inability to chew food, thin brittle fingernails and sparse hair, hypergonadotropic hypogonadism, delayed psychomotor development, skeletal deformities
Martsolf syndrome	1q41, RAB3GAP2 gene	AR	Mental retardation, microcephaly, hypogonadism in siblings of consanguineous parents, cataracts
Menkes syndrome	Xq21.1, ATP7A gene	XLR	Kinky hair (Menkes kinky hair), severe mental retardation, bone and connective tissue lesions, pronounced cupid's bow to upper lip, hypothermia, cataracts
Nance–Horan syndrome (Mesiodens-cataract syndrome, NHS)	Xp22Xp22.2.13-Xp22.1, NHS gene	XLD	Congenital cataract in almost 100% cases (bilateral, dense, mostly total), microcornea, microphthalmos, dental anomalies (Hutchinsonian teeth, supernumerary teeth with impacted teeth), facial dysmorphism (long, narrow, often rectangular face, long chin, prognathism, large nose, narrow nasal bridge, large protruding ears), mental retardation (in 30%). Cataracts: bilateral, asymmetrical and predominantly posterior lens opacities. Carrier females (heterozygous) have posterior Y-sutural cataracts with small corneas
Norrie disease	Xp11.3 NDP gene	XLR	Early childhood blindness, retinal dysplasia, mental disorder, sensorineural deafness, cataracts
Pollitt syndrome (Trichothiodystrophy 1—Sulfur deficient hair)	ERCC2 gene, 19q13.32	AR	Sparse brittle body hair, ichthyosis, developmental delay, growth retardation, dysplastic nails, photosensitivity, xeroderma pigmentosum, eczema, microcephaly, recurrent infections, receding chin, protruding ears, conjunctivitis, nystagmus, hypoplastic genitalia, bilateral central nuclear cataracts

(continued)

Table 1.7 (continued)

Syndrome	Genetic loci	Inheritance pattern	Phenotypic features
Smith–Lemli–Opitz (SLO) syndrome	11q13.4, DHCR7 gene	AR	Microcephaly, broad nasal tip with anteverted nostrils, micrognathia, ptosis of eyelids, epicanthal folds, cataracts, broad maxillary alveolar ridges, slanted or low set ears, syndactyly of second and third toes, cleft palate, cardiac defects, cryptorchidism in males
RSH syndrome			

Source: From OMIM—Online Mendelian inheritance in man
AD autosomal dominant, *AR* autosomal recessive, *XLD* X-linked dominant, *XLR* X-linked recessive

Table 1.8 List of systemic and facial features giving clue to syndromes of congenital cataract [34]

Facial dysmorphism	Down's syndrome
	Hallermann–Streiff–Francois syndrome
	Lowe's oculocerebrorenal syndrome
	Nance–Horan syndrome
	Smith–Lemli–Opitz syndrome
	Martsolf syndrome
Short stature	Chondrodysplasiapunctata (Conradi–Hünermann syndrome)
	Marinesco–Sjogren syndrome
	Pollitt syndrome
	Martsolf syndrome
Microcephaly	COFS
	AR congenital infection-like syndrome
	Early onset Cockayne syndrome
	Cri-du-chat syndrome
	Czeizel Lowry syndrome
	Edwards syndrome
	Martsolf syndrome
Digital abnormalities	Majewski syndrome
	Smith–Lemli–Opitz syndrome
Dermatological issues	Conradi–Hünermann syndrome
	Pollitt syndrome
	Menkes syndrome
Hydrocephalus or skull deformities	HEC syndrome
	Craniosynostosis
	Martsolf syndrome

1.7 Parent Counseling

Counseling is perhaps the most important step while planning any surgery. Parents/guardians need to be clearly explained about the child's problem. Postoperative visual gain may be poor subject to amblyopia which may have set in due to long-term visual deprivation, and abnormality of the posterior segment whose assessment may not have been possible preoperatively. Parents have to be counseled regarding abnormal eye movements, long-term implications thereof, and that the child will be dependent on spectacles lifelong for distance as well as near vision. Parents should be ready to monitor their children's use of spectacles and also if need be occlusion therapy for amblyopia and timely follow up.

The counseling should include information regarding possibility of VAO, need for resurgery, future need for IOL exchange. Sibling screening should also be highlighted.

1.8 Rehabilitation

Surgery should be immediately followed by prescription of glasses and amblyopia therapy. The suture removal and repeat refraction is done at 1 month postoperatively and again at 3 months. Contact lenses are more suitable in children with unilateral aphakia as spectacles cause aniseikonia. According to the Infant Aphakia Treatment Study, primary IOL implantation and contact lens did not show a significant difference in terms of final visual acuity in infants <7 months of age. The children who had IOL implantation had more adverse events and required more reoperations to clear visual-axis opacities. Hence, the use of contact lens is a good alternate to IOL implantation in such children.

In younger children, glasses are prescribed for near. In school going children, executive bifocal glasses with near add are prescribed after correcting for distance. In children <12 months of age, occlusion is given where both eyes are occluded depending on age (6-month-old child is given occlusion half of the waking hours per day in alternate eyes). A child aged >1 year is given occlusion in the better eye more than worse eye (3-year-old child is given occlusion 8 waking hours per day for 3 days in better eye and 1 day in the worse eye). The worse eye is occluded to avoid development of occlusion amblyopia in the better eye. Patients are followed up every 4–6 weeks initially and every 3 months thereafter to see for response of treatment. Occlusion is gradually tapered off once the desired effect is achieved. Levodopa, carbidopa, and citicoline have shown good results in modulating the plasticity [21].

1.9 Summary (Point Wise)

- Major signs for pediatric cataracts include leukocoria, strabismus, abnormal ocular movements and delayed visual milestones.
- Leukocoria can be due to opacity anterior to lens, in the lens or posterior to it.
- Family members especially siblings should always be screened.
- A detailed treatment history should be taken to rule out drug induced cataracts.
- Mother should be enquired about exanthematous fever during antenatal period in cases of suspected rubella.
- Bilateral cataracts have something abnormal in the body; unilateral cataracts have something abnormal in the eye.
- Small children can be examined in mother's lap or shoulder hold.
- Vision assessment is the most elementary investigation that can be done using specialized tests depending on the age of child.
- Ocular movement's evaluation is a crucial part of pediatric cataract assessment.
- Pupillary reactions give us a fair idea of neuronal status.
- Red reflex test helps us assess cataracts, squints and refractive errors and also provides a hint toward any possible posterior segment pathology.
- Cataract morphology should be assessed on distant direct ophthmoscopy as well as on slit lamp examination.
- Indirect ophthalmoscopy with scleral indentation is the gold standard for posterior segment evaluation wherever possible.
- Systemic investigations should be tailor cut and warranted only based on clinical clues.
- Ultrasound B-scan should be done in cases of total media opacity.
- Prefer 20% undercorrection in IOL power for infants less than 6 months, 15% for 6 months to 1 year, 10% for 1–2 years, 5% for 2–5 years, and emmetropic power thereafter.
- IOL should not be put in axial lengths less than 17 mm or white to white less than 9 mm.
- Posterior capsulotomy must be done in children upto 8 years of age with limited anterior vitrectomy in children upto 6 years of age to prevent VAO formation.
- Rehabilitation with contact lens or glasses with amblyopia therapy is the most important part in management of pediatric cataracts.

References

1. Foster A. Epidemiology of cataract in childhood: a global perspective. J Cataract Refract Surg. 1997;23:601–4.
2. Rahi JS, Dezateux C, British Congenital Cataract Interest Group. Measuring and interpreting the incidence of congenital ocular anomalies: lessons from a national study of congenital cataract in the UK. Invest Ophthalmol Vis Sci. 2001;42(7):1444–8.
3. Khokhar S, Agarwal T, Kumar G, Kushmesh R, Tejwani LK. Lenticular abnormalities in children. J Pediatr Ophthalmol Strabismus. 2012;49(1):32–7.
4. Kumar M, Agarwal T, Kaur P, Kumar M, Khokhar S, Dada R. Molecular and structural analysis of genetic variations in congenital cataract. Mol Vis. 2013;19:2436–50.
5. Khokhar SK, Dhull C. Atlas of pediatric cataract. Singapore: Springer Nature Singapore Pte Ltd; 2019. p. 22.
6. Khokhar SK, Dhull C. Atlas of pediatric cataract. Singapore: Springer Nature Singapore Pte Ltd; 2019. p. 128.

7. Liu Y. Pediatric lens diseases. Singapore: Springer Pte Ltd; 2017. p. 106.
8. Rabiah PK, Smith SD, Awad AH, Al-garni A, Al-mesfer SA, Al-turkmani S, et al. Results of surgery for bilateral cataract associated with sensory nystagmus in children. Am J Ophthalmol. 2002;134:586–91.
9. Wilson ME, Trivedi RH. Pediatric cataract surgery - techniques, complications and management. 2nd ed. Philadelphia, PA: Lippincott Williams and Wilkins, Wolters Kluwer; 2014. p. 34.
10. Boop JJ, van Dalen JT, Tyner GS. Assessment of the Catford drum in visual acuity testing and its use as a measurement of visual performance in low-vision patients. Br J Ophthalmol. 1987;71(10):797–802.
11. Sharma P. Strabismus simplified. 2nd ed. New Delhi: CBS Publishers and Distributors; 2016. p. 58.
12. Gole G. Visual acuity assessment in children. Clin Exp Ophthalmol. 1989;17:1–2.
13. Jay WM, Williams BB, De Chicchis A. Periodic alternating nystagmus clearing after cataract surgery. J Clin Neuroophthalmol. 1985;5(3):149–52.
14. Felius J, Busettini C, Lynn MJ, Hartmann EE, Lambert SR, Infant Aphakia Treatment Study Group. Nystagmus and related fixation instabilities following extraction of unilateral infantile cataract in the Infant Aphakia Treatment Study (IATS). Invest Ophthalmol Vis Sci. 2014;55(8):5332–7.
15. Mansour AM, Reinecke RD. The pop eye phenomenon: an extreme form of the oculodigital phenomenon. J Clin Neuroophthalmol. 1985;5(4):281–2.
16. Tongue A, Cibis GW. Bruckner test. Ophthalmology. 1981;88:1041–4.
17. Kothari MT. Can the Bruckner test be used as a rapid screening test to detect significant refractive errors in children? Indian J Ophthalmol. 2007;55:213–5.
18. Bhayana AA, Prasad P, Azad SV. Refractive errors and the red reflex - Bruckner test revisited. Indian J Ophthalmol. 2019;67:1381–2.
19. Bhayana AA. Response to comments on: using Brückner's test for gross keratometry screening. Indian J Ophthalmol. 2020;68:263.
20. Khokhar SK, Dhull C. Atlas of pediatric cataract. Singapore: Springer Nature Singapore Pte Ltd; 2019. p. 1.
21. Khokhar SK, Pillay G, Dhull C, Agarwal E, Mahabir M, Aggarwal P. Pediatric cataract. Indian J Ophthalmol. 2017;65:1340–9.
22. Dada T, Bhartiya S, Baig NB. Cataract surgery in eyes with previous glaucoma surgery: pearls and pitfalls. J Curr Glaucoma Pract. 2013;7(3):99–105.
23. Chandra P, Khokhar S, Kumar A. Bilateral total cataract after laser treatment of aggressive posterior retinopathy of prematurity. Indian Pediatr. 2016;53(Suppl 2):S157–8.
24. Khokhar S, Agrawal S, Gupta S, Gogia V, Agrawal T. Epidemiology of traumatic lenticular subluxation in India. Int Ophthalmol. 2014;34:197–204.
25. Khokhar SK, Dhull C. Atlas of pediatric cataract. Singapore: Springer Nature Singapore Pte Ltd; 2019. p. 129.
26. Dahan E, Drusedau MU. Choice of lens and dioptric power in pediatric pseudophakia. J Cataract Refract Surg. 1997;23(Suppl 1):618–23.
27. Enyedi LB, Peterseim MW, Freedman SF, Buckley EG. Refractive changes after pediatric intraocular lens implantation. Am J Ophthalmol. 1998;126:772.
28. Khokhar SK, Tomar A, Pillay G, Agarwal E. Biometric changes in Indian pediatric cataract and postoperative refractive status. Indian J Ophthalmol. 2019;67:1068–72.
29. Dave H, Phoenix V, Becker ER, Lambert SR. Simultaneous vs sequential bilateral cataract surgery for infants with congenital cataracts: visual outcomes, adverse events, and economic costs. Arch Ophthalmol. 2010;128(8):1050–4.
30. Roizen NJ, Mets MB, Blondis TA. Ophthalmic disorders in children with Down syndrome. Dev Med Child Neurol. 1994;36:594–600.
31. Bökenkamp A, Ludwig M. The oculocerebrorenal syndrome of Lowe: an update. Pediatr Nephrol. 2016;31:2201–12.
32. Mets MB. Eye manifestations of intrauterine infections. Ophthalmol Clin N Am. 2001;14:521–31.
33. Khokhar SK, Dhull C. Atlas of pediatric cataract. Singapore: Springer Nature Singapore Pte Ltd; 2019. p. 25.
34. Khokhar SK, Dhull C. Atlas of pediatric cataract. Singapore: Springer Nature Singapore Pte Ltd; 2019. p. 27.
35. Trumler AA. Evaluation of pediatric cataracts and systemic disorders. Curr Opin Ophthalmol. 2011;22:365–79.

2 IOL Power Calculation

Abdelrahman M. Elhusseiny and Bharti R. Nihalani

2.1 Introduction

IOL power calculation is relatively simple in adult eyes, requiring axial length (AL), corneal power—keratometry (*K*) values and IOL parameters. The constant size of the adult eye ensures the refraction remains stable. However, IOL power calculation is challenging in pediatric eyes [1, 2]. These eyes have shorter AL, steeper corneas with high *K*-values and shorter anterior chamber depth (ACD) compared to adults. The biometry measurements are performed under anesthesia in infants and young children where it is difficult to ensure central fixation making it less precise. IOL calculation formulas designed for adult eyes are used in pediatric eyes with varied accuracy [3–6]. None of the formulas encounter for the growth of pediatric eyes. The ocular growth has profound effects and results in large myopic shift as the child grows. To prevent this, most surgeons tend to undercorrect the IOL power depending on age of the child at cataract surgery. The rate of ocular growth of an aphakic or pseudophakic eye is further complicated by laterality of cataract, amblyopia, adherence to amblyopia treatment, and presence of other co-morbidities such as glaucoma. All these factors complicate the IOL power calculation in pediatric eyes.

In this chapter, we discuss the challenges of IOL power calculation that are encountered by a pediatric ophthalmologist and discuss current practices.

A. M. Elhusseiny
Department of Ophthalmology, Boston Children's Hospital, Harvard Medical School, Boston, MA, USA

Department of Ophthalmology, Harvey and Bernice Jones Eye Institute, University of Arkansas for Medical Sciences, Arkansas, USA

B. R. Nihalani (✉)
Department of Ophthalmology, Boston Children's Hospital, Harvard Medical School, Boston, MA, USA
e-mail: Bharti.Gangwani@childrens.harvard.edu

2.2 Eye Growth

The mean AL ranges from 16.6 to 17 mm in a full-term newborn eye. In a premature infant, AL increases from 15.38 ± 0.25 mm at the age of 33 weeks to 16.88 ± 0.59 mm at 41 weeks [7, 8]. Most of ocular growth occurs in the first few years of life resulting in significant refractive changes. Axial elongation occurs at a rate of 0.18 mm/week until 40 weeks postmenstrual age then at a rate of 0.15 mm/week till the age of 3 months. AL increases rapidly in the first 2 years of life then it slows down until it reaches the mean adult value of 23.5 mm in males (22.9 mm in females) at the age 16 years (Fig. 2.1) [9, 10]. The mean *K* power at birth is 51.2 diopters (D) (steeper corneal curvature) and as AL increases, the average *K* decreases until it reaches 43.5 D in

S. K. Khokhar, C. Dhull (eds.), *Essentials of Pediatric Cataract Surgery*,
https://doi.org/10.1007/978-981-16-0212-2_2

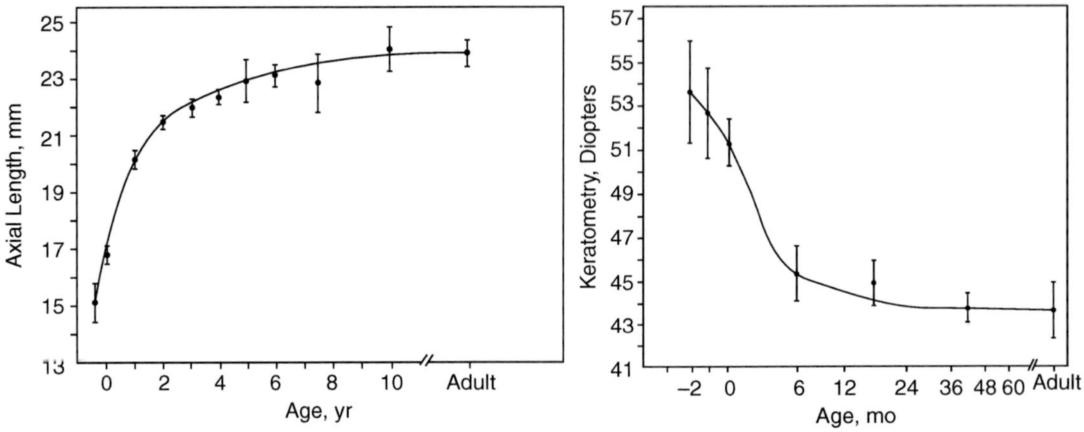

Fig. 2.1 Graph showing the change in keratometry and axial length from birth until it stabilizes and reaches the adult values. (Graph is taken from the landmark article. Gordon RA, Donzis PB. Refractive development of the human eye. Arch Ophthalmol 1985;103: 785–9)

adulthood. The changes in the diopteric power of the crystalline lens follows a triphasic pattern with marked reduction in the diopteric power by >10 D during the 12 months after birth then a slower rate of 3–4 D decrease from the age of 2 before stabilizing at the age of 10 years [7]. This process of developing and maintaining emmetropia with axial elongation and corneal flattening is referred to as emmetropization.

Ocular growth patterns differ in children with cataractous eyes. Axial elongation after pediatric cataract surgery is related to several factors such as age at time of surgery, presence of IOL or not, amblyopia and genetic factors. Lambert and colleagues as a part of the Infant Aphakia Treatment Study (IATS) have evaluated AL, *K*-readings and corneal diameter (CD) in children with unilateral cataract compared to the normal fellow eyes [11]. They reported that cataractous eyes have shorter AL of 18 ± 1.3 mm compared to 18.6 ± 0.9 mm in the normal fellow eye by an average of 0.6 mm [11]. A statistically significant difference in the rate of axial elongation was observed, by the age of 1 year, in eyes who underwent primary IOL implantation (0.24 mm/month) compared to eyes with aphakic contact lens correction (0.17 mm/month). Rates of axial elongation differed according to the timing of cataract surgery [11]. For the pseudophakic group, the mean AL at the age of 1 year was 19.5 mm for patients who underwent cataract surgery at the age of 1 month compared to 21.1 mm for patients operated on at the age of 6 months. For aphakic group with contact lens correction, the mean AL at the age of 1 year was 19 mm for patients operated on at the age of 1 month compared to 19.5 mm for patients operated on at the age of 6 months [11]. Cataractous eyes had significantly higher *K*-readings (46.4 ± 2.7 D compared to 45.5 ± 1.8 D) and smaller CD (10.5 ± 0.7 mm compared to 10.8 ± 0.6 mm) compared to normal fellow eyes [11]. Although Lambert and colleagues have demonstrated a difference in AL between the normal fellow eye (20.7 ± 0.6 mm) and pseudophakic or aphakic eyes at the age of 1 year, other authors have reported no significant difference between pseudophakic eyes and normal fellow eyes over time suggesting normal growth of pseudophakic eyes [12, 13]. Recently, Trivedi and colleagues developed a model to predict rate of axial elongation in patients undergoing bilateral cataract extraction aiming to help surgeons to select the appropriate IOL power for primary implantation [14]. They retrospectively evaluated 64 patients with a median age of 5.1 months at time of surgery and developed a multivariable generalized estimating equation regression model to predict individual future adult size AL for each child [14].

2.3 Biometry

Optical biometry using partial coherence interferometry has become the gold standard as it is highly accurate, easy to perform, noninvasive, and comfortable for the patients [15–18]. It carries the advantages of higher reproducibility and operator independence [15–17, 19]. However, it is not possible to get the measurements in young uncooperative children and in children with dense cataract, anterior and posterior capsular plaques that are commonly encountered in pediatric eyes. In our clinic, we try to perform optical biometry in all patients older than 4 years of age. Biometry is performed under general anesthesia (GA) on the day of surgery for infants and young children and in patients where optical biometry could not be obtained.

Keratometry is typically performed with portable autokeratometer. Errors in keratometric readings alter IOL power in a ratio of 1:1 [20]. Mittelviefhaus and Gentner have demonstrated that lack of fixation in young infants and children during keratometry under GA can lead to inaccurate *K*-readings with higher deviations of the predicted postoperative refraction, therefore multiple measurements are required to improve accuracy [21]. We consider a mean of at least 3 *K*-readings for IOL power calculation.

AL measurements are performed under GA in infants and children where it is difficult to ensure central fixation. Changes in AL alter IOL power by 2.5–3 D for each 1 mm error in measurement [22]. A-scan ultrasound biometry can be performed either by applanation or immersion technique. In applanation/contact technique, the ultrasound probe comes in direct contact with the cornea which may indent the corneal surface resulting in shorter AL and IOL power underestimation with subsequent myopic prediction error [23]. Too much tear film or too light a touch can cause erroneously long AL readings because it will include the thickness of the coupler. Absence of enough tear film will give poor quality, low intensity spikes. In contrast to applanation ultrasound biometry, immersion ultrasound uses a coupling fluid between the ultrasound probe and the cornea preventing corneal indentation. The main difference on appearance of the scan will be two corneal spikes representing the front and back surfaces of cornea (Fig. 2.2). Once the ultrasound probe is properly aligned with optical axis of the eye, a straight, steep retinal spike will be displayed on the screen, however if the probe is not perpendicular to the retina, the spike will be jagged slow-rising echo spike [23, 24]. It is important to look for good spikes on the scan, use adequate gain and take a mean of at least five measurements.

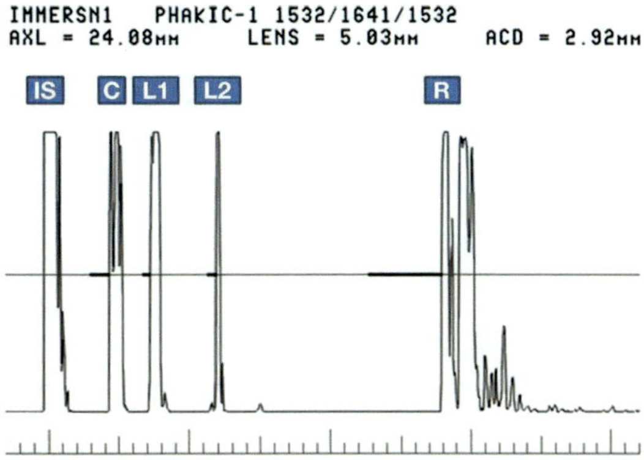

Fig. 2.2 Axial length tracing using immersion method showing twin corneal spikes representing front and back surfaces of the cornea. It is important to get straight, steep retinal spike with descending orbital fat behind the scleral echo. (Image taken with permission from AAO)

Ben-Zion and colleagues [24] retrospectively evaluated 203 children who underwent cataract extraction and primary IOL implantation comparing the accuracy of A-scan immersion biometry to applanation A-scan biometry. They reported no significant difference in the postoperative refractive results or IOL prediction errors between the two methods; however, Trivedi and Wilson reported that there is a statistically significant difference in the mean prediction errors between both methods, recommending immersion A-scan biometry for more accurate pediatric IOL power calculation [23].

2.4 IOL Power Calculation Formula

There are two categories of IOL calculation formulas, regression formulas such as the Sanders-Retzalff-Kraff (SRK I) formula and its modification with improved accuracy (SRK II) or theoretical formulas such as Hoffer Q, Holladay I, Holladay II, Haigis, T2, Barrett Universal I and II and Super formula. The regression SRK formula was subsequently modified and optimized for postoperative anterior chamber depth (ACD) prediction, AL correction and corneal refractive index creating a third generation nonlinear theoretic formula (SRK/T) [25]. Several studies have evaluated the predictability of these formulae in pediatric eyes.

Andreo and colleagues studied 47 consecutive pseudophakic pediatric patients, aged 3 months to 16 years and compared four formulas (SRK II, SRK/T, Holladay and Hoffer Q). They found no significant difference in accuracy between the formulas and reported the average initial postoperative refractive error between 1.2 and 1.4 D with all formulas [26]. Another study found that the mean difference between the predicted and the actual postoperative refractions was slightly more accurate using theoretic formulas (1.06 D vs. 1.22 D with regression formulas), though none of the formulas were satisfactory in achieving target refraction [27].

Nihalani and VanderVeen retrospectively evaluated 135 eyes of children <18 years of age who underwent cataract surgery and IOL implantation with a mean age of 6.4 years and mean AL of 22.16 mm at the time of surgery [5]. They compared four different formulas (Hoffer Q, Holladay I, SRK II, SRK/T) and reported a mean absolute prediction error (|predicted refraction minus actual refraction|) of 0.76 D, 0.76 D, 1.11 D, 0.84 D using Hoffer Q, Holladay I, SRK II and SRK/T formulas respectively. The minimum prediction error was achieved by Hoffer Q formula in 46% of eyes compared with 12.5% with Holladay I, 23% with SRK II, and 18.5% with SRK/T indicating that Hoffer Q was the most predictable for the highest number of eyes [5].

Neely and colleagues evaluated 101 eyes of children with pediatric cataract and concluded that SRK II was the least variable compared with Hoffer Q, Holladay I, SRK/T especially in patients with preoperative AL less than 19 mm [3], however 37% of study population had special types of pediatric cataract such as persistent fetal vasculature (PFV)-associated cataract and traumatic cataract [4]. Kekunnaya and colleagues evaluated 128 eyes of 48 children less than age of 2 years who underwent cataract extraction and primary IOL implantation and reported that SRK II was the most predictable IOL formula in their cohort [28].

Shuaib and colleagues retrospectively evaluated 235 pediatric cataract eyes and showed that SRK/T formula is significantly more predictive than Hoffer 1, Holladay I, and SRK II especially in patient with preoperative AL less than 25 mm [6]. VanderVeen and colleagues, as a part of IATS, evaluated 43 eyes with a mean age of 2.5 ± 1.5 months at time of surgery and mean preoperative AL of 18.1 ± 1.1 mm and showed that SRK/T and Holladay I had the lowest mean absolute prediction error of 1.4 ± 1.1 D and 1.7 ± 1.3 D, respectively [29].

SRK/T formula has been further modified by Sheard and colleagues to account for the nonphysiologic behavior in calculating AL and corneal height creating a new T2 formula which showed 9.7% less prediction error than SRK/T formula ($p < 0.0001$) [30]. In the IATS population, T2 had the lowest mean and median prediction error when compared to Haigis, Olsen, and Barret Universal formulas [31]. Holladay had added several factors such as white to white diameter, ACD, and preoperative lens thickness to his original formula to improve its accuracy (Holladay II). Trivedi and colleagues reported that Holladay II is more predictable when compared to other formulas (Holladay I, Hoffer Q, and SRK/T) especially for eyes with AL less than 22 mm even in absence of preoperative refraction [32].

In the largest to-date study comparing the predictability of six IOL calculation formulas (SRK II, SRK/T, Holladay I, Hoffer Q, T2, and Super formulas), Li and colleagues evaluated 377 eyes with pediatric eyes (<13 years) that underwent cataract extraction and primary IOL implantation with a mean AL of 22.48 ± 1.91 mm. They included only patients with congenital and developmental cataract excluding other causes like PFV, traumatic cataract or cataract associated with other anterior segment abnormalities. They reported that Hoffer Q and Holladay I, followed closely by Super formula had the best predictive values while SRK II had the highest mean absolute predictive errors compared to other formulas ($p < 0.001$) [3].

The prediction error should be zero in ideal scenario; however, most studies report a prediction error ranging from 0.7 to 1.5 D in pediatric eyes. Overall, there is no consensus regarding the IOL calculation formula that works in pediatric eyes. The factors that have been reported to result in high prediction errors in pediatric eyes include steep corneal curvature [33], younger age at time of cataract surgery [34] and shorter preoperative AL [32].

A-constant is used in SRK II and SRK/T formulas and is a theoretical value that relates the lens power to AL and *K*-values. It depends on multiple variables including IOL manufacturer, refraction index, style, and placement within the eye. Any change in the A-constant can change IOL power calculation with a ratio of 1:1. It varies among IOL models and is specified by the manufacturer on the lens case. A personalized A-constant can be calculated by measuring the postoperative refractions from last 20–50 patients to account for the calculation errors in the personal practice. Other constants used in the modern IOL formulas include the ACD value in Binkhorst and Hoffer Q formulas, the a0, a1, and a2 constants of the Haigis formula, and the Surgeon factor (SF) in Holladay formulas.

If the site of the IOL implantation needs to be changed after the start of surgery, an appropriate IOL power adjustment can be made without the need for re-evaluation. The IOL intended for capsular bag placement should be decreased by 1–2 D (depending on the IOL power; the higher the power, the greater the reduction), when placed in the ciliary sulcus.

2.5 IOL Power Selection

Various opinions exist regarding postoperative refractive goal. Most surgeons prefer to undercorrect and leave the patients with initial hyperopia that carries the advantage of less myopic shift at adulthood with continued axial growth, however, optical correction will be needed postoperatively which may be challenging in this age group carrying the risk of dense amblyopia associated with high uncorrected hyperopia. Other surgeons prefer initial emmetropia given that it may be helpful in amblyopia management in the immediate postoperative period however this needs to be balanced with risk of myopia in adulthood [35]. It is prudent to consider factors such as status of the fellow eye, density of amblyopia, likelihood of amblyopia treatment compliance, family history of myopia in addition to the primary factor aka age at surgery.

One of the commonly used principle for IOL power selection based on age at surgery was proposed by Enyedi and colleagues who recommended target refraction for various ages suggesting +6.00 for age 1 and aiming emmetropia at age 7. This is often referred to as the "Rule of 7." [13] Dahan and Drusedau suggested that IOL power should be chosen based on calculating a percentage of the IOL power required to achieve emmetropia recommending 20% undercorrection for children <2 years of age, and 10% undercorrection for children 2–8 years of age [36]. Table 2.1 shows these two studies whose formulas are commonly used for IOL power undercorrection.

The McClatchey Pediatric IOL Calculator is another useful tool that involves a computer program that calculates the IOL power to achieve desired refraction at age 20 years, based on a typical rate of refractive growth, and utilizes both axial length and age at surgery. However, to date no simple algorithm has been proposed that utilizes axial length and age together to suggest which IOL power implanted in early childhood could best achieve a final refraction of low myopia to near emmetropia in adulthood [37]. In our practice, we follow the rule of 7 for deciding the amount of undercorrection depending on the age at surgery.

Table 2.1 Commonly used methods for IOL power undercorrection in pediatric eyes

	Sample size	Mean refractive change with age	Suggested formula
Enyedi et al. [13]	83 eyes	0–2 years: −3.0 D over 2.5 years	Age + SRE = 7
		2–6 years: −1.5 D over 2.5 years	SRE = suggested refractive error
		6–8 years: −1.8 D over 3 years	(Age 1: +6 D; Age 2: +5 D; Age 3: +4 D; Age 4: +3 D; Age 5: +2 D; Age 6: +1 D; Age 7: Plano)
		>8 years: −0.38 D over 1.8 years	
Dahan and Drusedau [34]	156 eyes	0–1.5 years: -6.3 D	Undercorrection for IOL
		1.5–3 years: -2.7 D	<2 years: 20%
		3–8 years: -2.6 D	2–8 years: 10%

Table 2.2 Undercorrection in pediatric eyes using SRK II formula recommended by Khokhar et al. [38, 39]

Age	Undercorrection to IOL power calculated by SRK II formula
<6 months	20%
6–12 months	15%
1 year	10%
1.5 years	7%
2 years	5%
5 years	2%
>5 years	Nil

Axial growth may vary with population. A large sample size study (147 eyes) conducted in Indian population by Khokhar and colleagues showed median AL growth of 0.21 mm for 0–6 months, 0.18 mm for 6–18 months, and 0.06 mm from 18 to 60 months [38]. Mean IOL power under correction in 0–6, 6–18, and 18–60-month age groups was 15% 10.5% and 3.6% respectively. The under correction formula applied to SRK II for IOL power calculation recommended by Khokhar and colleagues is given in Table 2.2 [38, 39].

Gayton and Sanders suggested implanting two posterior chamber IOLs, one implanted in the capsular bag and the other one in the ciliary sulcus in children with microphthalmia to correct high hyperopia with intent to remove the sulcus-implanted IOL as the eye grows and myopia happens [40]. Wilson and colleagues retrospectively evaluated 15 eyes of 11 children implanted with piggyback IOLs below the age of 1 year and reported that 26% of these cases required re-operation for anterior segment complications [41]. Boisvert and colleagues have proposed a theoretical IOL power calculator that can be used to predict the postoperative refraction and help choosing the appropriate IOL power when piggyback IOL implantation is planned [42]. However, this approach is not widely accepted given the high risk of anterior segment complications that may be associated with implanting two IOLs in the limited space in small pediatric eyes along with the known risks of sulcus-implanted IOLs such as postoperative inflammation, pigment dispersion, uveitis, and glaucoma.

2.6 Myopic Shift

Rates of postoperative myopic shift differ among different studies with marked variability in postoperative refraction [43–46]. Plager and colleagues evaluated 38 eyes who underwent unilateral cataract extraction with posterior chamber IOL (PC-IOL) implantation with a mean follow-up of 6.1 years and reported a mean myopic shift of 4.6 D when surgery was done at age of 2–3 years, 2.3 D when surgery was done at age of 6–7 years, and 1.25 D when surgery was done at age 8–9 years [47]. In a prospective study including 42 eyes who underwent unilateral or bilateral cataract surgery between the age of 12 months and 18 years with a mean follow-up time of 5.45 years, Crouch and colleagues reported a mean myopic shift of 5.96 D in patients operated on at age of 1–2 years, 3.66 D in patients operated on at age of 3–4 years, 3.4 D in patients operated on at age of 5–6 years, 2.3 D at age of 7–8 years [46].

McClatchey and colleagues retrospectively compared the rates of refractive growth in children with or without IOL implantation with a minimum follow-up time of 3 years. They concluded that the rate of growth was significantly less in pseudophakic children (−4.6 D) compared to aphakic children (−5.7 D) (p = 0.03) [48]. Patients with unilateral pseudophakia had a lesser rate of growth (−4 D) compared to those with bilateral pseudophakia (−5.2 D) [48]. Superstein and colleagues evaluated rates of myopic shift in 233 aphakic eyes to 92 pseudophakic eyes. They reported a mean myopic shift of 1.5 D in pseudophakic eyes compared to 7.4 D in aphakic eyes [49]. Vasavada and colleagues evaluated rate of axial growth after congenital cataract surgery and found that it was higher in children ≤1 year of age and increases until the second year after surgery [50]. They also found that unilateral pseudophakia revealed accelerated growth compared to bilateral pseudophakia.

Weakley and colleagues evaluated myopic shift at 5 years of age after cataract extraction and IOL implantation in patients who were included in IATS. They reported a mean myopic change of 0.35 D/month from 1 month after cataract surgery to 1.5 years of age, 0.97 D/year after age of 1.5 years [51]. Another study showed that myopic shift may continue in the second decade of life with a mean myopic shift of 0.3 D/year [52]. Lambert and colleagues concluded that rate of refractive growth was similar in both aphakic and pseudophakic group, however higher rate of refractive growth was associated with worse visual outcomes in aphakic not pseudophakic group [53]. Gochnauer and colleagues also demonstrated that preoperative interocular AL difference as found in unilateral cataractous eyes increases the risk of poor postoperative best corrected visual acuity (BCVA) [54]. Glaucoma following cataract surgery (GFCS) can also be one of the contributing factors for axial elongation and myopic shift [55, 56].

The optics of the growing eyes are poorly understood till date, and there is no model of refractive growth or way to predict the ultimate refraction in aphakic or pseudophakic eyes.

2.7 Future Directions

There is a need for more normative database to better understand the growth of pediatric eye and to compare it with the growth of pediatric eye treated for congenital cataract with aphakia or pseudophakia. This will help us develop IOL power calculation formula that is specifically designed for pediatric eyes and tailored for each eye depending on various factors such as age at surgery, predicted ocular growth for that eye, and status of fellow eye to achieve best refractive outcomes.

2.8 Conclusion

The goal of pediatric cataract surgery is to promote the development of good visual acuity and achieve emmetropia by adulthood. IOL power choice is only one step in the path of this goal, which includes amblyopia management and refractive correction. Despite our best efforts, it may be that some of these children will get large myopic shifts, which will be the greatest in children having surgery in first few years of life. There is a need to develop simple IOL power calculation algorithms for use in young children undergoing cataract surgery.

2.9 Method of Literature Review

A literature review of PubMed, CENTRAL, Google Scholar, the Register of Controlled Trials, ClinicalTrials.gov (www.clinicaltrials.gov), Ovid MEDLINE In-Process, Ovid MEDLINE, EMBASE and other Non-Indexed Citations was performed. The databases were searched using the following terms: “predictability of intraocular lens calculation formula,” “pediatric cataract,” "refractive errors," "prediction errors," and "axial length.". There were no language or date restrictions.

Acknowledgment None

Funding: Children's Hospital Ophthalmology Foundation

Disclosure: No financial disclosures

References

1. Lambert SR, Lynn M, Drews-Botsch C, DuBois L, Wilson ME, Plager DA, Wheeler DT, Christiansen SP, Crouch ER, Buckley EG, et al. Intraocular lens implantation during infancy: perceptions of parents and the American Association for Pediatric Ophthalmology And Strabismus Members. J AAPOS. 2003;7(6):400–5.
2. Wilson ME Jr, Bartholomew LR, Trivedi RH. Pediatric cataract surgery and intraocular lens implantation: practice styles and preferences of the 2001 ASCRS and AAPOS memberships. J Cataract Refract Surg. 2003;29(9):1811–20.
3. Li J, Liu Z, Wang R, Cheng H, Zhao J, Liu L, Chen W, Wu M, Liu Y. Accuracy of intraocular lens power calculations in paediatric eyes. Clin Exp Ophthalmol. 2020;48:301.
4. Neely DE, Plager DA, Borger SM, Golub RL. Accuracy of intraocular lens calculations in infants and children undergoing cataract surgery. J AAPOS. 2005;9(2):160–5.
5. Nihalani BR, Vander Veen DK. Comparison of intraocular lens power calculation formulae in pediatric eyes. Ophthalmology. 2010;117(8):1493–9.
6. Shuaib AM, Elhusseiny AM, Hassanein DH, Zedan RH, Elhilali HM. Predictive value of intraocular lens power calculation formulae in children. J Am Assoc Pediatr Ophthalmol Strab. 2019;23(4):e54.
7. Gordon RA, Donzis PB. Refractive development of the human eye. Arch Ophthalmol. 1985;103(6):785–9.
8. O'Brien C, Clark D. Ocular biometry in pre-term infants without retinopathy of prematurity. Eye (Lond). 1994;8(Pt 6):662–5.
9. Fledelius HC, Christensen AS, Fledelius C. Juvenile eye growth, when completed? An evaluation based on IOL-master axial length data, cross-sectional and longitudinal. Acta Ophthalmol. 2014;92(3):259–64.
10. Eibschitz-Tsimhoni M, Archer SM, Del Monte MA. Intraocular lens power calculation in children. Surv Ophthalmol. 2007;52(5):474–82.
11. Lambert SR, Lynn MJ, DuBois LG, Cotsonis GA, Hartmann EE, Wilson ME. Axial elongation following cataract surgery during the first year of life in the infant aphakia treatment study. Invest Ophthalmol Vis Sci. 2012;53(12):7539–45.
12. Hutchinson AK, Drews-Botsch C, Lambert SR. Myopic shift after intraocular lens implantation during childhood. Ophthalmology. 1997;104(11):1752–7.
13. Enyedi LB, Peterseim MW, Freedman SF, Buckley EG. Refractive changes after pediatric intraocular lens implantation. Am J Ophthalmol. 1998;126(6):772–81.
14. Trivedi RH, Barnwell E, Wolf B, Wilson ME. A model to predict postoperative axial length in children undergoing bilateral cataract surgery with primary intraocular lens implantation. Am J Ophthalmol. 2019;206:228–34.
15. Roy A, Das S, Sahu SK, Rath S. Ultrasound biometry *vs.* IOL master. Ophthalmology. 2012;119(9):1937–1937.e1932.
16. Nakhli FR. Comparison of optical biometry and applanation ultrasound measurements of the axial length of the eye. Saudi J Ophthalmol. 2014;28(4):287–91.
17. Wang X-G, Dong J, Pu Y-L, Liu H-J, Wu Q. Comparison axial length measurements from three biometric instruments in high myopia. Int J Ophthalmol. 2016;9(6):876–80.
18. Packer M, Fine IH, Hoffman RS, Coffman PG, Brown LK. Immersion a-scan compared with partial coherence interferometry: outcomes analysis. J Cataract Refract Surg. 2002;28(2):239–42.
19. Hussin HM, Spry PG, Majid MA, Gouws P. Reliability and validity of the partial coherence interferometry for measurement of ocular axial length in children. Eye (Lond). 2006;20(9):1021–4.
20. Holladay JT. Standardizing constants for ultrasonic biometry, keratometry, and intraocular lens power calculations. J Cataract Refract Surg. 1997;23(9):1356–70.
21. Mittelviefhaus H, Gentner C. [Errors in keratometry for intraocular lens implantation in infants]. Ophthalmologe. 2000;97(3):186–8.
22. Prager TC, Hardten DR, Fogal BJ. Enhancing intraocular lens outcome precision: an evaluation of axial length determinations, keratometry, and IOL formulas. Ophthalmol Clin N Am. 2006;19(4):435–48.
23. Trivedi RH, Wilson ME. Prediction error after pediatric cataract surgery with intraocular lens implantation: contact versus immersion a-scan biometry. J Cataract Refract Surg. 2011;37(3):501–5.
24. Ben-Zion I, Neely DE, Plager DA, Ofner S, Sprunger DT, Roberts GJ. Accuracy of IOL calculations in children: a comparison of immersion versus contact a-scan biometery. J AAPOS. 2008;12(5):440–4.
25. Retzlaff JA, Sanders DR, Kraff MC. Development of the srk/t intraocular lens implant power calculation formula. J Cataract Refract Surg. 1990;16(3):333–40.
26. Andreo LK, Wilson ME, Saunders RA. Predictive value of regression and theoretical IOL formulas in pediatric intraocular lens implantation. J Pediatr Ophthalmol Strabismus. 1997;34(4):240–3.
27. Mezer E, Rootman DS, Abdolell M, Levin AV. Early postoperative refractive outcomes of pediatric intraocular lens implantation. J Cataract Refract Surg. 2004;30(3):603–10.
28. Kekunnaya R, Gupta A, Sachdeva V, Rao HL, Vaddavalli PK, Om Prakash V. Accuracy of intraocu-

lar lens power calculation formulae in children less than two years. Am J Ophthalmol. 2012;154(1):13–19.e12.
29. Vanderveen DK, Trivedi RH, Nizam A, Lynn MJ, Lambert SR. Predictability of intraocular lens power calculation formulae in infantile eyes with unilateral congenital cataract: results from the infant aphakia treatment study. Am J Ophthalmol. 2013;156(6):1252–1260.e1252.
30. Sheard RM, Smith GT, Cooke DL. Improving the prediction accuracy of the srk/t formula: the t2 formula. J Cataract Refract Surg. 2010;36(11):1829–34.
31. Vander Veen DK, Trivedi RH, Nizam A, Lynn MJ, Lambert SR. Reply: to PMID 24011524. Am J Ophthalmol. 2014;157(6):1332–3.
32. Trivedi RH, Wilson ME, Reardon W. Accuracy of the holladay 2 intraocular lens formula for pediatric eyes in the absence of preoperative refraction. J Cataract Refract Surg. 2011;37(7):1239–43.
33. Hoevenaars NE, Polling JR, Wolfs RC. Prediction error and myopic shift after intraocular lens implantation in paediatric cataract patients. Br J Ophthalmol. 2011;95(8):1082–5.
34. Moore DB, Ben Zion I, Neely DE, Plager DA, Ofner S, Sprunger DT, Roberts GJ. Accuracy of biometry in pediatric cataract extraction with primary intraocular lens implantation. J Cataract Refract Surg. 2008;34(11):1940–7.
35. Consultation section. Artificial lens implantation in the pediatric age group? J Cataract Refract Surg. 1991;17(4):512–8.
36. Dahan E, Drusedau MU. Choice of lens and dioptric power in pediatric pseudophakia. J Cataract Refract Surg. 1997;23(Suppl 1):618–23.
37. McClatchey SK. Intraocular lens calculator for childhood cataract. J Cataract Refract Surg. 1998;24(8):1125–9.
38. Khokhar SK, Tomar A, Pillay G, Agarwal E. Biometric changes in Indian pediatric cataract and postoperative refractive status. Indian J Ophthalmol. 2019;67(7):1068–72.
39. Khokhar SK, Tomar A, Pillay G, Agarwal E. Response to comments on: biometric changes in Indian pediatric cataract and postoperative refractive status. Indian J Ophthalmol. 2019;67(11):1907.
40. Gayton JL, Sanders VN. Implanting two posterior chamber intraocular lenses in a case of microphthalmos. J Cataract Refract Surg. 1993;19(6):776–7.
41. Wilson ME, Peterseim MW, Englert JA, Lall-Trail JK, Elliott LA. Pseudophakia and polypseudophakia in the first year of life. J AAPOS. 2001;5(4):238–45.
42. Boisvert C, Beverly DT, McClatchey SK. Theoretical strategy for choosing piggyback intraocular lens powers in young children. J AAPOS. 2009;13(6):555–7.
43. Brady KM, Atkinson CS, Kilty LA, Hiles DA. Cataract surgery and intraocular lens implantation in children. Am J Ophthalmol. 1995;120(1):1–9.
44. Inatomi M, Kora Y, Kinohira Y, Yaguchi S. Long-term follow-up of eye growth in pediatric patients after unilateral cataract surgery with intraocular lens implantation. J AAPOS. 2004;8(1):50–5.
45. Vasavada AR, Vasavada V, Shah SK, Praveen MR, Vasavada VA, Trivedi RH, Rawat F, Koul A. Five-year postoperative outcomes of bilateral aphakia and pseudophakia in children up to 2 years of age: a randomized clinical trial. Am J Ophthalmol. 2018;193:33–44.
46. Crouch ER, Crouch ER Jr, Pressman SH. Prospective analysis of pediatric pseudophakia: myopic shift and postoperative outcomes. J AAPOS. 2002;6(5):277–82.
47. Plager DA, Kipfer H, Sprunger DT, Sondhi N, Neely DE. Refractive change in pediatric pseudophakia: 6-year follow-up. J Cataract Refract Surg. 2002;28(5):810–5.
48. McClatchey SK, Dahan E, Maselli E, Gimbel HV, Wilson ME, Lambert SR, Buckley EG, Freedman SF, Plager DA, Parks MM. A comparison of the rate of refractive growth in pediatric aphakic and pseudophakic eyes. Ophthalmology. 2000;107(1):118–22.
49. Superstein R, Archer SM, Del Monte MA. Minimal myopic shift in pseudophakic versus aphakic pediatric cataract patients. J AAPOS. 2002;6(5):271–6.
50. Vasavada AR, Raj SM, Nihalani B. Rate of axial growth after congenital cataract surgery. Am J Ophthalmol. 2004;138(6):915–24.
51. Weakley DR Jr, Lynn MJ, Dubois L, Cotsonis G, Wilson ME, Buckley EG, Plager DA, Lambert SR. Myopic shift 5 years after intraocular lens implantation in the infant aphakia treatment study. Ophthalmology. 2017;124(6):822–7.
52. VanderVeen D.K. Selecting an Intraocular Lens Power. In: Lloyd I., Lambert S. (eds) Congenital Cataract. Springer, Cham; 2017. https://doi.org/10.1007/978-3-319-27848-3_8.
53. Lambert SR, Cotsonis G, DuBois L, Wilson ME, Plager DA, Buckley EG, McClatchey SK. Comparison of the rate of refractive growth in aphakic eyes versus pseudophakic eyes in the infant aphakia treatment study. J Cataract Refract Surg. 2016;42(12):1768–73.
54. Gochnauer AC, Trivedi RH, Hill EG, Wilson ME. Interocular axial length difference as a predictor of postoperative visual acuity after unilateral pediatric cataract extraction with primary iol implantation. J AAPOS. 2010;14(1):20–4.
55. Elhusseiny AM, El Sayed YM, El Sheikh RH, Gawdat GI, Elhilali HM. Circumferential Schlemm's canal surgery in adult and pediatric glaucoma. Curr Eye Res. 2019;44(12):1281–90.
56. Gouda J, Elhusseiny A, Tomairek RH, Elfayoumi D, Awadein A, Gawdat G, Elhilali H. Changes in intraocular pressure and anterior chamber angle after congenital cataract extraction. J Am Assoc Pediatr Ophthalmol Strab. 2019;23(4):e30–1.

Step Wise Surgical Treatment of Pediatric Cataract

3

Chirakshi Dhull and Sudarshan Kumar Khokhar

3.1 Introduction

Childhood cataracts differ from adult cataracts in their age of presentation and impact on visual development. In addition to this, the surgical technique also needs to be molded according to differences in anatomy, physiological factors and inflammatory response. The aim of pediatric cataract surgery is not just to clear visual axis but also to maintain clear visual axis for a long time. In this chapter, we will discuss steps of pediatric cataract surgery in detail individually which can be used in majority of pediatric cases. Special considerations required for difficult situations such as persistent fetal vasculature (PFV), preexisting posterior capsular defect, plaques, uveitis, etc. are discussed in subsequent chapters in detail.

Supplementary Information The online version of this chapter (https://doi.org/10.1007/978-981-16-0212-2_3) contains supplementary material, which is available to authorized users.

C. Dhull (✉)
Eye Q Hospital, Rohtak, Haryana, India

S. K. Khokhar
Professor Ophthalmology, Dr. RP Centre for Ophthalmic Sciences, All India Institute of Medical Sciences, New Delhi, India

3.2 Historical Aspect

Pediatric cataract surgery developed parallel to advances in adult cataract and vitreoretinal surgery. From early to mid-twentieth century, *needling* was performed for treatment of pediatric cataract. Since the technique was simple and lens matter in children being soft, would absorb over a few weeks' time; technique remained popular amongst many. During 1960s, complications due to intense inflammatory reaction were noted and almost all eyes developed media opacity and as much as 20% eyes were lost [1].

Scheie popularized the *aspiration procedure* where 2 mL syringe was used with 19 gauze needle to aspirate the lens matter after making an anterior capsular opening [2, 3]. Since posterior capsule was left intact, visual axis opacification was just as common as needling [3].

While adult cataract surgery progressed to extracapsular cataract surgery and phacoemulsification, *phacoaspiration* and *irrigation and aspiration* started being used for pediatric cataracts.

An important development in pediatric cataract surgery came with development of automated vitrectors. Peyman used *pars plicata approach* for congenital cataracts [4]. Since posterior capsule is removed, chances of visual axis opacification are significantly reduced. This technique was later refined where central opening was made in the posterior capsule with limited anterior vitrectomy where a peripheral rim of posterior capsule

S. K. Khokhar, C. Dhull (eds.), *Essentials of Pediatric Cataract Surgery*,
https://doi.org/10.1007/978-981-16-0212-2_3

is left behind [5, 6]. The advantage was clear media in most cases and it could be used in cases with ocular co-morbidities.

With pars plana surgeries, the posterior capsule was either removed completely or a narrow rim was left. **BenEzra** utilized the anterior route (limbal) to perform *posterior capsulotomy with anterior vitrectomy* [7]. BenEzra and Cohen compared limbal and pars plana route surgery with posterior capsulotomy and anterior vitrectomy with intact posterior capsule [8]. They found visual opacification in all children with intact capsule while both limbal and pars plana surgery where posterior capsulotomy and anterior vitrectomy was performed well.

Gimbal first described *posterior capsulorhexis* with optic capture of intraocular lens (IOL) for pediatric cataract [9].

IOL implantation was not a norm in pediatric cataract 30 years ago. Early trials with IOL were associated with frequent complication but as the surgical technique was refined with advent of bimanual automated aspiration and guillotine vitrectomy cutters, outcomes with IOL improved gradually. IOL implantation

3.3 Anesthesia Considerations

General anesthesia is required for ophthalmic surgery and serial examinations especially in young children. It is important for ophthalmologists to understand important aspects of anesthesia in children although the primary care is taken by the anesthesiologists. Optimal condition in addition to anesthetized child is still eye in central gaze with controlled intraocular pressure.

3.3.1 Perioperative Routine

Standard fasting/nil per oral (NPO) of 8 h for solids and 2 h for water or clear fluids before surgery without risk of aspiration is required [10, 11]. Prolonged fasting especially in an infant can cause dehydration or electrolyte balance. To avoid this, intravenous fluids including ringer lactate or D-5 (dextrose) can be used.

3.3.2 Anesthetic Agents

In children, induction of anesthesia can be performed by inhalational or intravenous (iv) route. In an infant or toddler, inhalational induction is carried out after which an iv line is placed. Sevoflurane having mild odor and minimal airway stimulation, is the drug of choice for children. Anesthesia can be maintained by sevoflurane, isoflurane, or desflurane with a mixture of the air and/or oxygen. Induction in older children cooperative for iv line can be performed with propofol which is rapidly acting. In developing countries, ketamine may be used for anesthesia if flurane gases are unavailable [11]. In these cases, periocular anesthesia can be used in addition to ketamine to reduce postoperative pain [11].

3.3.3 Muscle Relaxants

The requirement for anesthesia in ocular surgery includes immobility of eye and stability in central gaze. Deviation of eye has been described under anesthesia in the past [12, 13]. Deeping of anesthesia using additional propofol, opioids or dexmetodomine have been reported for maintaining central eye position [14–16]. Balanced anesthesia using muscle relaxants have been noted to provide good condition for surgeon's comfort [16–18]. In a study conducted at our center, we found balanced anesthesia with atracurium provided better surgical condition and good surgeon satisfaction which improved with increasing dose from 25% to 100% ED_{95} dose [19].

3.3.4 Surgeon Coordination with Anesthesiologist

Anticipation of approximate time duration for surgery is helpful to anesthesiologist in dose titration for anesthesia. A 10-min warning is always useful to avoid unnecessary delay in extubating. Patient positioning has to be done under supervised case so as not to displace endotracheal (ETA) tubes. Anesthesiologists take care of expected postoperative pain and nausea with appropriate medication. In cases, more pain or inflammation is expected; dexamethasone and/or ibuprofen or appropriate analgesic can be administered.

3.4 Timing of Surgery

The timing of surgery is determined by a variety of factors including age of the patient, laterality, and density of cataract. The ideal time to perform cataract surgery is when optimal visual outcome can be achieved with minimum risk of complications. Delay in surgery increases risk of stimulus deprivation amblyopia while early surgery is associated with higher risks of complications. There is evidence that risk of glaucoma reduces if cataract surgery is performed at older age [20, 21]. In addition, there is greater risk of anesthesia-related complications in younger children.

Visual outcome has been observed to be better in surgery at earlier age especially in cases of unilateral cataract [22, 23]. Birch et al. [22] identified a 6 week latent period for unilateral cataract, where there was no difference in visual outcome in this period. We have identified the ideal time for surgery in unilateral and bilateral cataract to be 6 weeks and 8 weeks, respectively [24]. In case of bilateral cataract, we prefer to perform sequential surgery within a week's time [24].

3.5 Stepwise Surgical Technique

The technique of surgery is ever evolving. The surgical steps are refined over time. Newer modalities are introduced and over time, replace the older modalities. We would like to emphasis the importance of surgical technique over technology. Good visual outcomes can be achieved by following standard surgical techniques and meticulous postoperative care.

3.6 Head Positioning

In adult cataract, topical anesthesia is used for most patients as they are cooperative for the procedure. Head and eye position can be adjusted before and during surgery. The same does not hold true for children. Pediatric cases require proper head positioning before beginning the surgery to ensure good exposure and comfort, as the child is under general anesthesia. Flexible LMA is generally used to enable adjustment of head position. We should not change the head position without the support of anesthesiologist.

Head ring of correct size can be used according to the age along with shoulder support. Size of the speculum in relation to palpebral aperture has to be taken intoconsideration (Fig. 3.1a–c). Correct size of the speculum aids in proper exposure and avoiding difficulty in instrumentation.

3.7 Incision Construction

3.7.1 Paracentesis

One or two paracentesis wound are constructed in uniplanar fashion (stab incision) at the limbus. We prefer two incisions almost 180° apart as we perform bimanual surgery in most cases. Microvitreoretinal (MVR) blade of 0.9 mm (20 gauze) is used. Twenty or 21 gauze bimanual irrigation and aspiration cannula can be used via these incisions to aspirate 360° of the cortex while avoiding leak from the incisions. Ideally 20 gauze vitrector cannula with irrigation should be used although 23 gauze vitrector also works well with minimal or no leakage. We should match the size the instrument with the size of the port.

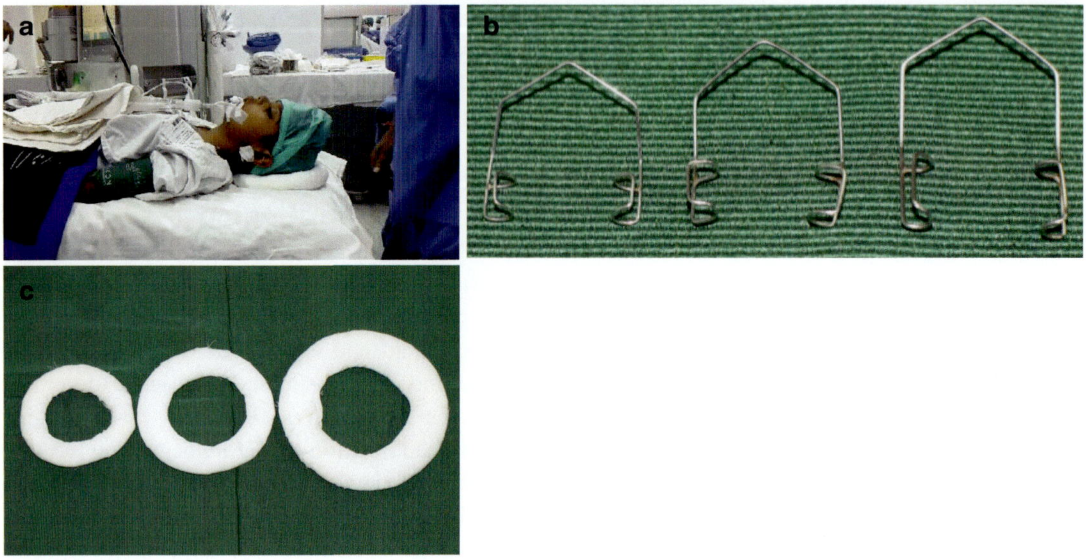

Fig. 3.1 (**a**) Ideal Head position after intubation with head ring and shoulder roll for appropriate exposure. (**b**) Various sizes of head rings. (**c**) Various size of eyelid speculum

3.7.2 Main Wound Construction

We prefer limbal incision to scleral tunnel in most cases of pediatric cataract. It is a personal choice based on surgeon comfort and both incisions work equally well in children. We construct a 2.2 or 2.8 mm biplanar limbal incision if IOL implantation is planned. It can be constructed at the time of capsulorhexis if utrata forceps is used. If microincision forceps is used, it can be constructed at the time of IOL implantation. We make two paracentesis nasal and temporal; and construct superior 2.2 mm/2.8 mm wound.

3.7.3 Considerations for Wound Construction

- *Wound construction technique*: Both scleral or corneal (limbal) tunnel are considered suitable for pediatric cataract surgery. Both have advantages and disadvantages. Limbal incision is quick, avascular, associated with less inflammation, cosmetically better and conjunctiva is left undisturbed for future glaucoma surgery if at all required [25, 26]. Scleral incision heals faster, is self-sealing and generally does not require suturing.
- *Surgically induced astigmatism (SIA)*: It has widely accepted that for larger incision 5.5 or 6 mm size, scleral tunnel causes lesser SIA as compared to corneal incisions. Larger incisions are made when rigid IOLs are implanted. In most cases, foldable IOLs are implanted. For these incisions, SIA has been reported to be similar in scleral and limbal incisions [27].
- *Site*: Superior incisions are preferred in children as they are protected by the brow as well as the bell's phenomena. Children are more prone to trauma; hence temporal incisions are avoided.
- *Size*: Size depends on the IOL used. For foldable IOLs, 2.2 or 2.75 mm incision can be made depending on the IOL cartridge and surgeon's preference. Standard surgical keratome blades are available in these sizes, which can be used for construction of incision. For rigid

IOLs, 5.5 or 6 mm incision is required. A crescent knife is required in these cases for scleral tunnel construction.

- *Astigmatism*: In older children, incisions can be placed at the steep axis to cause flattening and reduce astigmatism [28]. However, in smaller children who are not cooperative keratometry can be difficult especially the accuracy of axis [29]. In addition, corneal astigmatism changes with age in children. These factors make reducing astigmatism difficult. Most surgeons prefer superior surgical incision irrespective of the steeper meridian

3.7.4 Pars Plana Port

We perform surgery from anterior route in most cases of congenital cataract. Nevertheless, it is important to learn construction of pars plana ports for all pediatric cataract surgeons as it may be required for primary surgery or management of visual axis opacification. It is considered as a rule of thumb, that port is made 4 mm from limbus in children older than 4 years. In younger children, distance from limbus is followed as given in Table 3.1 [30].

Ports can be made using 23 gauge trocar system. Since scleral rigidity in children is very low, care has to be taken at the time of port construction. Oblique placement of trocars may not be possible due to thin sclera. Trocar has to enter parallel to the visual axis to avoid trauma to lens or posterior capsule. Before entry, wounds have to be sutured and anterior chamber has to be well formed. After completion of anterior vitrectomy, port should be sutured with absorbable suture. Leaving port sutureless may increase risk of infection.

Table 3.1 Recommendation of scleral entry from the limbus [30]

Age in months	<3	3–6	6–12	12–24	>24
Distance in mm	1.5	2	2.5	3	3.5

3.7.5 Suturing

Main incision should be sutured with absorbable or nonabsorbable sutures. The survey conducted by Wilson et al. showed that only 3% of surgeons in AAPOS and 20% in ASCRS left all wounds sutureless. The advantage of suturing the main wound is prevention of possible leak, which may reduce risk of infection. Children may rub their eyes and suturing can prevent wound leak in such situation. Paracentesis wound may be hydrated or sutured. If there is a suspicion of leak after hydration, wounds should be sutured.

Choice of absorbable and nonabsorbable suture needs various factors to be taken into consideration. Absorbable sutures may incite inflammation and suture granuloma formation. Non absorbable suture such as 10-0 nylon monofilament have excellent tensile strength and elasticity but it requires examination under anesthesia (EUA) for removal at 6 weeks. Since in most children, EUA is required at that time for change in prescription of glasses, intraocular pressure (IOP) measurement AND assessment of visual axis; suture can be removed at this time. Advantage of absorbable suture such as 10-0 vicryl is that there is no need for removal. If not removed, nylon sutures may be associated vascularization. Bar Sela et al. compared vicryl to mersilene sutures with no suture removal and found vicryl to be associated with no complications [31]. One patient with mersilene suture developed endophthalmitis after suture removal. Matalia et al. compared 10-0 vicryl and 10-0 nylon sutures in pediatric cataract surgery [32]. They found less chances of vascularization, loosening and need for suture removal with vicryl suture. With time, there has been gradual shift toward absorbable sutures.

3.8 Ophthalmic Visco Surgical Device (OVD)

OVD are used to maintain anterior chamber, perform anterior capsulorhexis, posterior capsulorhexis and IOL insertion. There is large range

Table 3.2 Commonly used OVD with their properties. *MW* molecular weight, *Da* Dalton, V_0 zero sheer viscocity, *mPs* milli-Pascal seconds, *M* million, *K* thousand, *NaHa* sodium hyaluronate, *CDS* chondroitin sulfate

OVD	Contents	MW (Da)	V_0 (mPs)	Type
Healon	1% NaHa	4.0 M	230 K	Visco-cohesive
Healon GV	1.4% NaHa	5.0 M	2.0 M	Visco-cohesive
Viscoat	3% NaHa, 4% CDS	500 K, 25 K	50 K	Visco-dispersive
Healon 5	2.3% NaHa	4.0 M	7.0 M	Visco-adaptive

of OVDs available which differ in their molecular weight and viscocity (Table 3.2). Anterior capsule in children is highly elastic and heavier visco-cohesive OVD such as Healon GV (AMO) can be used to flatten the capsule and can aid in the capsulorhexis by pressure equalization. Visco-adaptive OVDs such as Healon 5 which have both dispersive and cohesive property can be used in cases with small pupil to maintain dilatation [33]. For posterior capsulorhexis, OVD is required in anterior chamber only. After IOL implantation, visco-cohesive OVDs can be removed easily and quickly. If visco-dispersive OVD is used to coat endothelium or prevent vitreous prolapse, longer time is required for visco aspiration.

3.9 Anterior Capsule Management

3.9.1 Properties of Anterior Capsule

Anterior capsule differs in pediatric age group as compared to adults. It is thinnest at birth (about 4 mm) and keeps increasing in thickness both at equator and centrally throughout life till 75 years of age [34, 35]. Anterior capsule is highly elastic and its extensibility decreases by 0.5% per year (108–40%) [34]. There is progressive decrease in tensile strength with age as well [34]. Due to these anatomical factors much more sheering force is required to create capsulorhexis.

3.9.2 Manual Anterior Continuous Curvilinear Capsulorhexis (ACCC)

ACCC is considered the standard of care in adult cataract surgery since its development in 1990 [36]. However, it is much more difficult in children. Once completed, ACCC has minimal or no risk of tearing or extension during surgery. The sclera is less rigid and there may be added upthurst of well-formed vitreous. It is important to utilize the understanding of anatomy while performing ACCC.

Anterior capsular staining is required in cases of total cataract or where glow is absent. Trypan blue dye used for staining has an additional advantage of reducing capsular elasticity and hence can be used to an advantage especially in younger children [37]. Anterior chamber is filled with heavy visco-cohesive OVD for flattening of anterior capsule. This will reduce the chances of rhexis run off. We should aim for a 0.5 to 1 mm smaller size of capsulorhexis as at completion it is usually larger than it appears during the process. The nick requires greater force in children. After nick is given, utrata's forceps or microincision capsulorhexis forceps can be used to hold the edge of the rhexis. Frequent regrasps are required and aim should be to pull the rhexis toward the center rather than in circular fashion [5, 6] (Fig. 3.2). This will avoid inadvertent tearing or enlargement of rhexis. A callisto assist tool may be used to access the size of capsulorhexis (Fig. 3.3a–c). The instruments used for capsulorhexis are shown in (Fig. 3.3d–f) Alternately, there are multiple size guides available on the surface or intraocular. A well-centered circular ACCC is important for centration of IOL and prevention of posterior capsular opacification (PCO).

3.9.3 Vitrectorhexis

In certain cases where manual capsulorhexis is not possible, a vitrectorhexis can be planned. Management of special cases such capsular

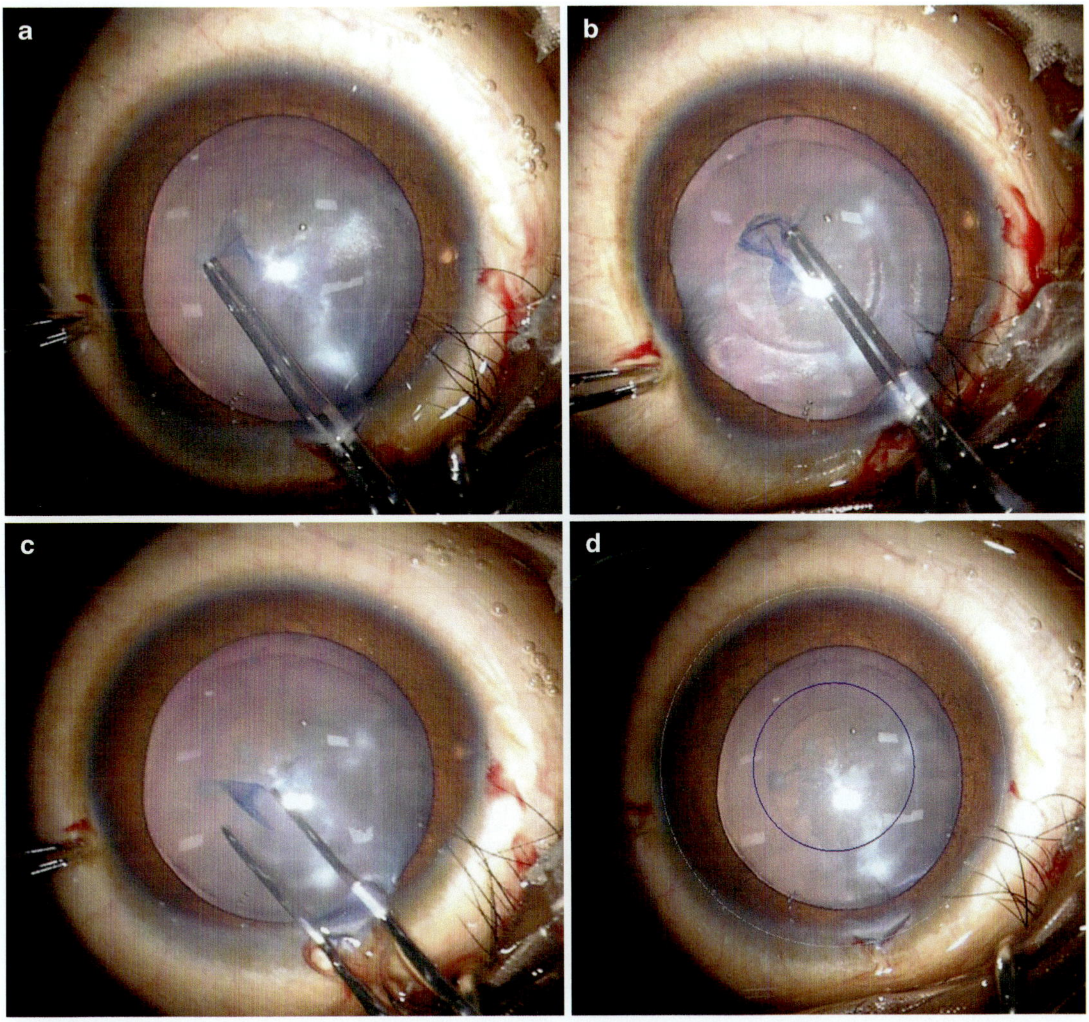

Fig. 3.2 Steps of anterior capsulorhexis (**a**, **b**) After nick of capsule, sheering edge of the capsulorhexis is held with capsulorhexis forceps with frequent regrasp. (**c**) Capsulorhexis is completed in circular fashion. (**d**) Relative size and centration in relation to limbus using capsulorhexis assist of Zeiss Lumera 700 microscope

plaques, persistent fetal vasculature (PFV), microphthalmos, etc. are discussed in respective chapters. Vitrectomy cutter can be used in Cut IA mode even in an uncomplicated pediatric cataract surgery. After intial cut with the cutter upside down, central opening is made in a spiral fashion. It is easier compared to the manual ACCC. The margin regularity and strength is inferior to manual ACCC which remains the gold standard for children.

Various other methods including use of diathermy, fugo blade, femtosecond laser, etc. for creation of capsulorhexis are also available and can be selected for specific cases [38–43].

3.10 Hydrodissection

Multiple quadrant cortical cleaving gentle hydrodissection is recommended for pediatric cataracts [24, 44]. It should be performed under OVD as it provides better cleavage of the cortex from capsule. The fluid wave passes more easily under OVD. It should be avoided in cases of pre-

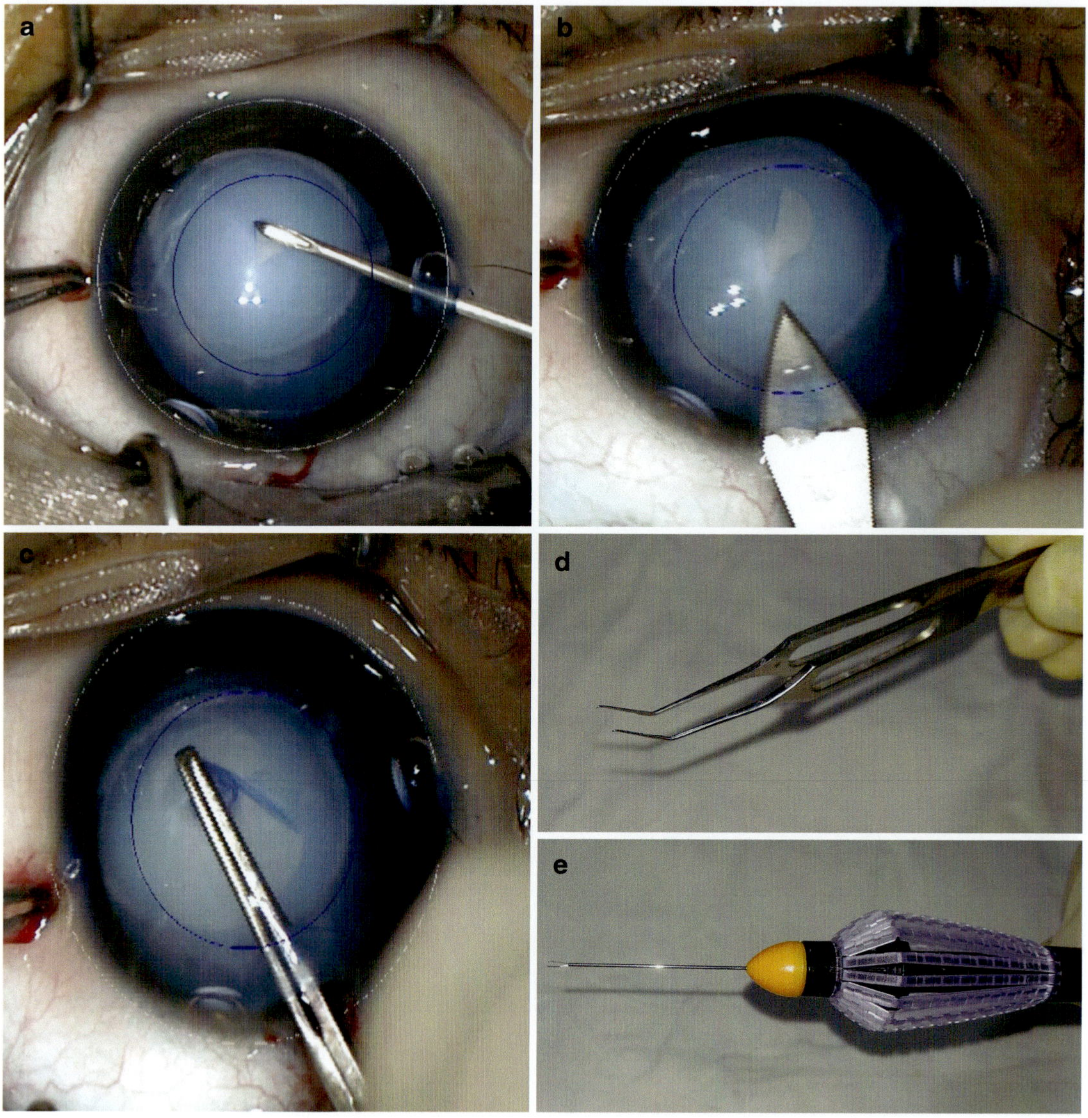

Fig. 3.3 Anterior capsulorhexis using capsulorhexis assist of Zeiss Lumera 700 microscope. (**a**) Nick is given to anterior capsule. (**b**) Nick is extended to 1 mm short of intented rhexis size and wound is extended. (**c**) Capsulorhexis is completed using Utrata capsulorhexis forceps. (**d**) Utrata capsulorhexis forceps. (**e**) Intravitreal forceps which can be used in place of microincision capsulorhexis forceps

existing posterior capsular defect, posterior polar cataract or traumatic cataract with suspected posterior capsular opening. Good hydrodissection reduces surgical durations, ensures complete removal of lens matter and reduced PCO formation. Caution is recommended if anterior capsulotomy has irregularities or small tear as it may get extended.

3.11 Lens Aspiration

3.11.1 Bimanual Technique

Bimanual technique uses two separate probes for irrigation and aspiration (Fig. 3.4). It is a quick and effective technique. The probes can be used via paracentesis incisions and do not require a

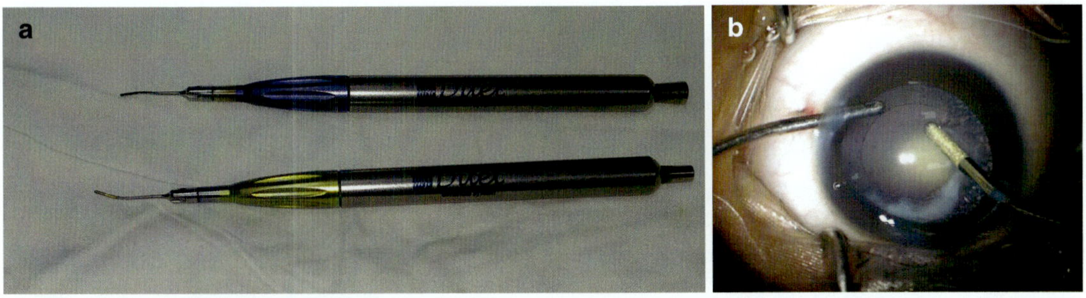

Fig. 3.4 (**a**) Bimanual Irrigation and aspiration instrument. (**b**) Intraoperative picture of bimanual Irrigation and aspiration in total cataract

large opening. The chamber remains more stable throughout surgery. Irrigation should be started before entry in the anterior chamber. Complete removal of lens matter can be performed including the difficult sub-incisional lens matter by using both hands for aspiration alternately. Irrigation probe can also be used for maintain centration of the eye if immobilization effect of anesthesia is insufficient.

3.11.2 Coaxial Techniques

If bimanual probes are unavailable, coaxial technique can also be used. There may be some discomfort in sub-incisional cortical matter removal; good hydro dissection and central adequate size capsulorhexis can provide ease with that. The aspiration tip should be under surgeon's visualization to avoid inadvertent damage to posterior capsule. The advantage is that thorough capsular polish can be performed with coaxial probe.

3.11.3 Vitrectomy Cutter

Vitrectomy cutter can be used for bimanual irrigation and aspiration in IA Cut mode (Low cut rate and high vacuum) of the vitrectomy system. It can be used in special cases such as microphthalmos, pre-existing posterior capsular defect, etc. where multiple instrumentation should be avoided.

3.12 Posterior Capsulorhexis

3.12.1 Rationale

The aim of pediatric cataract surgery is to not just provide clear visual axis but also maintain it for as long as possible. Visual axis opacification (VAO) is very common in young children if posterior capsule is left intact. The factors involved are discussed in detail in the respective chapter. Posterior capsulorhexis with or without anterior vitrectomy has been used for reduce VAO formation since 1980s [45]. This has been advocated over and again and is now considered standard of care for pediatric cataract surgery [46–49]. We recommend posterior capsulorhexis in children upto 8 years of age and anterior vitrectomy in children upto 6 years of age [24, 50]. This limit can be extended further in mentally challenged children or those with nystagmus.

3.12.2 Manual Posterior Capsulorhexis (PCC)

Posterior capsule is thinner than the anterior capsule. It is more elastic in children compared to adults. Like ACCC, manual PCC has strong margins and is unlikely to extend or tear off easily. It can support IOL well.

The technique PCC is different than ACCC in pediatric cataract (Fig. 3.5). Anterior capsule is filled with heavy visco-cohesive OVD. OVD

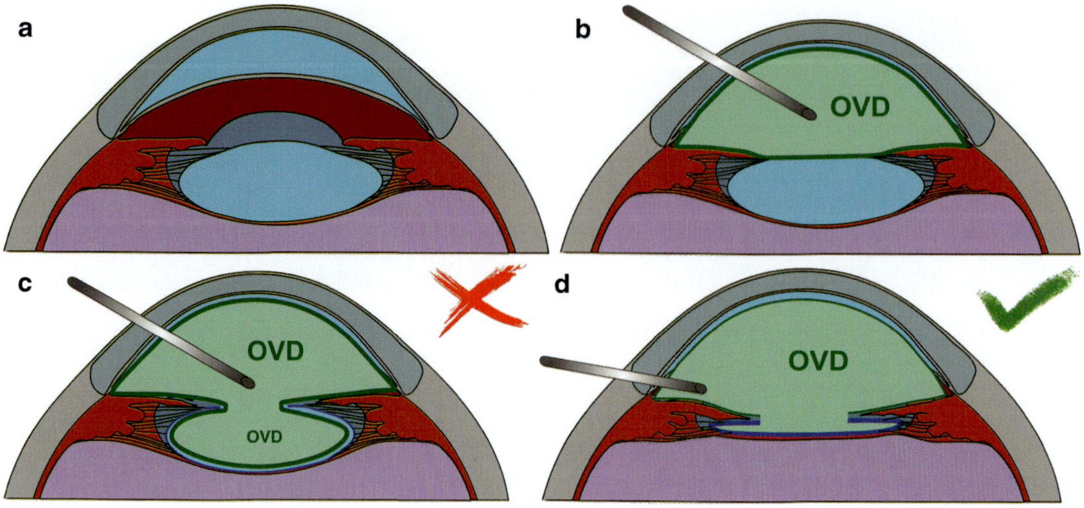

Fig. 3.5 Tricks for anterior and posterior capsulorhexis (**a**) Sketch diagram showing lens and its capsule before capsulorhexis (**b**) Anterior chamber showing flattening of anterior lens capsule after insertion of OVD (ophthalmic viscosurgical device) for anterior capsulorhexis. (**c**) For posterior capsulorhexis, OVD, if filled inside the capsular bag would lead to bulging of posterior capsule (PC), which may lead to run out of posterior capsulorhexis. (**d**) For posterior capsulorhexis, OVD should be filled in anterior chamber only, to avoid bulging of posterior capsule (PC). A flat PC maintained by just adequate vitreous pressure is desirable for good posterior capsulorhexis

is not injected in the bag. By avoiding OVD in the bag, a convexity of posterior capsule can be retained due to vitreous thrust. Capsule becomes lax and easy to manipulate. Similar to ACCC, nick is given in the center of the capsule. Since posterior capsule is farther away than anterior capsule, a longer and thinner instrument may be preferred. PCC is performed from the nick in a circular fashion with frequent regrasps (Fig. 3.6). For PCC, forceps can be sheering in a circular manner rather than toward the center only. Size for PCC should be around 4–4.5 mm, 1 mm smaller than ACCC. To achieve this, 1 mm small PCC should be aimed at, as the capsule is lax and after anterior vitrectomy it falls back and stretches; thus increasing in size.

3.12.3 Posterior Capsulotomy with Cutter

In cases where manual PCC is not possible such as in case of plaques or is not under surgeon's expertise, posterior capsulotomy of adequate size can be performed with vitrectomy cutter. Like ACCC, the disadvantage is irregular margins which may extend while IOL insertion.

3.12.4 Posterior Capsulotomy After IOL Insertion

Many surgeons prefer posterior capsulotomy using pars plana port after IOL insertion with adequate wound closure. IOL implantation becomes easy with intact capsule. Adequate size opening can be created in children without fear of extension as IOL serves as a guide for sizing. This is one of the most commonly employed techniques for surgery. We prefer manual PCC for it greater strength and regularity. The advantage of posterior capsulotomy after IOL insertion is that a bigger opening can be created. In our experience, manual PCC is just as easy and size can be controlled without additional effort.

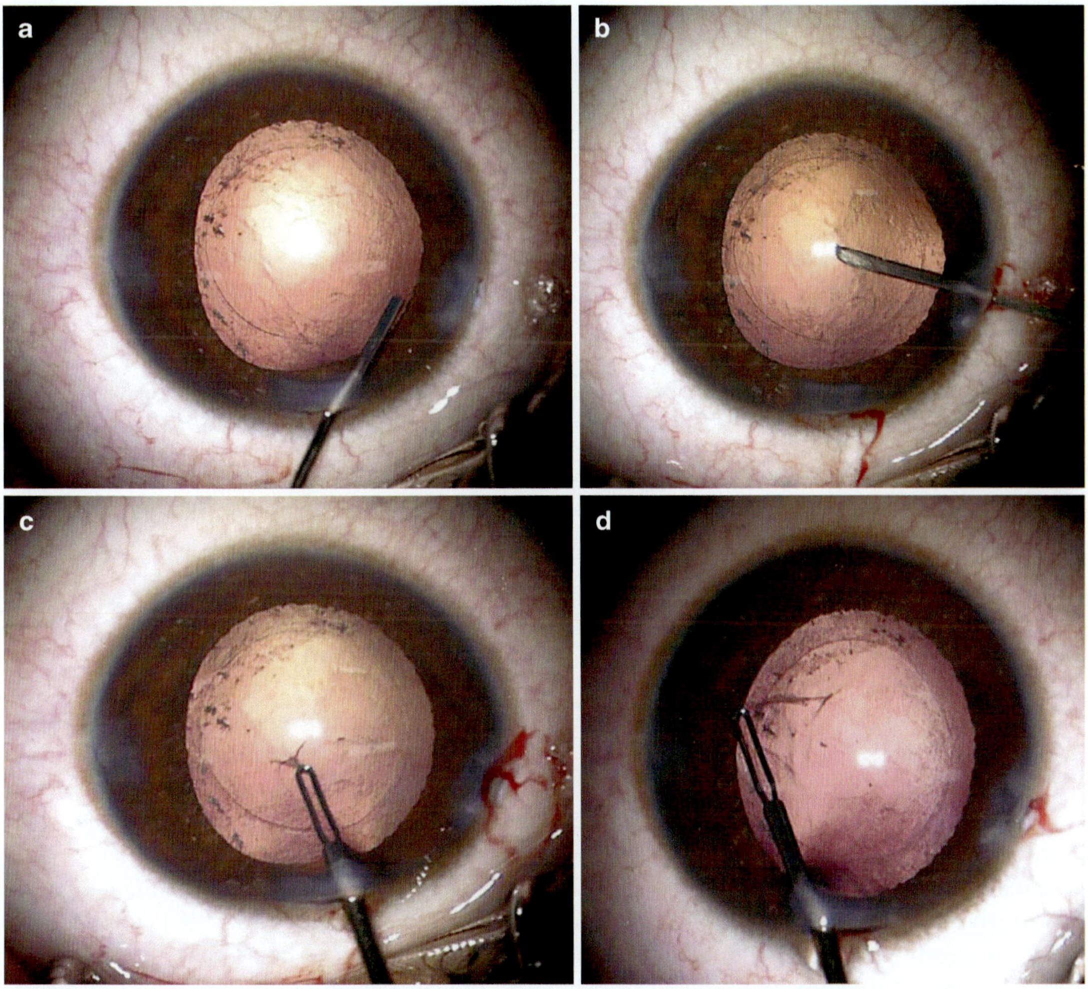

Fig. 3.6 Posterior capsulorhexis. (**a**) Anterior chamber is formed with viscoelastic devices. (**b**) Nick is given to anterior capsule. (**c**) Capsulorhexis started using microincision forceps. (**d**) Capsulorhexis is completed

3.13 Anterior Vitrectomy

3.13.1 Rationale

Anterior vitrectomy should be performed in smaller children to remove scaffold for proliferation of epithelial cells. This reduces VAO formation.

3.13.2 Machine Settings

Automate guillotine vitrectomy cutters are used currently for limited anterior vitrectomy. Based on the machine, cut rate and settings may vary. Current vitrectomy systems have better control and high cut rate. Vitrectomy can be performed using same machine as that for lens aspiration like centurion or separate machine like constellation. There are two mode of vitrectomy in a standard machine such as centurion (Fig. 3.7). Cut IA mode where cut rate is high (4000 cpm) and vacuum is kept low. It is meant for cutting tissues followed by aspiration such as vitreous, capsule etc. This does not cause any traction. Other mode is IA Cut mode, where cut rate is low (100–400 cpm) and vacuum and aspiration rate is high. It is meant for aspiration of tissue such as lens matter followed by cutting

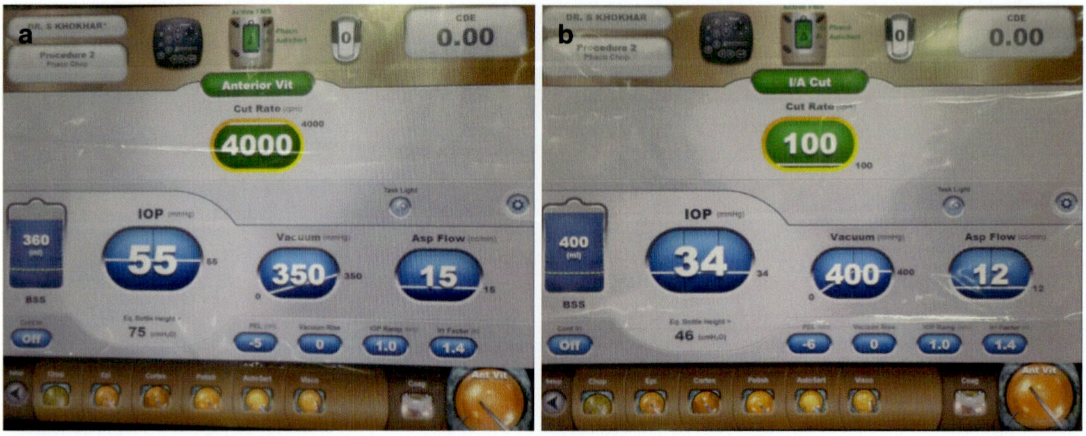

Fig. 3.7 Setting for vitrectomy machine (Centurion system @Alcon). (**a**) For anterior vitrectomy, use high cut rate and low vacuum. (**b**) For lens matter or viscoelastic removal keep low cut rate and more vacuum

if required. It can cause vitreous traction hence used for lens aspiration but not anterior vitrectomy (Fig. 3.8).

3.13.3 Technique

After performing PCC, localized anterior vitrectomy can be performed. Vitreous is well formed in children and the purpose of vitrectomy is to remove the scaffold for VAO formation. This allows surgeons to perform vitrectomy in the area of visualization. Vitrectomy should be performed not just in the center but also under the margins of posterior capsulotomy. This can be achieved by turning the cutter opening downwards away from capsular edge and 360° vitrectomy under margin can be performed. A bimanual technique can be used and hands can be switched in between to ensure complete limited anterior vitrectomy. There is no need to dip the probe deep and 2 cm depth of vitrectomy below capsule is generally sufficient. At the end point, posterior capsule should be free and opening should be circular with no tenting or peaking of capsule. Triamcinolone can be used as a negative stain to visualize residual vitreous [51].

3.14 IOL Insertion

3.14.1 Indication

There has been controversy related to IOL implantation especially in younger children <2 years of age. Infant aphakia treatment study (IATS) was a multicentric trial which compared IOL with contact lens in unilateral cataract patients. They reported similar visual outcome but greater complications in IOL group [52]. IOL implantation has been reported to be associated with greater risk of glaucoma in pediatric patients [53, 54].

With time, there has been a gradual shift toward use of IOL in pediatric cataracts [55]. The IoLunder2 Cohort Study was a non-randomized study for unilateral and bilateral cataract. It found better visual acuity in primary IOL group in bilateral cataracts although complications were more frequent [56]. Negalur et al. found encouraging results with primary IOL implantation in children under 6 months of age with good safety [57]. We recommend judicious decision making for IOL implantation in both unilateral and bilateral cataracts. IOL can be implanted in eyes with AL > 17 mm and white to white distance >10 mm [24].

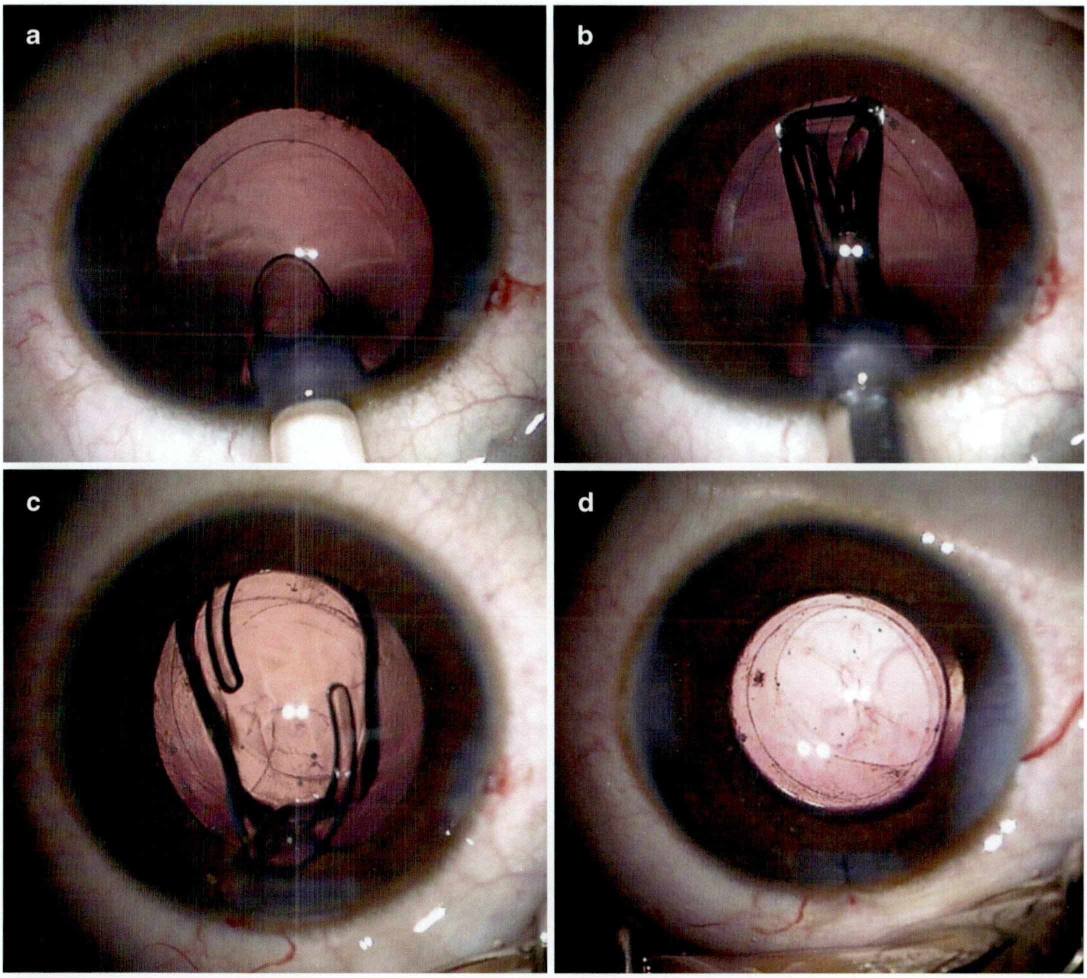

Fig. 3.8 Safe technique of IOL insertion in bag with posterior capsule opening. (**a**) Tip of IOL cartridge is inserted in anterior chamber via slightly larger incision. (**b**) Leading haptic of the IOL is gently inserted in the bag against the bag surface of the anterior capsule. (**c**) Allow IOL to open. (**d**) Final position of IOL after tucking trailing haptic

3.14.2 IOL Type

Most surgeons prefer hydrophobic acrylic IOL for children as well as adult [58]. A survey of AAPOS members showed that 93% respondents preferred in-the-bag fixation, hydrophobic acrylic IOLs [59]. In developing countries, there may be cost concerns related to IOL. Pediatric ophthalmologists have reported fair outcomes with hydrophilic IOL as well [60].

3.14.3 Technique

Insertion of IOL is challenging in cases of open posterior capsule. We have described a safe technique of IOL injection in pediatric cases [61]. Incision slightly larger than the size of injector system is made. In this technique, instead of wound assisted IOL injection, we prefer IOL injection where cartridge is in the anterior chamber. In a properly loaded IOL, both haptics are folded on the top of the lens. IOL is gently injected in the anterior chamber such that the folded leading haptic opens just under the anterior capsule. Once the leading haptic is secure in the bag, trailing haptic is gentle tucked in the bag using IOL dialer or sinsky's hook (Fig. 3.8). IOL should not be dialed vigorously instead the trailing haptic is nudge under the anterior capsule. Throughout this technique, there is no excess force on the posterior capsule. In-the-bag IOL implantation is the most preferred technique in children.

Alternately, technique of optic capture [62] can be used in pediatric cataract. This has been used to reduce the incidence of VAO formation [63, 64]. Multipiece IOL is used for optic capture technique. Optic capture (OC) includes fixation of IOL with capsulorhexis margin, hence it can with IOL in sulcus and capture with anterior capsule, OC with IOL in bag and capture with anterior capsule (reverse capture) or posterior capsule or most preferred technique where IOL is captured with both anterior and posterior capsule. When capture with both capsules is performed, they fuse together and prevent migration of cells behind IOL and hence prevent PCO formation [64]. It is simple technique and can be used in cases where anterior or posterior capsule is not intact.

3.15 Conclusion

To summarize, cataract surgery in children poses greater surgical challenge as compared to adults due to difference in anatomy and higher risk of complications. Special considerations and meticulous surgical technique for primary surgery can helps in achieving optimal outcome.

References

1. Chandler PA. Surgery of congenital cataract. Am J Ophthalmol. 1968;65:663–74.
2. Scheie HG. Aspiration of congenital or soft cataracts: a new technique. Am J Ophthalmol. 1960;50:1048–56.
3. Scheie HG, Ewing MQ. Aspiration of soft cataracts. Int Ophthalmol Clin. 1977;17:51–8.
4. Peyman GA, Raichand M, Goldberg MF. Surgery of congenital and juvenile cataracts: a pars plicata approach with the vitrophage. Br J Ophthalmol. 1978;62:780–3.
5. Taylor D. Choice of surgical technique in the management of congenital cataract. Trans Ophthalmol Soc U K. 1981;101:114–7.
6. Parks MM. Posterior lens capsulectomy during primary cataract surgery in children. Ophthalmology. 1983;90:344–5.
7. Benezra D. The surgical approaches to paediatric cataract. Eur J Impl Refract Surg. 1990;2:241–4.
8. Benezra D, Cohen E. Posterior capsulectomy in pediatric cataract surgery: the necessity of a choice. Ophthalmology. 1997;104:2168–74. https://doi.org/10.1016/S0161-6420(97)30045-1.
9. Gimbal H. Posterior continuous curvilinear capsulorhexis and optic capture of the intraocular lens to prevent secondary opacification in pediatric cataract surgery. J Catar Ref Surg. 1997;23(Suppl 1):652–6. https://doi.org/10.1016/S0886-3350(97)80049-1.
10. Gayer S, Tutiven J. Anesthesia for pediatric ocular surgery. Ophthalmol Clin N Am. 2006;19(2):269–78.
11. Cote CJ. NPO guidelines: children and adults. In: McGoldrick KE, editor. Ambulatory anesthesiology. Baltimore, MD: Williams & Wilkins; 1995. p. 20–32.
12. Rossiter JD, Wood M, Lockwood A, Lewis K. Operating conditions for ocular surgery under general anesthesia: an eccentric problem. Eye (Lond). 2006;20:55–8.
13. Mindel JS, Eisenkraft JB, Raab EL, Teutsch G. Succinyldicholine and the basic ocular deviation. Am J Ophthalmol. 1983;95:315–26.
14. Wei LX, Deng XM, Wang L, Sui JH, Zhang YM, Tong SY, et al. Induction of tracheal intubation without muscle relaxant by target controlled infusion of propofol combined with remifentanil in children. Zhongguo Yi Xue Ke Xue Yuan Xue Bao. 2011;33:440–4.
15. James I. Anesthesia for paediatric eye surgery. Contin Educ Anaesth Crit Care Pain. 2008;8:5–10.
16. Hopster K, Ohnesorge B, von Borstel M, Rohn K, Kästner S. Influence of atracurium on cardiovascular parameters in horses undergoing vitrectomy during general anesthesia, and on recovery duration and quality. Tierarztl Prax Ausg G Grosstiere Nutztiere. 2013;41:371–7.
17. McMurphy RM, Davidson HJ, Hodgson DS. Effects of atracurium on intraocular pressure, eye position, and blood pressure in eucapnic and hypocapnic isoflurane-anesthetized dogs. Am J Vet Res. 2004;65:179–82.
18. Martini E, Bressan F, Benvenuti S, Rizzo L, La Torre MS, Novelli GP. Anesthesia with sevoflurane and orotracheal intubation for pediatric ophthalmic surgery of medium length in day hospital. Minerva Anestesiol. 2000;66:807–10.
19. Darlong V, Garg R, Pandey R, Khokhar S, et al. Evaluation of minimal dose of atracurium for cataract surgery in children: a prospective randomized

double-blind study. Saudi J Anaesth. 2015;9(3):283–8. https://doi.org/10.4103/1658-354X.154711.
20. Beck AD, Freedman SF, Lynn MJ, Bothun E, Neely DE, Lambert SR. Glaucoma-related adverse events in the Infant aphakia treatment study: 1-year results. Arch Ophthalmol. 2012;130:300–5.
21. Freedman SF, Lynn MJ, Beck AD, et al. Glaucoma-related adverse events in the first 5 years after unilateral cataract removal in the infant aphakia treatment study. JAMA Ophthalmol. 2015;133:907–14.
22. Birch EE, Stager DR. The critical period for surgical treatment of dense congenital unilateral cataract. Invest Ophthalmol Vis Sci. 1996;37:1532–8.
23. Hartmann EE, Lynn MJ, Lambert SR, Infant Aphakia Treatment Study G. Baseline characteristics of the infant aphakia treatment study population: predicting recognition acuity at 4.5 years of age. Invest Ophthalmol Vis Sci. 2015;56:388–95.
24. Khokhar SK, Pillay G, Dhull C, Agarwal E, Mahabir M, Aggarwal P. Pediatric cataract. Indian J Ophthalmol. 2017;65(12):1340–9.
25. Broadway DC, Grierson I, Hitchings RA. Local effects of previous conjunctival incisional surgery and the subsequent outcome of filtration surgery. Am J Ophthalmol. 1998;125:805–18.
26. Dick HB, Schwenn O, Krummenauer F, et al. Inflammation after sclerocorneal versus clear corneal tunnel phacoemulsification. Ophthalmology. 2000;107:241–7.
27. Bar-Sela SM, Spierer A. Astigmatism outcomes of scleral tunnel and clear corneal incisions for congenital cataract surgery. Eye (Lond). 2006;20:1044–8.
28. Matsumoto Y, Hara T, Chiba K, et al. Optimal incision sites to obtain an astigmatism-free cornea after cataract surgery with a 3.2 mm sutureless incision. J Cataract Refract Surg. 2001;27:1615–9.
29. Noonan CP, Rao GP, Kaye SB, et al. Validation of a handheld automated keratometer in adults. J Cataract Refract Surg. 1998;24:411–4.
30. Meier P, Wiedemann P. Surgery for pediatric vitreoretinal disorders. Surgical considerations and techniques – posteriorsegment surgical techniques. In: Ryan SJ, editor. Surgical retina. Part 1. 5th ed. Amsterdam: Elsevier; 2013. p. 3; (Sec. 3. 1936–1939).
31. Bar-Sela SM, Spierer O, Spierer A. Suture-related complications after congenital cataract surgery: vicryl versus mersilene sutures. J Cataract Refract Surg. 2007;33:301–4.
32. Matalia J, Panmand P, Ghalla P. Comparative analysis of non-absorbable 10-0 nylon sutures with absorbable 10-0 vicryl sutures in pediatric cataract surgery. Indian J Ophthalmol. 2018;66:661. https://doi.org/10.4103/ijo.IJO_654_17.
33. Jhanji V, Sharma N, Vajpayee RB. Management of intraoperative miosis during pediatric cataract surgery using healon 5. M E Afr J Ophthalmol. 2011;18(1):55–7.
34. Krag S, Olsen T, Andreassen TT. Biomechanical characteristics of the human anterior lens capsule in relation to age. Invest Ophthalmol Vis Sci. 1997;38:357–63.
35. Seland JH. Ultrastructural changes in the normal human lens capsule from birth to old age. Acta Ophthalmol. 1974;52:688–706.
36. Gimbel HV, Neuhann T. Development, advantages, and methods of the continuous circular capsulorhexis technique. J Cataract Refract Surg. 1990;16:31–7.
37. Dick HB, Aliyeva SE, Hengerer F. Effect of trypan blue on the elasticity of the human anterior lens capsule. J Cataract Refract Surg. 2008;34(8):1367–73. https://doi.org/10.1016/j.jcrs.2008.03.041.
38. Comer RM, Abdulla N, O'Keefe M. Radiofrequency diathermy capsulorhexis of the anterior and posterior capsules in pediatric cataract surgery: preliminary results. J Cataract Refract Surg. 1997;23(Suppl 1):641–4.
39. Kloti R. Anterior high frequency capsulotomy. I. Experimental study. Klin Monbl Augenheilkd. 1992;200:507–10.
40. Fugo RJ, Delcampo DM. The Fugo Blade: the next step after capsulorhexis. Ann Ophthalmol. 2001;33:13–20.
41. Khokhar S, Tejwani LK, Kumar G, Kushmesh R. Approach to cataract with persistent hyperplastic primary vitreous. J Cataract Refract Surg. 2011;37:1382–5.
42. Palanker DV, Blumenkranz MS, Andersen D, et al. Femtosecond laser assisted cataract surgery with integrated optical coherence tomography. Sci Transl Med. 2010;2:58–85.
43. Toropygin SG, Krause M, Akkaya A, et al. Experimental femtosecond laser-assisted nanosurgery of anterior lens capsule. Eur J Ophthalmol. 2011;21:237–42.
44. Vasavada AR, Trivedi RH, Apple DJ, et al. Randomized, clinical trial of multiquadrant hydrodissection in pediatric cataract surgery. Am J Ophthalmol. 2003;135:84–8.
45. Parks MM. Management of the posterior capsule in congenital cataracts. J Pediatr Ophthalmol Strabismus. 1984;21:114–7.
46. Ben Ezra D, Cohen E. Posterior capsulectomy in pediatric cataract surgery the necessity of a choice. Ophthalmology. 1997;104:2168–74.
47. Vasavada A, Desai J. Primary posterior capsulorhexis with and without anterior vitrectomy in congenital cataracts. J Cataract Refract Surg. 1997;23(Suppl 1):645–51.
48. Alexandrakis G, Peterseim MM, Wilson ME. Clinical outcomes of pars plana capsulotomy with anterior vitrectomy in pediatric cataract surgery. J AAPOS. 2002;6:163–7.
49. Guo S, Wagner RS, Caputo A. Management of the anterior and posterior lens capsules and vitreous in pediatric cataract surgery. J Pediatr Ophthalmol Strabismus. 2004;41:330–7.
50. Lin AA, Buckley EG. Update on pediatric cataract surgery and intraocular lens implantation. Curr Opin Ophthalmol. 2010;21:55–9.

51. Burk SE, Da Mata AP, Snyder ME, et al. Visualizing vitreous using Kenalog suspension. J Cataract Refract Surg. 2003;29:645–51.
52. Plager DA, Lynn MJ, Buckley EG, Wilson ME, Lambert SR. Complications, Adverse Events, and Additional Intraocular Surgery 1 Year after Cataract Surgery in the Infant Aphakia Treatment Study. Ophthalmology. 2011;118:2330–4.
53. Freedman SF, Lynn MJ, Beck AD, Bothun ED, Orge FH, Lambert SR. Glaucoma-related adverse events in the first five years after unilateral cataract removal in the Infant Aphakia Treatment Study. JAMA Ophthalmol. 2015;133(8):907–14.
54. Yagev R, Khatib N, Barrett C, Lior Y, Lifshitz T, Tsumi E. Intraocular lens implantation as an isolated risk factor for secondary glaucoma in pediatric patients. Can J Ophthalmol. 2019;54(5):621–5. https://doi.org/10.1016/j.jcjo.2019.01.003.
55. Kumar P, Lambert SR. Evaluating the evidence for and against the use of IOLs in infants and young children. Expert Rev Med Devices. 2016;13(4):381–9. https://doi.org/10.1586/17434440.2016.1153967.
56. Solebo AL, Russell-Eggitt I, Cumberland PM, Rahi JS. Risks and outcomes associated with primary intraocular lens implantation in children under 2 years of age: the IoLunder2 cohort study. Br J Ophthalmol. 2015;99:1471–6.
57. Negalur M, Sachdeva V, Neriyanuri S, Ali MH, Kekunnaya R. Long-term outcomes following primary intraocular lens implantation in infants younger than 6 months. Indian J Ophthalmol. 2018;66(8):1088–93. https://doi.org/10.4103/ijo.IJO_182_18.
58. Wilson ME Jr, Bartholomew LR, Trivedi RH. Pediatric cataract surgery and intraocular lens implantation: practice styles and preferences of the 2001 ASCRS and AAPOS memberships. J Cataract Refract Surg. 2003;29:1811–20.
59. Wilson ME, Trivedi RH. Choice of intraocular lens for pediatric cataract surgery: survey of AAPOS members. J Cataract Refract Surg. 2007;33:1666–8.
60. Kleinmann G, et al. Pediatric cataract surgery with hydrophilic acrylic intraocular lens. J AAPOS. 2013;17(4):367–70. https://doi.org/10.1016/j.jaapos.2013.04.007.
61. Khokhar S, Sharma R, Patil B, Sinha G, Nayak B, Kinkhabwala RA, et al. A safe technique for in-the-bag intraocular lens implantation in pediatric cataract surgery. Eur J Ophthalmol. 2015;25:57–9.
62. Gimbel HV, DeBroff BM. Intraocular lens optic capture. J Cataract Refract Surg. 2004;30:200–6.
63. Raina UK, Gupta V, Arora R, et al. Posterior continuous curvilinear capsulorhexis with and without optic capture of the posterior chamber intraocular lens in the absence of vitrectomy. J Pediatr Ophthalmol Strabismus. 2002;39:278–87.
64. Zhou HW, Zhou F. A meta-analysis on the clinical efficacy and safety of optic capture in pediatric cataract surgery. Int J Ophthalmol. 2016;9:590–6.

4 Bag in the Lens

Marie-José Tassignon and Luc Van Os

Cataract surgery in adults is one of the most performed surgical procedures worldwide with a success rate of around 75% to 85% in achieving target refraction using a standard cataract surgical technique, which varies very little form case to case. In contrast, cataract surgery in babies and children requests a case per case approach. Different ocular or systemic parameters may influence the surgical procedure and ultimately the surgical outcome. Axial length and corneal curvature in children under the age of two have not yet reached final biometrical measures to allow a routine surgery or to implant a precise power of the Intra Ocular Lens (IOL) that will guarantee emmetropia at adulthood. An easily changeable IOL should therefore be preferred.

At the department of the University hospital of Antwerp, a novel surgical approach was developed to compensate for these drawbacks and allow surgical procedures with intraocular IOL implantation without anterior vitrectomy (except in special cases) in babies and children under the age of two and that is easily exchangeable. This technique is known as the Tassignon method or even better known as the Bag-In-the-Lens (BIL) surgical technique of lens implantation [1]. It is based on the insertion of the capsular bag, after performing an anterior and posterior capsulorhexis, within a peripheral groove defined by the anterior and posterior elliptic shaped haptic flanges confined around the central optic. Based on this particular implantation method, the name of bag-in-the-lens was given to this IOL.

The reputation of this IOL being difficult to implant is based on the fact that the BIL requires a more precise surgical technique since both the anterior and posterior capsulorhexes must be alike in shape and size in order to prohibit the remaining lens epithelial cells to proliferate toward the visual axis as it is described after Lens-In-the-Bag implantation technique. This more complex surgery will finally result in a better outcome at the long term.

To encompass this exercise, a foldable caliper ring of a precise diameter was developed and patented [2]. This is the smallest intraocular device available on the market allowing a sized and centered anterior capsulorhexis. It can be inserted through a 1.2 mm clear cornea incision. This is particularly interesting in case of cataract in children. We all agree that keeping the anterior seg-

M. J. Tassignon has an intellectual proprietary interest in the bag-in-the-lens and ring caliper, licensed to Morcher-Germany.

Supplementary Information The online version of this chapter (https://doi.org/10.1007/978-981-16-0212-2_4) contains supplementary material, which is available to authorized users.

M.-J. Tassignon (✉) · L. Van Os
Department of Ophthalmology of the University Hospital of Antwerp, The Antwerp University, Edegem-Antwerp, Belgium
e-mail: marie-jose.tassignon@uza.be

S. K. Khokhar, C. Dhull (eds.), *Essentials of Pediatric Cataract Surgery*,
https://doi.org/10.1007/978-981-16-0212-2_4

ment closed is preferred by all surgeons not only to reduce surgical induced astigmatism but also to avoid iris prolapse and to keep the pressure in the anterior segment balanced with the pressure of the posterior segment. Only Femtosecond laser can perform a sized anterior and posterior capsulorhexis prior to performing a corneal incision. Centration in the visual axis is not yet guaranteed in most of currently available machines.

The BIL-IOL was patented in 1997 and licensed to Morcher, Germany. The aim of this new device is to eradicate Posterior Capsule Opacification (PCO). It was approved by the Belgian Government in 2004. The clinical trial following the 2006 ISO normation for IOLs was published in 2011 [3]. The BIL was further affined with the aim of using this IOL in more complex cases like in cases with corneal astigmatism [4] but also in more difficult cases like in sub-luxated crystalline lenses, traumatic cases with torn capsules or eyes with extreme biometrical parameters. Bean shaped ring fixation segments have been developed for the purpose of BIL IOL centration in complex cases with loose zonules [5, 6]. The adult shape of BIL has a total diameter of 7.5 mm and an optic of 5 mm. The reason for this choice was dictated by the knowledge of the retrolenticular space (Berger space) diameter which in adults is typically 8 mm in width.

When starting the BIL in babies in the year 2000, we were convinced that a BIL of smaller diameter would have be superior for the purpose of implantation in children with small eyes as we expected smaller retrolenticular spaces. With increased expertise and the added value of the intraoperative OCT [7] we were able to evaluate the variations in dimensions of the retrolenticular space. We described a new entity of congenital cataract based on dysgenesis of the vitreolenticular anterior interface [8]. This study evolved in a better understanding of what can go wrong due to underdevelopment of the vitreous during embryological development of the eye.

Our aim is to equip most eyes with a BIL-IOL and to optimally respect the existing anatomy of the eye and the compartmentation between anterior and posterior segment of the eye.

This chapter will discuss three different clinical conditions of congenital cataract.

- CASE 1 shows a BIL procedure and the implantation in an 18-month-old child with Down syndrome presenting with a developmental cataract.
- CASE 2 shows a BIL procedure in an anterior subcapsular plaque in a 11 months old child without any predisposing factors for congenital or syndromal cataract.
- CASE 3 shows the viscodissection of the anterior hyaloid from the posterior capsule until the ligament of Wieger is reached.

4.1 Case 1

We perform currently a clinical trial for the use of Mydrane (Théa Pharma-France) to dilate the pupil of the babies and children on the operating table. This off-label, study-based, approach avoids ocular manipulation of the patient prior to the narcosis. Dilation is often quick and optimal except in patients with iris pathologies (e.g., synaechiae or neurotrophic iris). The benefit of this drug is multiple. Most important is that the child cannot crying out the dilation drops anymore and is more relaxed when entering the surgical facilities in the parent's arms.

A 1 mm corneal incision is performed while avoiding small vessels to bleed (systemic absorption of the drug!) prior to injecting very slowly 0.12 mL Mydrane. Dispersive heavy molecular weight Healon (Johnson & Johnson Vision—USA) is then injected to further sustain pupil dilation and counteract vitreous pressure. The caliper ring (Morcher—Germany 4.5 internal mm) is injected using a dedicated caliper guide manufactured by EyeTech-UK Fr2268. Centration of the ring is based on first and fourth Purkinje reflexes. The ring is then firmly pushed in contact with the anterior capsule by means of a heavy weight cohesive OVD and a final centration control is made by means of a self-made eye cage (EyeTech-UK LCD305B). The outer rim of this cage is centered on the limbus so that the inner ring will guide the surgeon to adapt once more the final centration of the ring caliper. The younger the child the more elastic the capsule will be. We therefore prefer to puncture the anterior capsule with a 27G needle before initiating the anterior capsulorhexis with the capsulorhexis Ikeda forceps (EyeTech Fr2268). The anterior capsulorhexis is a crucial step in the BIL technique and should be performed slowly but accurately by the surgeon. This step is essential since the posterior capsulorhexis will be performed by using the anterior capsulorhexis as a guide.

Depending on the patient age or eye condition, the lens content will be removed with a bimanual method or using a coaxial aspiration-irrigation probe. In our particular case, a bimanual irrigation-aspiration of the lens content is used.

Once the lens content is completely removed the anterior chamber is filled again with high molecular weight cohesive OVD taking care that the capsular bag is absolutely not inflated but on the contrary that both anterior and posterior capsule remain closely collapsed against each other and pushed back until both capsules have reached a horizontal position. This position is ideal to perform the posterior capsulorhexis after having punctured the posterior capsule by means of a 27G needle.

All these maneuvers can now be observed by means of the OCT of the Lumera microscope (Zeiss-Germany). It is well visible on OCT how closely the anterior hyaloid is located to the posterior capsule in eyes of children or babies with normal crystalline anatomy. The space defined within the area of the posterior capsule and the anterior hyaloid and surrounded by the ligament of Wieger, is quasi virtual in children and babies. In case of dysgenesis of that space a posterior plaque will be present. This was obviously not the case in this particular child. We thus can conclude that the anterior interface in this child is intact and follows the expectation of a mature tertiary vitreous development.

Once the posterior capsulorhexis is performed, we usually separate the anterior hyaloid even further to ensure a proper bag-in-the-lens implantation with a total diameter of 7.5 mm.

This video (Video 4.1) illustrates very well that we did not pay enough attention to optimize the sizing of the Berger space. The BIL can still be properly inserted but we had to try and retry again before total insertion of the capsule within the lens groove was achieved. We therefore use ever since a bimanual push-pull technique of the capsulorhexis opening taking care that we dilate this opening widely by reducing the width of the Wieger ligament until we are sure the posterior haptic can take full position within the Berger's area.

Once the BIL is implanted, the lens can eventually be rotated within the rhexis opening to assure the optimal position of the lens (not shown in this video).

We then reclose the pupil with diluted Miostat (Alcon) in the dilution: 0.5 cc Miostat: 2 mL with BSS.

All incisions are carefully closed with vicryl 10/0 for children older than 2 years or by Nylon 10/0 in younger children.

The incisions are then inflated with Aprokam 0.1 mL (Théa Pharma-France) to close the case.

4.2 Case II

This case presents the difficult task to perform a sized and centered anterior capsulorhexis in the presence of a retro-capsular plaque.

Corneal incision, insertion of the 4.5 internal diameter ring caliper are identical to CASE I. We used vision blue to enhance the visibility of the anterior capsule. This case shows beautifully that the anterior capsule is totally independent of the subcapsular plaque, which is an excellent condition to perform a precise anterior capsulorhexis.

The lens content and the plaque are then removed by means of a bimanual irrigation-aspiration technique.

Here again both capsules are kept collapsed and pushed back by means of high molecular weight cohesive OVD until they achieved a horizontal position.

To visualize the anterior hyaloid separation of the posterior capsule from the anterior hyaloid using the OCT, we now face the problem that the reflection of the cornea prohibits the visualization of the anterior interface. This is due to the very small anterior chamber depth.

The use of the OCT in childhood cataract using the Lumera has some limitations as in case of small anterior chamber depth and movements of the eye with the child breathing because of the intubation.

The posterior capsulorhexis is further performed as explained in CASE I.

In this video (Video 4.2) we show an alternative technique to ensure proper capsules insertion within the lens groove. We called this the bimanual implantation technique, which is done by positioning the BIL on top of the remaining capsule but with the longest axis of the posterior haptic in the surgeon's 6–12 o'clock position. The insertion of the posterior haptic is then initiated by first inserting both capsules at the surgeon's 6 o'clock position in the lens groove followed by little pushing maneuvers until half of the capsule rim is inserted. Then the left hand holds a blunt instrument, which is positioned between both IOL haptics while the right hand keeps a lens positioner in such way that this ball shaped hook is glided behind the posterior lens haptic. The hook retracts then both capsules and helps their positioning into the BIL groove.

The case is ended by constricting the pupil with Miostat dilution as explained in CASE I, followed by cleaning the OVD out of the anterior chamber, suturing the corneal incisions and hydrating the incisions with Aprokam as explained in CASE I.

4.3 Case III

This case shows an OCT clip of a 2-year-old child demonstrating the progressive viscodissection of the anterior hyaloid from the posterior capsule until the ligament of Wieger is reached. Further insisting to fill the Berger space with OVD might result in blowing up the puncture performed in the posterior capsule to initiate the posterior capsulorhexis.

4.4 In Conclusion

Increasing the precision of the surgical procedure and using the BIL technique of implantation, allowed us to discover quite some interesting details about the anatomy of the anterior interface in children. Still more is to be described by using this technique in more cases around the world.

The beauty of this technique is that it not only controls PCO but it also reduces secondary surgical procedures [9], it is easy to exchange and it helped us to discover a new cause for congenital cataract due to anterior interface dysgenesis.

Other centers are studying the benefit of this technique like less inflammation [10] and less postoperative instillation of corticosteroid drugs. Our postoperative regimen consists of 4 instillations daily up to a maximum of 6 times per day during the first postoperative week to be tapered down over the following 4 weeks. This can undeniably be considered a child and parent friendly postoperative treatment. More information about the bag-in-the-lens implantation technique can be found in the book published in 2019 by Springer Nature in the series Innovative Implantation Technique: Bag-in-the-lens Cataract Surgery [11].

References

1. Tassignon MJ. Morcher GmbH, assignee. Intraocular lens and method for preventing secondary opacification. US patent 6 027 351, 2000.
2. Tassignon M, Rozema JJ, Gobin L. Ring-shaped caliper for better anterior capsulorhexis sizing and centration. J Cataract Refract Surg. 2006;32:1253–5.
3. Tassignon MJ, Gobin L, Mathysen D, Van Looveren J, De Groot V. Clinical outcomes of cataract surgery after bag-in-the-lens intraocular lens implantation following ISO standard 11979-7:2006. J Cataract Refract Surg. 2011;37(12):2120–9.
4. Tassignon M-J, Gobin L, Mathysen D, Van Looveren J. Clinical results after spherotoric intraocular lens implantation using the bag-in-the-lens, J. Cataract Refract. Surg. 2011;37:830–7.
5. Altenburg A, Dhubhghaill SN, Tassignon MJ. Bean-shaped ring segments as a capsule enhancement tool in complex bag-in-the-lens intraocular lens implantation. J Refract Surg. 2017;33(7):454–9.

6. Dhubhghaill SN, Dogaroiu AC, Zakaria N, Tassignon MJ. Modified bean-shaped ring segments for suture fixation of the bag-in-the-lens intraocular implant. J Cataract Refract Surg. 2017;43:1003.
7. Tassignon MJ, Dhubhghaill SN. Real time intraoperative optical coherence tomography imaging confirms older concepts about the Berger space. Ophthalmic Res. 2016;56(4):222–6.
8. Van Looveren J, et al. Pediatric bag-in-the-lens intraocular lens implantation: long-term follow-up. J Cataract Refract Surg. 2015;41:1685–92.
9. Nyström A, Almarzouki N, Magnusson G, Zetterberg M. Phacoemulsification and primary implantation with bag-in-the-lens intraocular lens in children with unilateral and bilateral-cataract. Acta Ophthalmol. 2018;96:364–70.
10. Auchère Lavayssiere C, Lux AL, Beraud G, Degoumois A, Billotte C, Denion É. Bag-in-the-lens implantation helps avoid posterior synechiae of the iris after phacovitrectomy. J Cataract Refract Surg. 2019;45(10):1386–92.
11. Tassignon MJ, Dhubhghaill SN, Van Os L, editors. Innovative implantation technique: bag-in-the-lens cataract surgery. Cham: Springer Nature; 2019. https://doi.org/10.1007/978-3-030-03086-5.

Secondary IOL in Congenital Cataract Surgery

5

M. Edward Wilson and Rupal H. Trivedi

5.1 Introduction

Primary intraocular lens (IOL) implantation can be done at any age, including early infancy. However, in the first 6 months of age, the preferred approach is to leave the child aphakic and implant an IOL at a later date when the child is older and the remaining refractive growth is easier to predict. There is a higher incidence of reoperations for visual axis opacification when IOLs are implanted in the first 6 months of life compared to leaving the child aphakic [1]. These results have resulted in more children being left aphakic when operated in infancy. Most of these children will eventually undergo secondary IOL implantation. For the initial aphakia after infantile cataract surgery, timely refractive correction is necessary to preserve monocular vision and binocularity and to protect against stimulus deprivational amblyopia. Conservative management may include correction with glasses or contact lenses, although these measures are not possible for all children. Aphakic spectacles are an option for bilateral aphakic children but often undesirable for social and optical reasons.

5.2 General Considerations

Secondary implantation of an IOL is generally recommended when traditional spectacle or contact lens correction of aphakia is unsuccessful or becomes a barrier to the child's development and activities of daily living. If sufficient capsular support for capsular bag or ciliary sulcus fixation is present, we offer secondary IOL implantation soon after we notice contact lens/spectacle wear becomes difficult or fails.

5.3 IOL Fixation Sites

Most commonly, secondary IOL implantation in our patients is performed between the ages of 4 and 6 years, a period when contact lens compliance can be difficult to maintain and yet there is still hope to reverse amblyopia. Due to relatively slower growth of eye after this age, IOL power calculation is also more predictable. We use SilSoft contact lens or aphakic glasses to treat aphakia prior to secondary IOL placement. SilSoft contact lenses are well tolerated in very young children but the material is less well tolerated as children get older. The silicone contact lenses develop more deposits and the lens coat-

Supplementary Information The online version of this chapter (https://doi.org/10.1007/978-981-16-0212-2_5) contains supplementary material, which is available to authorized users.

M. E. Wilson · R. H. Trivedi (✉)
Storm Eye Institute, Medical University of South Carolina, Charleston, SC, USA
e-mail: wilsonme@musc.edu; trivedi@musc.edu

S. K. Khokhar, C. Dhull (eds.), *Essentials of Pediatric Cataract Surgery*,
https://doi.org/10.1007/978-981-16-0212-2_5

ing breaks down more quickly when worn in older children. Rather than change to a non-silicone contact lens material, some parents will opt to have a secondary IOL implanted at that point.

If capsular support is not available, every effort to correct aphakia using spectacles or contact lens should be exhausted before deciding on secondary IOL implantation. Risk must be minimized but amblyopia must not be left untreated or undertreated. Nowhere is that balance more difficult than when there is inadequate capsular support in the face of contact lens and aphakic spectacle intolerance.

The technical success of secondary implantation depends mainly on how much capsular support was left behind at the time of primary cataract surgery. Ultrasound biomicroscopy (UBM) may help to detect residual capsular support and image the ciliary sulcus when viewing it directly is difficult. Three hundred sixty degree visibility of the fused edge of the posterior and anterior capsulectomy from the previous surgery increases the chances of achieving successful posterior segment implantation of an IOL. In the office, if the posterior capsule is not initially visible at the slit lamp, having the patient look in extremes of gaze while maintaining the slit lamp chin position may allow the capsular remnant to be seen under the iris. Sometimes, examination through a peripheral iridectomy (if present) is useful to look for capsular remnants. There are times, however, when uncertainty about how much capsular support is present remains until surgery when a push–pull instrument or hook can be used to look directly under the iris in all quadrants.

When performing infantile cataract surgery without a primary IOL implantation, an adequate capsular rim should be left for subsequent posterior segment IOL placement. We urge surgeons to plan for the next surgery when performing the initial lensectomy. A 4.5-mm central matching anterior and posterior capsulectomy is ideal. This size is adequate to prevent subsequent closure and reopacification of the visual axis but assures an adequate rim of support when secondary IOL implantation is elected.

5.3.1 In the Bag

If capsular support is available, the IOL should be placed in the posterior segment either in-the-bag or in the ciliary sulcus. The most desirable position for the IOL is within the reopened capsular bag. However, if the capsular leaflets are sealed to one another without re-proliferated cortex (Soemmering ring) to maintain anterior and posterior leaflet separation in the lens equator, ciliary sulcus fixation is an acceptable and safe choice [2].

Despite the above recommendation, poor capsular support is often seen in pediatric aphakic eyes, particularly after removal of congenital cataracts, traumatic cataract, or ectopia lentis. In the absence of sufficient lens capsule support, choosing the best site for the IOL in a child is more difficult and controversial. Sutured or intrascleral fixated posterior chamber IOLs, an open-loop flexible anterior chamber IOL or the Artisan (Ophtec) iris-claw lens are available options. In the absence of capsular support and in the presence of a disrupted iris, sutured transcleral or non-sutured intrascleral fixated posterior chamber IOL are the only viable options.

The technique of in-the-bag secondary IOL implantation in children was reported in 1999 by one of us (MEW) [3]. Our updated experience with this technique was published in 2005 and 2011 [4, 5]. In-the-bag fixation is more consistently achieved in eyes made primarily aphakic during early infancy. This young age at surgery leads to a higher tendency for an exuberant Sommering ring formation. The Sommering ring lens cortex fills the capsular bag equator and prevents the anterior and posterior capsule remnants from sealing to one another and closing the capsular bag remnant. Removing the contents of the Sommering ring and replacing them with an ophthalmic viscosurgical device (OVD), allows in-the-bag IOL placement to occur more predictably. An odds ratio analysis revealed that within our study group, eyes originally operated before 6 months of age were 8.7 times more likely to receive a secondary in-the-bag than those patients who were remained aphakic after the age of 6 months [5]. In a subsequent study, we noticed that all of the eyes that received in-the-bag IOL insertion had a cataract extraction within the first 4 months of life [4].

During surgery, it is important to assess whether it is possible to reopen the capsular bag leaflets. The key is to locate one area in which the anterior capsule edge is not strongly adherent to the posterior capsule [6]. Using the entry point, an OVD can be very useful in the separation of the capsular layers. A combination of dissection techniques using intraocular scissors, a micro vitreoretinal knife, and, most commonly, the 25-gauge vitrector handpiece are used to create a new anterior capsule edge and reopen the capsular bag for 360°. The Soemmering ring cortical material is then removed by bimanual irrigation/aspiration and a secondary IOL is placed into the capsular bag.

5.3.2 Ciliary Sulcus Fixation

If in-the-bag fixation is not possible, ciliary sulcus fixation is an acceptable alternative if technically possible [2–5, 7–9]. Awad et al. [10] performed UBM on the ciliary sulcus in 10 eyes after secondary IOL implantation. The structure of the sulcus in the implanted eye appeared similar to the sulcus in the contralateral normal eye. However, ciliary sulcus-fixated IOLs are more prone to develop pupillary capture, pigment dispersion, ciliary body erosion, decentration, unstable loop fixation, and lens tilt than IOL with bag fixation [11]. A study of adult eyes reported that even more than 2 years after cataract surgery, anterior chamber flare counts in eyes with sulcus IOL fixation were significantly higher than in eyes with in-the-bag fixation [12]. The three-piece Acrysof (Alcon, Fort Worth, Tx) is appropriate for sulcus fixation as well as in-the-bag positioning. It does not have a propensity to cause pigment dispersion when placed in the ciliary sulcus, although it does decenter at times unless optic capture is done. Non-angulated single-piece acrylic IOLs are not usually recommended for ciliary sulcus fixation. However, we have found that the Rayner C-*flex (570-C)* IOL is an exception. It is well tolerated by pediatric eyes when it placed in the ciliary sulcus. Optic capture through fused anterior and posterior capsule and haptics in the ciliary sulcus is another viable option for keeping the three-piece Acrysof IOL centered and stable. At the time of this writing, the Rayner C-*flex (570-C)* is our preferred IOL for sulcus placement when optic capture is not also being done. The three-piece acrylic lenses are still used by us in the ciliary sulcus but mostly when we are planning either monocapsular or bicapsular optic capture.

In a patient with bilateral aphakia, we recommend implanting the eye with the worst capsular support first. If it is not feasible to safely achieve implantation, bilateral aphakia can still be chosen. This approach can help avoid an IOL in one eye and aphakia in the other. While corneal tunnel incisions are usually utilized for secondary IOL implantation, a scleral tunnel incision should be considered when the capsular support is limited. After the posterior synechiae are severed, a change to a PMMA IOL, if available, may be warranted to provide a stable bridge across a large posterior capsule opening. This change can be accomplished more easily from a scleral incision.

5.3.3 ACIOL

In absence of capsular support, the implantation of an open-loop anterior chamber IOL (AC IOL) is the simplest surgical procedure for surgical aphakic correction. Modern, flexible AC IOLs have a much lower incidence of complications compared to the poorly tolerated rigid closed-loop AC IOLs of the past. The current designs of AC IOLs remain a viable alternative to sutured IOLs when there is an absence of capsular support. However, AC IOLs are used with caution in children. The most common complication seen in children relate to sizing of an angle-supported AC IOL in an eye that is still growing. Lens rotation over time (lens is too short after growth) can cause ovaling of the pupil and iris entrapment. A lens that is too long can cause corneal contact and iris atrophy. Correct sizing for AC angle width is critical to prevent IOL rotation and/or corneal contact or iris entrapment and chronic inflammation. Traditionally, surgeons have used the corneal white-to-white measurement +1 mm as a guide for correct AC IOL sizing. A relatively large incision of at least 6 mm is required for currently available AC IOLs. A surgical peripheral iridectomy should be performed superiorly. A meta-analysis performed as part of the OTAC series revealed that insufficient evidence exists to demonstrate the superiority of a posterior versus an anterior chamber IOL in adults [13]. Anterior chamber intraocular lens implantation is contraindicated in the presence of extensive damage to the iris and anterior chamber angle, preexisting glaucoma, peripheral anterior synechiae (PAS), low endothelial cell count and shallow anterior chamber [14]. With the availability of iris-claw lenses, we no longer implant angle-supported AC IOLs in any children.

5.3.4 Iris-Claw IOL

Iris-claw IOLs, which are lenses placed in the anterior chamber and attached to the iris with small claw-like haptics, have been described to correct aphakia in adults and children, with good visual results (Fig. 5.1). These lenses have been available in most parts of the world for several years and are now being implanted in 20 sites in the USA under a compassionate-use FDA investigational device exemption. The aphakic Artisan IOL (Ophtec, Groningen, The Netherlands) is a peripheral "iris bridge" supported lens. The standard aphakic Artisan IOL is made of Perspex-CQ UV (a type of PMMA) and is 8.5 mm in overall diameter. The optic size is 5.0 mm and the overall body diameter is 5.4 mm. Implantation requires a 5.5 mm incision. Two smaller IOL sizes for microphthalmic eyes are manufactured at 6.5 mm and 7.5 mm in overall diameter with optic sizes of 4.4 mm. These smaller IOLs are not yet available in the USA. The fixation points for all of the Artisan IOLs are in the immobile peripheral iris. The IOL has a central oval shaped optic having an anterior vault (minimizes iris damage) and two fixation arms (haptics) that have a cut in them that provides a claw-grasping mechanism.

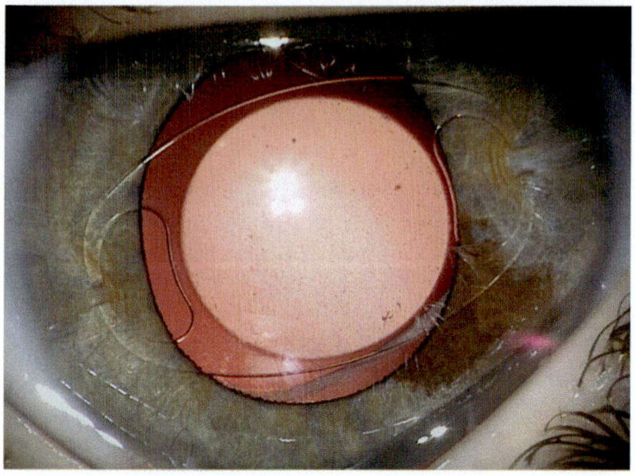

Fig. 5.1 Secondary Artisan IOL in an aphakic child with insufficient capsular support—note there is a small amount of capsule at the bottom of the picture but inadequate for posterior chamber support

Ideal method of iris-claw fixation includes: centrally placed optic, passing of an adequate amount of iris tissue through the claws of the lens, not pulling the iris root, not pulling the sphincter muscle/pupil margin toward the claw, and no injury to corneal endothelium. Advantages of artisan IOL implantation includes: The iris bridge protects the endothelium from touching the PMMA; There are no restrictions to pupil dilation or constriction; Excellent centration stability once fixated; The IOL has maximal visibility, accessibility, and controllability; Virtually cosmetically invisible; Easy to reposition and is reversible and exchangeable; No interference with vascular iris physiology; No sizing is normally needed—one size fits all. Disadvantage of artisan IOL includes: Requires surgical skill to position properly and create the ideal iris bridge but the learning curve is short. Implantation requires an incision of 5.5 mm ideally located at the limbus since the IOL is grasped through the incision when the iris bridge fixations are created. Early astigmatism is high but fades with healing. Wounds need to be sutured.

The Artisan IOL can also be fixated in a retropupillary manner if desired [15]. To accomplish this, the pupil is not initially constricted. The IOL is inserted with the convex side down (upside down) and held behind the pupil with the IOL implantation forceps through the corneal tunnel. As the lens is being inserted behind the pupil, a miotic should be injected into the anterior chamber to constrict the pupil. The lens is lifted and tilted slightly to show the contour of the claws through the iris stroma. A fins spacula is inserted through a paracentesis to exert gentle pressure on the slotted center of the lens haptic to perform the enclavation. The same maneuver is repeated on the other side. Late dislocation of the lens can occur when one of the enclavation sites becomes dislodged, most often due to trauma. Prevention of this complication involves being meticulous about getting the proper amount of iris enclavated into each claw of the IOL. Late endothelial decompensation is expected to be very rare with the Artisan lens but ongoing long-term monitoring continues.

Posterior chamber intraocular lens (PCIOL) offer several advantages and many authors recommend them even in eyes lacking capsular or zonular support [16]. Scleral fixation of PCIOL is a method to overcome the lack of capsular support but is technically more difficult and time-consuming compared to ACIOL or Artisan IOL implantation. Due to its anatomic location in the eye, PCIOL is often reserved for patients with low endothelial cell counts, peripheral anterior synechiae (PAS) and cystoid macular edema (CME) [17]. Transscleral sutured IOL fixation can be considered in cases with inadequate capsular support or in cases with compromised anterior chamber structure. Shuaib and colleagues compared the results of transscleral IOL fixation to retropupillary iris-claw lens implantation in cases of pediatric aphakia without capsular support. This study concluded that both techniques yielded comparable visual outcome. Retropupillary iris-claw lens fixation is a shorter procedure and technically easier than sutureless transscleral fixation, but the risk of disenclavation should be considered especially in younger age groups. Scleral fixation is the only option in cases of severe iris damage [15]. Scleral suture fixation can be performed by either Ab externo (passing needle from outside to inside) or ab interno approach (inside to out). The ab externo approach is preferred by many. A disturbing late complication of transscleral suture fixation of IOLs is the spontaneous breakage of the polypropylene suture leading to IOL displacement, especially in young patients [18, 19]. Buckley [20] reviewed the literature on transscleral sutured IOLs in children. He reported the outcome of 33 eyes with an average follow-up of 61 months (range 9–200 months). Twenty-one of the eyes had greater than 3 years of follow-up and 14 eyes (42%) had more than 5 years of follow-up. Four patients had spontaneous suture breakage at 38, 66, 96, and 107 months after implantation. An additional 13 cases of 10.0-prolene suture breakage in children were uncovered by a survey of pediatric ophthalmologists. In addition to slow biodegradation of the suture, there are other factors that may contribute to the higher probability of suture breakage in children. These include globe enlargement with age, continuous eye rubbing, and higher probability of eye trauma due to more active lifestyle. To reduce the chance of suture breakage, it is important to consider the use of multiple sutures on each haptic, thicker sutures [21] (such as the 9–0 polypropylene mentioned above), or a different suture material such as GORE-TEX (W. L. Gore & Associates, Newark DE).

In adult eyes, iris-sutured IOLs have been used successfully to correct aphakia. The application of these techniques in the pediatric age group has been limited. The iris-sutured IOL fixation is preferred by some surgeons over the transcleral IOL fixation techniques because it is technically less demanding [22], and requires a shorter operative time. It also believed that the risk for cystoid macular edema, IOL tilt, and late suture breakage is lower in iris-fixated IOLs [23, 24]. Another potential advantage of iris suturing is a lower risk of suture erosion, and diminished risk of suture wick endophthalmitis [25–29]. Condon and associates suggested that the lower risk of late suture breakage may be the result of the fact that the elasticity of the peripheral iris provides a more forgiving suspension system than the sclera, which, in a transsclerally sutured IOL, is fixated to a rigid IOL spanning the posterior segment [30]. Iris fixation of a PCIOL is an alternative for secondary IOL placement in pediatric aphakic patients without capsular support in the short-term, but should be approached with caution. Overall, in posterior chamber IOL suture techniques, the complication rate seems to be decreasing over the years, probably due to the increasing experience of surgeons in these difficult techniques. In addition, transscleral suturing techniques are now being replaced by intrascleral sutureless fixation techniques. With these methods, the IOL haptics are externalized and then tucked back into either an intrascleral tunnel beneath a glued scleral flap or tucked back after a cautery-induced mushroom cap has been fashioned at the tip of each haptic.

While secondary IOL power can be estimated using the aphakic refraction [31, 32], the estimate is less accurate than biometry [33]. If biometry cannot be obtained in the clinic setting due to poor cooperation and if biometry is not available in operating room, the aphakic refraction can be used to estimate IOL power. A change of the IOL fixation site may require adjusting the *IOL power*. If a decision is made to place the IOL in the ciliary sulcus, rather than the capsular bag, a decrease in lens power is often necessary. This is due to the fact that as the optic is shifted more anterior (moved closer to the cornea), its "effective power" increases. The amount of this change is dependent on the "base power" of the IOL. The greater the power of the IOL, the greater the difference in its effective power when it is placed in the ciliary sulcus instead of the capsular bag. If an IOL power calculated for the capsular bag needs to be changed to the ciliary sulcus, substract 1.5 D for ≥28.5 D, 1 D for 28.0 to 17.5, 0.5 D for 17.0 to 9.5 D. No substraction is required if power at capsular bag is <9 D (http://www.doctor-hill.com/iol-main/bag-sulcus.htm).

Simultaneous eye muscle and IOL implantation surgery in patients with strabismus and aphakia has been reported [34]. Combining IOL implantation and strabismus repair may reduce the number of surgical and anesthetic procedures, speed rehabilitation, and offer financial benefit to the patient and third-party payors. However, concern may arise regarding a potential increased risk of postoperative infection, anterior segment ischemia, or excessive discomfort for the patient. Determining the ocular alignment in eyes with poor vision may be difficult. We typically offer secondary IOL implantation surgery first (if indicated), wait for vision to recover, start amblyopia treatment, evaluate for strabismus, and offer strabismus surgery as a separate procedure.

5.4 Complications

Some postoperative complications after secondary IOL implantation are worth mentioning here. We reported that eyes with preexisting glaucoma were more likely to develop an IOP spike during the early postoperative period [35]. We recommend additional topical antiglaucoma medication or oral acetazolamide for children undergoing secondary IOL implantation with the preoperative diagnosis of aphakic glaucoma. Decentration of the IOL was the most common complication reported in our series. Clinically significant decentration was noted in 4 (5.2%), while dislocation of the IOL was reported in 2 (2.6%) eyes; and pupillary capture requiring repositioning of the IOL in 1 (1.3%) eye. Clinically significant decentration requiring surgical intervention was noted only in eyes with sulcus-fixated foldable IOLs (28.6%; 4/14). None of the 29 eyes with sulcus-fixated polymethylmethacrylate (PMMA) IOL implantation developed decentration. Perhaps the rigidity of PMMA IOLs helped to avoid decentration. Foldable IOLs in the sulcus have been noted to be at risk for decentration and dislocation [36]. Decentration/dislocation was responsible for 21% of explanted three-piece hydrophobic acrylic IOLs in a 2001 survey [37]. All the decentrations were in an inferior direction and occurred more often in the eyes of male patients [5]. Perhaps this is due to the higher incidence of trauma among males. Another possible reason is that male eyes have been noted to have a longer axial length than female eyes. Eyes with an axial length of >23 mm were 4 times more likely to develop decentration if implanted with a sulcus-fixated foldable IOL when compared with eyes measuring <23 mm. We hypothesized that longer eyes may also have a "wider" anterior segment. A wider sulcus-to-sulcus distance may promote IOL decentration [5]. Another recent study has reported decentration in 6% of eyes after secondary placement of foldable Acrysof IOLs in the ciliary sulcus [38]. Jacobi and associates noted decentration of a scleral fixation of a secondary foldable monofocal or multifocal IOL implant in 19.2% of eyes of children and young adults [39]. We have now begun to use the Rayner *C-flex (570C)* IOL in the ciliary sulcus more often than the Acrysof MA-60 IOL, especially in eyes longer than 23 mm in globe axial length and when optic capture is not easily achieved.

A higher incidence of *cystoid macular edema* with secondary IOL implantation in adults in whom vitreous loss occurred at the time of initial cataract surgery has been reported. Other studies, however, reported excellent results when a careful and controlled vitrectomy was performed with secondary IOL implantation. Although we did not perform angiography, we did not observe clinically significant cystoid macular edema after secondary implantation in our series of pediatric eyes [5].

5.5 Conclusion

In summary, in the presence of adequate capsular support, secondary IOL implantation can be safely achieved in pediatric eyes. In-the-bag fixation is preferred over ciliary sulcus fixation but either is acceptable. When leaving an infant aphakic in the first months of life, the surgeon should plan for the secondary IOL placement by carefully leaving 360° of capsular support and matching anterior and posterior capsulotomy edges at 4 to 4.5 mm centrally. With this plan, an easy and safe secondary IOL surgery can be offered when these children reach preschool or grade-school age. In the absence of available capsular support, scleral-supported IOLs, iris-claw lenses, or ACIOLs can be used, depending on the surgeon's preference, the ocular environment, and IOL availability. Each of these options require careful follow-up over an extended period of time. As opposed to when adequate capsular support is present, these alternative implantation strategies should be performed only after the surgeon and parents are convinced that visual rehabilitation of the patient cannot be achieved with a contact lens or a safer surgical procedure. Because of the possibility of late complications such as dislocation of IOL in these children without capsular support, they should be observed regularly.

References

1. Lambert SR, Aakalu VK, Hutchinson AK, Pineles SL, Galvin JA, Heidary G, et al. Intraocular lens implantation during early childhood: a report by the American Academy of ophthalmology. Ophthalmology. 2019;126(10):1454–61.
2. DeVaro JM, Buckley EG, Awner S, Seaber J. Secondary posterior chamber intraocular lens implantation in pediatric patients. Am J Ophthalmol. 1997;123(1):24–30.
3. Wilson ME Jr, Englert JA, Greenwald MJ. In-the-bag secondary intraocular lens implantation in children. J AAPOS. 1999;3(6):350–5.
4. Wilson ME Jr, Hafez GA, Trivedi RH. Secondary in-the-bag intraocular lens implantation in children who have been aphakic since early infancy. J AAPOS. 2011;15(2):162–6.
5. Trivedi RH, Wilson ME Jr, Facciani J. Secondary intraocular lens implantation for pediatric aphakia. J AAPOS. 2005;9(4):346–52.
6. Steinert RF, Arkin MS. Secondary intraocular lens implantation and stabilization. In: Steinert RF, editor. Cataract surgery. 3rd ed. Amsterdam: Elsevier; 2011.
7. Biglan AW, Cheng KP, Davis JS, Gerontis CC. Results following secondary intraocular lens implantation in children. Trans Am Ophthalmol Soc. 1996;94:353–73; discussion 74-9.
8. Biglan AW, Cheng KP, Davis JS, Gerontis CC. Secondary intraocular lens implantation after cataract surgery in children. Am J Ophthalmol. 1997;123(2):224–34.
9. Nihalani BR, Vanderveen DK. Secondary intraocular lens implantation after pediatric aphakia. J AAPOS. 2011;15(5):435–40.
10. Awad AH, Mullaney PB, Al-Hamad A, Wheeler D, Al-Mesfer S, Zwaan J. Secondary posterior chamber intraocular lens implantation in children. J AAPOS. 1998;2(5):269–74.
11. Apple DJ, Mamalis N, Loftfield K, Googe JM, Novak LC, Kavka-Van Norman D, et al. Complications of intraocular lenses. A historical and histopathological review. Surv Ophthalmol. 1984;29(1):1–54.
12. Amino K, Yamakawa R. Long-term results of out-of-the-bag intraocular lens implantation. J Cataract Refract Surg. 2000;26(2):266–70.
13. Wagoner MDCT, Ariyasu RG, Jacobs DS, Karp CL. Intraocular lens implantation in the absence of capsular support. Ophthalmology. 2003;110:840–59.
14. Malinowski SM, Mieler WF, Koenig SB, Han DP, Pulido JS. Combined pars plana vitrectomylensec-

tomy and open-loop anterior chamber lens implantation. Ophthalmology. 1995;102:211–6.
15. Shuaib AM, El Sayed Y, Kamal A, El Sanabary Z, Elhilali H. Transscleral sutureless intraocular lens versus retropupillary iris-claw lens fixation for paediatric aphakia without capsular support: a randomized study. Acta Ophthalmol. 2019;97(6):e850–e9.
16. Girard L. PC IOL implantation in the absence of posterior capsule support. Ophthalmic Surg Lasers Imaging. 1988;19:680–2.
17. Johnston RCD, Horgan S, Cooling R. Combined pars plana vitrectomy and sutured posterior chamber implant. Arch Ophthalmol. 2000;118:905–10.
18. Vote BJ, Tranos P, Bunce C. Long-term outcome of combined pars plana vitrectomy and scleral fixated sutured posterior chamber intraocular lens implantation. Am J Ophthalmol. 2006;41:308–12.
19. Assia EI, Nemet A, Sachs D. Bilateral spontaneous subluxation of scleral-fixated intraocular lenses. J Cataract Refract Surg. 2002;28:2214–6.
20. Buckley EG. Safety of transscleral-sutured intraocular lenses in children. J AAPOS. 2008;12(5):431–9.
21. Price MO, Price FW Jr, Werner L, Berlie C, Mamalis N. Late dislocation of scleral-sutured posterior chamber intraocular lenses. J Cataract Refract Surg. 2005;31(7):1320–6.
22. Kaiura TL, Seedor J, Kopline R, Rhee M, Ritterband D. Complications arising from iris-fixated posterior chamber intraocular lenses. J Cataract Refract Surg. 2005;31:2420–2.
23. Condon GP, Masket S, Kranemann C, Crandall AS, Ahmed II. Small-incision iris fixation of foldable intraocular lenses in the absence of capsule support. Ophthalmology. 2007;114(7):1311–8.
24. Dureau PMP, Edelson C, Caputo G. Iris fixation of foldable intraocular lenses for ectopia lentis in children. J Cataract Refract Surg. 2006;32:1109–14.
25. Epley KD, Shainberg MJ, Lueder GT, Tychsen L. Pediatric secondary lens implantation in the absence of capsular support. J AAPOS. 2001;5(5):301–6.
26. Bardorf CM, Epley KD, Lueder GT, Tychsen L. Pediatric transscleral sutured intraocular lenses: efficacy and safety in 43 eyes followed an average of 3 years. J AAPOS. 2004;8(4):318–24.
27. Heilskov TJB, Olsen KR, Blankenship GW. Late endophthalmitis after transscleral fixation of a posterior chamber intraocular lens. Arch Ophthalmol. 1989;107:1427.
28. Ozmen ATDM, Erturk H, Ozcetin H. Transsclerally fixated intraocular lenses in children. Ophthalmic Surg Lasers. 2002;33:394–9.
29. McCluskey PHB. Long-term results using scleral-fixated posterior chamber intraocular lenses. J Cataract Refract Surg. 1994;20:34–9.
30. Condon GPMS, Kranemann C, Crandall AS, Ahmed IIK. Small-incision iris fixation of foldable intraocular lenses in the absence of capsule support. Ophthalmology. 2007;114:1311–8.
31. Hug T. Use of the aphakic refraction in intraocular lens (IOL) power calculations for secondary IOLs in pediatric patients. J Pediatr Ophthalmol Strabismus. 2004;41(4):209–11.
32. Khan AO, AlGaeed A. Paediatric secondary intraocular lens estimation from the aphakic refraction alone: comparison with a standard biometric technique. Br J Ophthalmol. 2006;90(12):1458–60.
33. Abdel-Hafez G, Trivedi RH, Wilson ME, Bandyopadhyay D. Comparison of aphakic refraction formulas for secondary in-the-bag intraocular lens power estimation in children. J AAPOS. 2011;15(5):432–4.
34. Ticho BH, Ticho KE, Kaufman LM. Combined strabismus and lens surgery. J AAPOS. 2006;10(5):430–4.
35. Trivedi RH, Boden JH, Mickler C, Wilson ME. Intraocular pressure elevation during early postoperative period after secondary intraocular lens implantation in children and adolescents. J Cataract Refract Surg. 2012;38(9):1633–6.
36. Mamalis N. Explantation of intraocular lenses. Curr Opin Ophthalmol. 2000;11(4):289–95.
37. Mamalis N, Spencer TS. Complications of foldable intraocular lenses requiring explantation or secondary intervention—2000 survey update. J Cataract Refract Surg. 2001;27(8):1310–7.
38. Crnic T, Weakley DR Jr, Stager D Jr, Felius J. Use of AcrySof acrylic foldable intraocular lens for secondary implantation in children. J AAPOS. 2004;8(2):151–5.
39. Jacobi PC, Dietlein TS, Jacobi FK. Scleral fixation of secondary foldable multifocal intraocular lens implants in children and young adults. Ophthalmology. 2002;109(12):2315–24.

6 Intraoperative and Postoperative Complications

Rupal H. Trivedi and M. Edward Wilson

Cataract surgery in children is more difficult and the rate of complications is higher when compared to adult surgery. The rate of intraoperative and postoperative complications is inversely proportional to the age at surgery. In addition to age, surgical technique can influence the rate of complications (e.g., primary intraocular lens implantation vs. aphakia). Higher intraoperative complications in children may be attributed to the common occurrence of an immature iris that results in poor pupil dilation. In addition, the eyes of young children are small and soft. Even small and well-constructed surgical wounds leak when not sutured securely. The anterior capsule in children is highly elastic and difficult to predictably tear into a circular and centered capsulorhexis. Scleral collapse and a formed, non-liquified, vitreous body create the upthrust commonly referred to as posterior vitreous pressure. Postoperative complications are also higher due to an intense inflammatory response and poor compliance to postoperative topical anti-inflammatory drops. The detection of postoperative complications can be challenging because of the difficulties encountered in performing detailed postoperative examinations in children, who may be uncooperative.

6.1 Intraoperative Complications

Innovations in surgical technique (e.g., closed chamber techniques using bimanual irrigation/aspiration) and technology (e.g., high viscosity viscosurgical devices, improvement in intraocular lens materials and designs, advances in vitrectomy instruments, etc.) have helped us to minimize surgical trauma such as iris manipulation and improve the overall intraoperative performance. The rate of intraoperative complications is higher in eyes receiving primary intraocular lens (IOL) implantation as compared to aphakia. In the Infant Aphakia Treatment Study (IATS), intraoperative complications were observed in 11% (6/57) of eyes in the *no IOL group* versus 28% (16/57) of eyes in the *IOL group* [1].

Iris prolapse is more frequently observed during pediatric cataract surgery as compared to adult surgery as a result of poorly developed iris tissue and the nearly universal finding of a floppy iris. Over-filling of the anterior segment with ophthalmic viscosurgical device (OVD), to counteract the collapsibility of the soft eyes, may contribute to the frequency of iris prolapse. Incisions should be constructed to provide a snug

Supplementary Information The online version of this chapter (https://doi.org/10.1007/978-981-16-0212-2_6) contains supplementary material, which is available to authorized users.

R. H. Trivedi (✉) · M. E. Wilson
Storm Eye Institute, Medical University of South Carolina, Charleston, SC, USA
e-mail: trivedi@musc.edu

S. K. Khokhar, C. Dhull (eds.), *Essentials of Pediatric Cataract Surgery*,
https://doi.org/10.1007/978-981-16-0212-2_6

fit for the instruments that pass into the anterior chamber. This concept of a tight-fit, closed chamber, is much more important in pediatric surgery than it is when operating on adults. In IATS, iris prolapse during surgery was observed in 4% (2/57) of eyes in the *no IOL* group and 21% (12/57) of eyes in the *IOL group* ($P = 0.008$) [1]. The authors attributed this fivefold increase in the IOL group to a larger wound size and the greater intraocular manipulation required to implant an IOL in a small, soft and often microphthalmic infant eye [1].

A pupil may fail to dilate preoperatively if the iris is immature and lacking the smooth muscle development needed for an active dilation response to mydriatic drugs. The iris may also be fibrotic and adherent to the lens capsule. During surgery, a well-dilated pupil may constrict due to surgical iris manipulation or touch. Miosis from iris manipulation occurs in a more robust fashion in children as compared to adults. Use of 0.5 mL of 1:1000 non-preserved, bisulfite-free adrenaline (epinephrine) in 500 mL of irrigating fluid has been in standard use for pediatric cataract surgery for decades. Intracameral epinephrine helps to maintain pupillary dilation throughout the surgery. The use of OVD can also help to improve or maintain pupil dilation in children. As described in adult eyes, the intraoperative floppy-iris syndrome (IFIS) includes a triad of intraoperative signs: *iris billowing and floppiness, iris prolapse, and progressive miosis* [2, 3]. We reported pediatric IFIS in a 4-month old child when epinephrine was inadvertently omitted during cataract surgery [2]. Intracameral phenylephrine and ketorolac (1%/0.3%), known as Omidria (Omeros, Seattle, WA) is now FDA approved in the USA for adults and children to help maintain pupil diameter during cataract surgery and reduce postoperative pain. A direct comparison study of non-preserved epinephrine and Omidria in pediatric eyes has not, to our knowledge, been conducted.

Fluctuation of anterior chamber depth (anterior chamber "bounce") occurs frequently in soft pediatric eyes and can result in more inflammation via the iris stimulation that the bounce induces. Bimanual irrigation/aspiration through tight-fit wounds with minimal leaking helps to maintain a consistent deep anterior chamber throughout the lens aspiration, thus avoiding anterior chamber fluctuation. Some surgeons prefer to use an anterior chamber maintainer rather than holding both instruments as in bimanual surgery. An unstable anterior chamber usually results from too much leak around the instruments that are placed in the anterior chamber. Venturi-pump machines often have a fluid pump that can be increased to offset the leak. Gravity-fed irrigation systems are not as effective. The surgeon must also learn to balance the aspiration with the irrigation in a way that does not repeatedly shallow the anterior chamber during surgery.

It is no longer a secret that anterior capsulotomy is notoriously difficult in infants and young children because of the extreme elasticity of the anterior capsule. The capsulotomy is made even more challenging when there is poor dilation of the pupil and positive vitreous pressure. Rarely, an anterior capsule tear may be observed as soon as the anterior chamber is opened, caused by the sharp tip of the entrance knife, especially when the anterior chamber is very shallow. The availability of better operating microscopes, microsurgical instruments, higher-viscosity OVDs and the use of trypan blue are helpful. However, a "runaway rhexis" or a tear extending out toward the equator is still frequently encountered. For manual continuous curvilinear capsulorhexis (CCC)—it occurs mainly during the formation of the anterior capsulotomy. Once a manual CCC is achieved, the edge is very strong and will withstand intraocular gymnastics very efficiently. When a tear occurs during manual CCC, the surgeon should stop tearing, place more OVD, regrab close to the tear edge, and pull toward the center of the pupil. If this does not recover the capsulotomy easily, conversion to a vitrectorhexis or to a Kloti diathermy capsulotomy has been successful for us. For vitrectorhexis and Kloti diathermy—a tear is more likely to occur during IOL implantation or irrigation/aspiration or after OVD removal. Care should be taken to avoid right-angled edges, which is a weak point and likely to tear during intraoperative maneuvering. If a right-angled edge is seen during the capsulotomy, it should be rounded out manually or by using the vitrector before completion of the capsulotomy. The sudden flat anterior chamber that can occur after the OVD is removed but before the wounds are sutured can cause the IOL to move anteriorly and place stress on the capsulotomy edge. We compared the rate of inadvertent anterior lens capsular tears with CCC or vitrectorhexis in pediatric cataract and IOL implantation surgery [4]. Of the 339 eyes, 19 eyes (5.6%) were noted to develop an anterior capsule tear (vitrectorhexis, 12 of 226 eyes, 5.3%; CCC, 7 of 113, 6.2%). These tears occurred during anterior capsulotomy in seven eyes, hydrodissection in one, cataract removal in three, and IOL insertion/manipulation in eight. In eyes operated for cataract at or before 72 months of age, the manual CCC technique was more likely to develop a tear (relative risk, 3.09) compared with eyes of older children (>72 months of age), where the vitrectorhexis technique was more likely to develop a tear (relative risk, 3.14).

Inappropriate size and shape are also complications of the anterior capsulotomy that are seen more often with children than with adults. Surgeons are urged to go slow and pay particular attention to size, shape, and centration each time the capsulotomy edge is released. If the capsulotomy opening is too small, it can be enlarged after the IOL is inserted. If it is too large or poorly shaped, take care to get the haptics of the IOL under the capsulorhexis edge and place the haptics where the capsulotomy edges can be most easily seen.

A high intraoperative vitreous pressure is produced as a result of scleral collapse due to low scleral rigidity, which results in forward movements of the iris lens diaphragm. In pediatric eyes, the posterior capsule is often convex rather than concave from the surgeon's viewpoint. We often remove the peripheral lens cortex first, leaving the central nucleus of the lens until last since it holds the posterior capsule back in a more flat or concave configuration. Use of a high viscosity OVD (e.g., Healon-GV) helps to maintain a deep anterior chamber and keep the iris lens diaphragm back.

An inadvertent posterior capsule tear may not be as devastating to the pediatric cataract surgeon as it is to adult cataract surgeon, because pediatric cataract removal often includes posterior capsulotomy/capsulectomy with or without a vitrectomy. However, an uncontrolled posterior capsule tear may still compromise the ability of the surgeon to safely place an IOL into the capsular bag. Posterior capsule tears may occur in children due to preexisting posterior capsule abnormalities that are common in posterior polar cataracts and posterior lentiglobus. The surgeon can recognize a *torn posterior capsule* during lens aspiration by signs such as a sudden deepening of the anterior chamber. This occurs instantaneously as a rent appears in the capsule. As this occurs, the pupil will dilate in response to the deepening anterior chamber. Finally, during aspiration, lenticular particles/residual cortical matter falls away from, and will not come toward, the tip of the aspirator. This occurs because the tear in the posterior capsule alters the flow dynamics in the anterior chamber. Sometimes the presence of vitreous in the anterior chamber may also indicate a torn posterior capsule. The posterior capsule can tear during hydrodissection, irrigation and aspiration, capsular polishing, lens insertion, and OVD removal. Posterior capsule tear can also occur during incision enlargement with the sharp tip of the keratome.

In all cases, if the posterior capsular tear is entirely within view, a posterior capsulorhexis can be attempted. If the vitreous face is intact, this is done by placing OVD above and below the tear, pushing the vitreous face back, and allowing room to grasp the torn capsule. If the vitreous face is already broken, OVD is necessary only to stabilize the anterior chamber and make room for the forceps. Using a capsulorhexis forceps, the capsule is then gently torn to create a 360° posterior capsulorhexis. Failed attempts may result in extension of the tear and, if not already present, vitreous loss.

Alternatively, the vitrector handpiece can be used to round out the posterior capsule tear, remove residual cortex, and remove prolapsed vitreous. Pediatric surgeons are more likely to use this approach since the use of the vitrector is often more familiar than the use of a capsulorhexis forceps on the posterior capsule. Care should be taken to begin with a low flow so that the anterior chamber dynamics are not changed drastically when the instruments are placed in the eye. This could lead to an extension of the posterior capsule tear. Once rounded out, the posterior vitrectorhexis can be quite stable and resistant to further tearing. The advantage of the vitrector handpiece is that it can safely remove cortex when it is mixed with vitreous. It can also cut the capsule and vitreous simultaneously without undue traction on the vitreous base or the retina. A Venturi-pump-driven vitrector handpiece works best when used in this way.

Anterior vitreous face (AVF) disturbance during posterior capsule rupture is well recognized in adult cataract surgery. However, in children, this is less of a problem because anterior vitrectomy has become an integral part of the surgical strategy. However, some surgeons prefer to err on the conservative side and avoid anterior vitrectomy in children 2–8 years of age. When performing a PCCC without vitrectomy, surgeons should watch for signs of AVF disturbance, and if seen, a vitrectomy should be performed. The subtle signs are a vitreous strand in the anterior chamber, vitreous strands attached to the capsule flap, and distortion of the anterior and posterior capsulorhexis [5]. Intracameral Triamcinolone can be used in suspected cases of AVF disturbance to detect AVF disturbance. Some surgeons choose to use miotics to look for peaking of the pupil.

Intraoperative hyphema may occur and may or may not need to be cleared before wound closure [6]. A small hyphema will clear spontaneously. Hyphema was noted in approximately 5% of eyes in the IATS study [1]. Vascularized plaques or patent hyaloid artery remnants may lead to intraoperative vitreous hemorrhage. Another less commonly encountered complication is bleeding into the vitreous cavity. When exiting the pars plana, the vitrector cutter must be turned off before the handpiece is withdrawn. If not, the cutter may engage the tip on a ciliary process during handpiece withdrawal, causing profuse bleeding. If this occurs, intraocular cautery will likely not be needed but a full core vitrectomy may be needed to clear the blood. A retinal specialist will need to be consulted unless the surgeon is experienced in core vitrectomy techniques.

The most common intraoperative complication related to the IOL is malplacement or malpositioning of the implant on entry into the eye. When polymethylmethacrylate (PMMA) IOLs were used, asymmetrical fixation was common, especially in infants—the leading haptic could be placed easily into the capsular bag, but often there was unintended placement of the trailing haptic into the ciliary sulcus. Placing an oversized rigid IOL into a small soft eye was a real challenge. After the leading haptic entered the capsular bag, the OVD often exited the eye through the large wound, the pupil became miotic, and the surgeon was pleased just to get the trailing haptic somewhere posterior to the iris. Posterior vitreous upthrust made dialing the lens into the capsular bag more difficult. The modern-day use of foldable IOLs has made this complication less frequent. The trailing haptic of commonly used single-piece acrylic IOLs can now be manually placed under the capsulotomy edge using a push–pull instrument with great certainty. A second hook can be used to pull the iris edge back for better visualization if needed. Care should be taken to place the haptics into the capsular bag before they have unfolded completely. Once the haptics have unfolded outside the capsular bag, they are more difficult to place into proper position manually. This is especially true when a multi-piece acrylic IOL is used. If this happens, the IOL optic should be displaced eccentrically within the capsular bag as much as possible before an attempt is made to pull the haptic out of the ciliary sulcus. These lenses do not dial as easily in children as they do in adults.

Some pediatric surgeons choose to perform a primary posterior capsulotomy and an anterior vitrectomy prior to, rather than after, implantation of an IOL. An OVD is then used to inflate the remaining capsular "tire." The IOL must be carefully aimed at entry so that it enters the capsular bag. Fearing the deep entry, some surgeons aim too anteriorly and the IOL enters the ciliary sulcus. Unlike the situation mentioned earlier, where IOLs dial up into the ciliary sulcus due to vitreous upthrust, IOLs often dial through the posterior capsulotomy when a vitrectomy has already been performed. Even gentle dialing and gentle posterior force on the optic may send a soft foldable IOL through an even modestly sized posterior capsulotomy. In this situation, the IOL is best lifted entirely into the anterior chamber and then reinserted, rather than dialed. To avoid this complication and make IOL insertion easier, we recommend IOL insertion into an intact capsular bag prior to the posterior capsulotomy. The IOL haptics should be oriented 90° away from the wound. This allows the vitrector to be placed under the IOL optic more easily for OVD removal or for primary posterior capsulotomy and anterior vitrectomy. To avoid the possibility of dragging a strand of vitreous back to the wound, we recommend removing the OVD after the IOL is in place but performing the primary posterior capsulotomy and anterior vitrectomy through the pars plana, leaving the irrigation cannula in the anterior chamber.

Other less common complications include loss or disruption of a portion of the zonule, cloudy cornea, iris sphincterotomy, retained cortex, and lens fragments in the vitreous. Each of these was reported as an intraoperative complication in the IATS study cohort.

6.2 Postoperative Complications

Postoperative complications may be seen during the early postoperative period (e.g., wound leak, intraocular pressure (IOP) spike, corneal edema, anterior uveitis), after a few months but within a few years (posterior capsule opacification, glaucoma), or several years after cataract surgery (glaucoma, retinal detachment, high myopia).

Indications, risk factors and the rate of an unanticipated return to the operating room within 3 months of pediatric cataract-related intraocular surgery has been reported recently [7]. The overall reoperation rate was 3.3% within 90 days after cataract surgery. Reasons for reoperation included visual axis opacification (VAO), elevated IOP, vitreous wick to the cataract surgery wound, synechaie, uveitis unresponsive to topical anti-inflammatory medications, retained lens cortex, traumatic iris prolapse and foreign body in the anterior chamber. Factors that increased the risk for reoperation were a history of a traumatic cataract (relative risk 2.55) or age <1 year at the time of first surgery (relative risk 3.02). In the absence of these risk factors, the rate of reoperation during the first 90 days postoperative period was 1.1% [7]. The Toddler Aphakia & Pseudophakia Study (TAPS) recently reported outcomes of unilateral cataracts in infants and toddlers 7 to 24 months of age [8]. The Study authors concluded that the incidence of complications, reoperations, and glaucoma was low when surgery was performed between 7 to 24 months of age and compared favorably with same-site IATS data for infants undergoing surgery before 7 months of age. IOL implantation is relatively safe in children older than 6 months.

Posterior capsule opacification is inevitable in the very young child after cataract surgery if the posterior capsule is left intact. To prevent opacification and visual deprivation, posterior capsulectomy and anterior vitrectomy are performed (Fig. 6.1) [9]. Even after primary posterior capsulectomy and vitrectomy, eyes operated on during the first year of life are predisposed to develop VAO in the form of lens

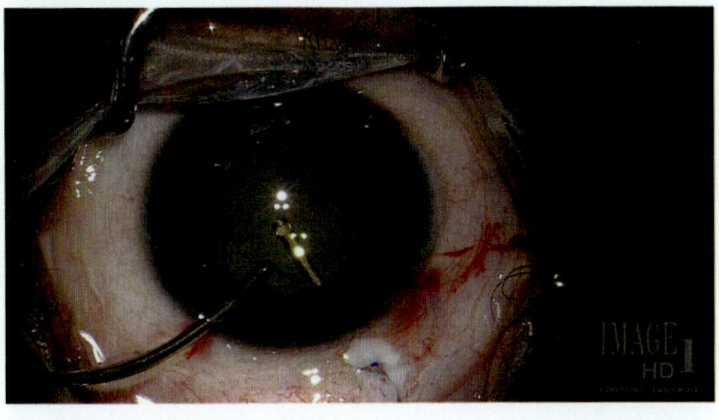

Fig. 6.1 To reduce the incidence of PCO or VAO, a pars plana posterior capsulotomy is being done after IOL insertion in this 12-month-old child

proliferation into the visual axis (defined as lens regrowth extending into the pupillary space and interfering with vision) or pupillary membrane (Figs. 6.2 and 6.3) [10]. Five-year results of the Infant Aphakia Treatment Study (IATS) reported 2 (4%) eyes with lens proliferation obscuring the visual axis in the contact lens group and 23 (40%) in the primary IOL group [10]. Pupillary membranes were observed in 2 (4%) eyes in the contact lens group versus 16 (28%) in the IOL group. TAPS investigators also reported that VAO was more common in pseudophakic (32%) than aphakic (8%) eyes (P = 0.009) in infants operated for bilateral cataract surgery [11]. In addition to age at surgery, the type of IOL used may also be a risk factor for developing a secondary opacification after cataract surgery. Different types of IOLs may have different lengths of time until opacification. For example, secondary opacification formed more quickly when PMMA lenses were implanted compared to acrylic lenses [12]. Eyes with traumatic cataract are more likely to develop PCO as compared to eyes without traumatic cataract [13]. If PCO does develop, YAG laser capsulectomy or surgical membranectomy can be performed [9].

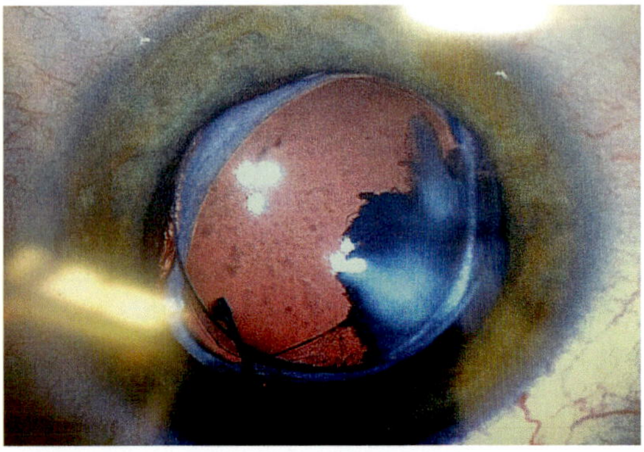

Fig. 6.2 Visual axis opacification despite the use of optic capture of a multi-piece IOL in a young child

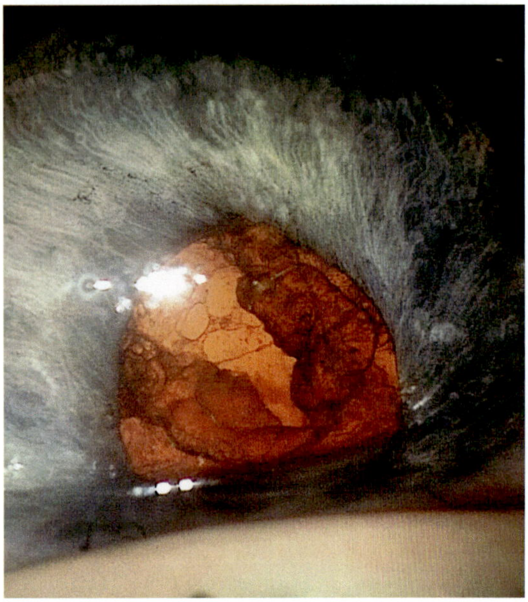

Fig. 6.3 Visual axis opacification in an eye with an immature iris and synechia

Glaucoma after pediatric cataract surgery may develop during early postoperative period or decades after cataract surgery. Late-onset glaucoma is typically open-angle and can often be diagnosed while patients are still asymptomatic. There have been numerous studies aimed at detecting factors in patients that predispose them to developing glaucoma. There is much disagreement, but age at surgery and age at diagnosis are the two most widely agreed upon factors. Previous studies have found the risk of glaucoma decreases with increasing months of age at the time of cataract extraction [14]. The highest risk is in infants who underwent cataract surgery at age 4 weeks or younger [15]. The multivariate analysis of infants enrolled in IATS showed that only younger age at surgery increased the risk of developing glaucoma (3.2 times) [15]. Some studies reported that the risk for developing postoperative glaucoma is decreased with primary IOL implantation [16–18]. We reported that this appearance of protection may be merely a selection bias, with older and more developed eyes receiving the IOLs and younger, less developed eyes being left aphakic [19]. Recently published randomized clinical trial results of IATS at five-years of age concur with our observations. Glaucoma was reported in 9 (16%) eyes with contact lens and 11 (19%) eyes with primary IOL implantation [15]. The IATS found that eyes with smaller corneal diameter ($\leq$10 mm) at cataract removal were not at higher risk for glaucoma within the

1 to <7 month age group [15]. TAPS investigators reported that younger age at surgery and smaller (<9.5 mm) corneal diameter at surgery conferred an increased risk for glaucoma or glaucoma-suspect designation [11].

Central corneal thickness should be measured during follow-up visits of children operated for cataract during infancy [20, 21]. Glaucoma is especially difficult to diagnose in children because it is harder to do detailed examination. It is particularly important to attempt regular IOP measurements in children after cataract surgery to stop disease progression before significant damage occurs. It is equally important to continue monitoring for many years, as there may be a lifelong risk of developing secondary glaucoma. If reliable IOP measurements cannot be obtained in the clinic, examinations under anesthesia (EUA) should be conducted at a yearly interval [22]. Different anesthetics will variably affect IOP, but AL will not be affected by anesthetics and should be included in the standard evaluation for glaucoma. The rebound tonometer (Icare USA, Raleigh, NC) may be used as a clinical tool for children who cannot withstand the traditional exam for measuring IOP. When using this tonometer, it is not necessary to administer a topical anesthetic, which leads to increased compliance in children. This instrument facilitates more frequent clinical IOP measurements and thus fewer EUAs. Any elevated IOP reading from the icare must be verified with a second device, such as a Tonopen. Treatment for glaucoma should ideally be early and effective to prevent ongoing damage to the eye. Treatment is typically topical medical management or surgical procedures. Open-angle glaucoma treatment for pediatric aphakic patients is different than pediatric congenital glaucoma. While initial treatment is usually surgical in congenital cases, the first line of treatment for glaucoma in aphakic and pseudophakic eyes is medical. Timolol 0.25% topical therapy is often the first-line medication. It should be avoided in children with asthma or heart conditions. Topical carbonic anhydrase inhibitors such as Drozolamide 2%/Trusopt 1%/Azopt also reduce aqueous humor production. Topical agents are not as efficacious as oral agents, but have fewer side effects. Phospholine iodide/echothiophate iodide 0.125% is also very effective in glaucoma after pediatric cataract surgery. This older and more difficult to get medication is rarely used in phakic patients because it may be associated with cataract formation. However, this is not a concern in aphakic or pseudophakic children, and it works well for managing pediatric secondary glaucoma [23]. Prostaglandin analogs such as Latanoprost 0.005%, Travoprost 0.004%, and Bimatoprost 0.03% are used as a secondary or tertiary option in secondary glaucoma. Prostaglandins increase outflow of aqueous humor, but are less efficacious in aphakic or pseudophakic children compared to adults. Aphakic patients refractory to medical management may need a surgical procedure such as a tube shunt implantation, trabeculectomy with mitomycin C (TMMC), trabeculotomy, goniotomy, or one of the cyclodestructive procedures, such as endoscopic cyclophotocoagulation. Though rare, children who are pseudophakic are more likely to develop closed-angle or pupillary block glaucoma. Surgical or laser iridectomy is the standard of care in these patients, both of which are followed by medical therapy in most cases.

A frequent complication of pediatric cataract surgery is early postoperative increased IOP. A study conducted by the Childhood Cataract Program of the Chinese Ministry of Health found IOP typically peaks at 1 week after surgery and remains elevated for an average of 30 days [24]. A possible explanation for an early postoperative spike in IOP is retained cohesive OVD, particularly in patients with marginally controlled glaucoma who are undergoing secondary IOL implantation [25]. Other explanations include damage to the iris during surgery [26]. Postoperative topical steroids can also cause an increase in IOP but this so-called "steroid response" type of ocular hypertension usually subsides soon after discontinuation of topical steroids. Ultimately, increased IOP that is untreated or does not return to baseline can result in pain, corneal edema, and optic nerve damage. Increased IOP is seen more frequently in patients who already have glaucoma and are undergoing secondary IOL implantation. The IOP spike can be treated with topical or systemic glaucoma medications. As in adults, retained viscous OVD can cause a marked postoperative IOP elevation after surgery for childhood cataracts. Englert and Wilson [25] have suggested the need for more meticulous removal of the OVD. We reported a high incidence of symptomatic early IOP spikes in patients with aphakic glaucoma undergoing secondary IOL implantation and we recommended the use of prophylactic topical and/or systemic glaucoma medications to help prevent or minimize the IOP spike. Monitoring during the early postoperative period was also suggested in these higher risk cases [27].

Toxic anterior segment syndrome (TASS) is a rare inflammatory condition usually observed within the first 2 days after anterior segment surgery [28–31]. The most common finding is a diffuse corneal edema. Fibrin in the anterior chamber and increased anterior chamber inflammation, often resulting in sterile hypopyon, can occur. With intense topical corticosteroid treatment, most cases resolve over a period of weeks to months. Ari and colleagues evaluated 893 eyes of patients undergoing pediatric cataract surgery [32]. TASS was observed in 19 eyes. In all TASS cases, it was noted that ethylene oxide-sterilized vitrectomy packs were used for anterior vitrectomy. After the abolition of use of this material, the authors did not have any new TASS cases [32]. A task force of the American Society of Cataract Refractive Surgery (ASCRS) has made a number of recommendations for cleaning and sterilizing intraocular surgical instruments to prevent TASS [28].

Endophthalmitis is one of the most severe complications that can occur following cataract surgery. Improved surgical conditions and early diagnosis has improved outcomes, but rates vary worldwide. Melo et al. reported an incidence rate between 0.05% and 0.4% worldwide [33]. Wheeler, Stager, and Weakley reported a rate of 0.071% following pediatric intraocular surgery for cataracts and congenital glaucoma [34]. The most common infectious organisms are *Staphylococcus* and *Pseudomonas* [35]. Additionally, the incidence of methicillin resistant *Staphylococcus aureus* (MRSA) infections is increasing [36]. Prophylaxis and treatment for endophthalmitis in pediatric cataract surgery is similar to adult cataract surgery. We strongly recommend the use of intracameral antibiotics at the end of the cataract surgery in children.

Transient corneal edema is a common problem after cataract surgery. Recent studies have asserted it is the most common complication on the first postoperative day [37]. The edema may be localized or diffuse. Localized edema is due to trauma to the corneal endothelium and resulting inflammation, and diffuse edema causes increased IOP. Steroids may be used to treat inflammation and thus decrease pressure inside the eye [38]. The IATS described corneal edema as an adverse postoperative complication only if it persisted for more than 30 days. This was observed in only 1 of 57 eyes in the IOL group [1]. Contact lens associated corneal problems include bacterial keratitis, corneal opacity due to tight contact lenses, corneal vascularization, and corneal abrasion [22]. The IATS study reported a corneal abrasion in only 1 eye of the 57 in the contact lens group. Cataract surgery may also result in increased corneal thickness and corneal endothelial cell loss. Increased corneal thickness is due to surgical manipulation and the corneal incisions. The thickest areas typically correlate with instrument incision points. Endothelial cell loss occurs after cataract surgery and is dependent upon cataract type, AL, anterior chamber depth, and surgical factors. Cell loss is greatest at 3 months after surgery. Endothelial cell loss is best measured with specular microscopy, and children receiving a secondary IOL, Artisan iris-claw IOL, or angle-supported anterior chamber IOL should be routinely measured [22].

A shallow or flattened anterior chamber may be observed during the early postoperative period and a peaked pupil may accompany this finding. This finding is usually from a wound leak caused by the child rubbing eye and forcing fluid out of the sutured wound. The chamber will usually need to be reformed and the wound may need to be re-sutured. Although the chamber will usually deepen on its own, failure to surgically reform the chamber and reposition the iris may lead to a peaked pupil that chronically sticks in place and is not easily repaired later.

Fibrinous uveitis due to increased tissue reactivity is a more common complication during the early postoperative period in eyes undergoing pediatric cataract surgery compared to adults. However, modern surgical techniques that limit iris manipulation and ensure capsular bag fixation of the IOL have resulted in less postoperative inflammation/fibrinous uveitis even in small children. Frequent topical steroids and even systemic steroids may be needed in selected cases to reduce uveitis-related complications.

A new hyphema occurring postoperatively (as opposed to residual hyphema from an intraoperative bleed) is uncommon, but it can occur [6]. Recurrent hyphema in an aphakic child has been reported [39].

Triamcinolone disappears from the anterior chamber in most eye within days after surgery, however, it may persist, especially if it reaches the vitreous cavity (Fig. 6.4). We don't leave triamcinolone in aphakic eyes since it deposits in the vitreous and is too slow to clear. In these aphakic eyes, if it is used to help visualize the vitreous, then it is removed before the end of the surgery. When an IOL is implanted in a young child, triamcinolone can be left in the anterior chamber to control postoperative inflammation. We commonly use 1 or 2 mg of triamcinolone placed anterior to the IOL just prior to intracameral antibiotic injection.

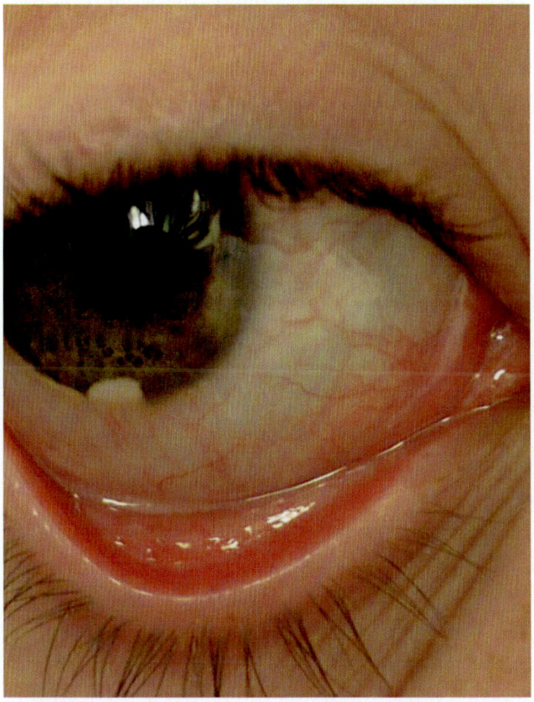

Fig. 6.4 Intracameral triamcinolone persisting in the inferior portion of the anterior chamber at 1 week after surgery

Postoperative iris and pupil abnormalities are observed after cataract surgery, more commonly after IOL implantation. Corectopia was reported in 2% eyes in the *no IOL* group versus 19% of eyes in the IOL group in the IATS study [1]. Posterior synechia are usually the reason for the observed corectopia although iris damage can also occur at the time of iris prolapse or during surgical manipulation. Younger age at the time of cataract surgery increases the risk for synechiae formation. Trivedi et al. [40] noted that synechiae were seen in 31% of eyes having surgery in the first year of life. Type of IOL also influence rate of synechiae. Wilson et al. [41] noted posterior synechiae in 5 of 110 AcrySof® (Alcon, Fort Worth, TX) lenses (4.5%), compared with 23 of 120 PMMA lenses (19.2%). Evaluating single-piece IOLs in children, we noted synechiae in five eyes (11.9%) [42]. None produced enough corectopia to cause a noticeable cosmetic deformity. Vasavada et al. [43] noted posterior synechiae in 13.6%.

Heterochromia iridis is an asymmetry of iris color in one eye in relation to the other. Summer and Letson reported it in 9% of patients [44]. Cataract surgery stimulates a prostaglandin release resulting the darkening of iris color, which may occur through the same or a similar mechanism by which latanoprost causes darkening of iris color. The darkening effect occurs more often when surgery is done in infancy. Lenart and colleagues evaluated 15 children [45]. Photographs were taken of both eyes. Masked examiners reviewed the photographs and compared, in each patient, the iris color of the eye that was operated and the eye that was not operated. Thirteen of 15 children had darker iris color in the operated eye relative to the non-operated eye.

Early hypotony may indicate a wound leak. Once this is ruled out, sustained hypotony may accompany a postoperative retinal detachment (RD). In glaucoma and uveitis patients, sustained hypotony can be an impending sign of phthisis bulbi. Hypotonous maculopathy may also be present. In patients with nanophthalmos, mild hypotony may be associated with large choroidal effusions. These usually resolve with time.

Excessive anterior capsule fibrosis and shrinkage of the CCC opening can lead to difficulty with retinoscopy and with examining the retinal periphery and, occasionally, decentration of the IOL.

Precipitates composed of pigment, inflammatory cells, fibrin, blood breakdown products, and other elements are often seen during the postoperative period on the surface of an IOL optic implanted in a child (Fig. 6.5). The deposits can be pigmented or nonpigmented but are usually not visually significant. They occur much more commonly in children with a dark iris and when compliance with postoperative medications has been poor. Sulcus-fixated IOL would likely have more deposits compared to bag-fixated IOL. In addition, Vasavada and Trivedi [46] found that the incidence of deposits was higher in eyes with the IOL optic captured through the posterior CCC in comparison with in-the-bag fixated IOLs. The type of IOL also influences IOL deposits. Wilson and colleagues [41] reported that IOL cell deposits were seen in 7 of 110 (6.4%) hydrophobic acrylic lenses, compared with 26 of 120 (21.75%) PMMA lenses. In addition, the incidence of deposits is inversely proportional to age at surgery.

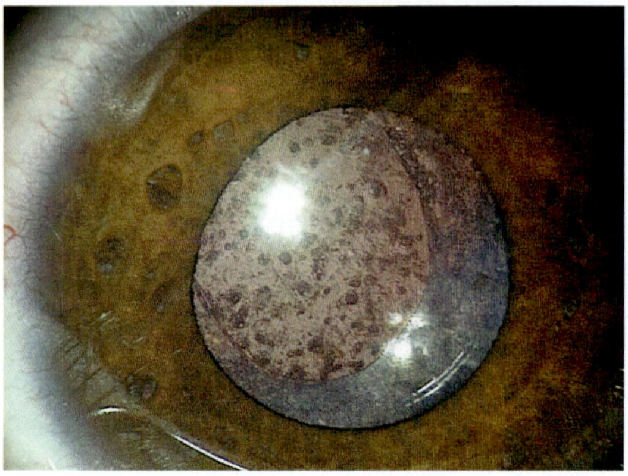

Fig. 6.5 Marked cell deposits on an IOL in a child with poor compliance with postoperative steroid drops

In a recent review from Toronto, IOL repositioning was required in 4/55 eyes [47]. Placing the IOL in the capsular bag with an anterior capsulotomy smaller than the IOL optic helps to prevent pupillary capture, a complication that is much more common in children than in adults. It often occurs in association with posterior synechiae formation and PCO. Pupillary capture occurs most often in children <2 years of age, when an optic size <6 mm is used and the lens is placed in the ciliary sulcus. Pupillary capture can be left untreated if it is not associated with decreased visual acuity or glaucoma. However, surgical repair recreates a more round pupil shape and IOL centration. Fixation of PCIOLs in the capsular bag (whenever possible) is recommended to decrease the incidence of this complication. Also, the anterior capsulotomy should be continuous and smaller than the IOL optic for 360 degrees, if possible. Prolapsing the optic of a secondary sulcus–fixated IOL through the anterior capsulorhexis opening can also prevent pupillary capture.

Excessive capsular fibrosis and asymmetric IOL fixation are the most common causes of a decentered IOL. Decentration of an IOL can also occur because of traumatic loss of a portion of the zonule and/or inadequate capsular support. Capsular bag placement of the IOL is the most successful way to reduce this complication. Posterior capture of the IOL optic also resulted in better centration of the implanted IOL [46]. Explantation or repositioning of the IOL may be necessary in some cases presenting with significant decentration/dislocation.

Late postoperative opacification of some specific IOL models in adults has been reported widely in the literature. Kleinmann and associates [48] reported the clinicopathological and ultrastructural features of three hydrophilic acrylic IOLs, manufactured from two different biomaterials, explanted from children who had visual disturbances caused by progressive postoperative opacification of the lenses' optic component. These lenses were explanted at 20, 22, and 25 months postoperatively, from children aged 10, 36, and 20 months, respectively, at lens implantation. Pehere and colleagues [49] reported that the deposits were found to be composed of calcium, phosphate, and silicone.

Mullner-Eidenbock et al. [50] noted glistening in both eyes of one patient 1 week postoperatively. The glistening increased during the first 2 postoperative years to a degree of 3+ and then remained stable until the last follow-up at 40 months. Glistenings are commonly observed on postoperative slit lamp examination when a single-piece AcrySof IOL (Alcon, Fort Worth, TX) has been implanted. They appear to be visually insignificant but some surgeons argue that they may have some yet unproven deleterious effect on visual performance.

Retinal detachment is a well-known late complication of pediatric cataract surgery, historically reported to occur 20 years or more after cataract surgery, with only a third of cases occurring in the first 10 years after surgery [51]. The incidence of RD following pediatric cataract surgery appears to have decreased markedly as surgical techniques have advanced and evolved. The use of a modern high-speed vitreous cutter and more frequent use of pars plana approach reduces vitreoretinal traction. During surgery, wound sweeping and scissors cutting ("Weck-cell vitrectomy") should be avoided. This technique can remove vitreous from the wound but it invariably induces acute vitreoretinal traction. Similarly, if a vitreous wick is seen attached to one of the anterior cataract wounds (corneal tunnel or paracentesis) during a postoperative examination, it should be removed as soon as possible to relieve any traction on the retina at the vitreous base. In children without associated ocular anomalies, the incidence of RD is reported as 3.2% after a mean follow-up of 6.8 years [52], 0.8% at 5 years [53], and 2.5% at 5 years [54]. The median interval between pediatric cataract surgery and RD is reported as 6.8, 9.1, and 5.8 years after pediatric cataract surgery [52–54]. High myopia (long axial length) has been reported as significant risk factor for postoperative RD [52, 54]. Intellectual disability has also been reported to greatly increase the risk of RD [53, 54]. Long-term follow-up is critical in children, as RD can occur many years after cataract surgery. A detailed retinal examination is recommended after cataract surgery at least yearly. This is especially important for those eyes at higher risk for RD by virtue of a long axial length for age, persistent fetal vasculature, Stickler syndrome, traumatic cataract, ectopia lentis, or intellectual disability associated with self-injurious behavior.

Cystoid macular edema (CME) is a rare complication following pediatric cataract surgery, probably because of the healthy retinal vasculature and formed vitreous in children. Ahmadieh et al. evaluated 45 eyes of 31 children undergoing cataract surgery and IOL implantation, using intravenous fluorescein and fundus fluorescein angiography, and did not detect CME in any eye at 6 weeks after surgery [55]. Rao et al. [56] performed a similar evaluation 4 to 6 weeks after surgery, using oral fluorescein and angioscopy, in 25 eyes of children and did not detect CME in any of them. CME occurs with unknown frequency after pediatric cataract extraction, in part due to the difficulty in detecting CME in the pediatric patient because of the challenges of performing macular examination, inability to visualize CME with the indirect ophthalmoscope or RetCam, the sedation issues associated with fluorescein angiography, and the inability of young children to position for ocular coherence tomography (OCT). If detected and visually significant, the treatment should parallel guidelines for adult pseudophakic CME, including topical corticosteroids and nonsteroidal anti-inflammatory medications.

To increase safety during wound healing, pediatric cataract surgeons typically place sutures. Since children rub their eyes after surgery and the wounds are prone to leaking, the sutures are placed and tied tight. This can induce large amounts of surgically induced astigmatism in the immediate postoperative period. However, relaxation of a large amount of this suture-induced astigmatism occurs in children having cataract surgery when the wound heals and the Vicryl suture dissolves [57–65].

High postoperative myopia can occur with axial eye growth after early IOL implantation. Optical rehabilitation with contact lens, spectacles, or IOL exchange will be necessary. Alternatively, secondary implantation of a piggyback lens in the ciliary sulcus or corneal refractive surgery can be performed. Secondary Artisan phakic IOL for correction of progressive high myopia in a pseudophakic child has also been reported [66]. IATS study reported phthisis bulbi in 1 eye of the 57 who did not receive an IOL [1]. Other rare complication included ptosis [67].

In summary, intraoperative complications are uncommon but occur in pediatric cataract surgery more commonly than in adult surgery. Also, postoperative complications may develop in the early postoperative period or after many years. Therefore, it is crucial to follow children closely on a long-term basis after pediatric cataract surgery.

References

1. Infant Aphakia Treatment Study G, Lambert SR, Buckley EG, Drews-Botsch C, DuBois L, Hartmann EE, et al. A randomized clinical trial comparing contact lens with intraocular lens correction of monocular aphakia during infancy: grating acuity and adverse events at age 1 year. Arch Ophthalmol. 2010;128(7):810–8.
2. Wilson ME Jr, Trivedi RH, Mistr S. Pediatric intraoperative floppy-iris syndrome. J Cataract Refract Surg. 2007;33(7):1325–7.
3. Motley WW, Melson AT. Pediatric intraoperative floppy iris syndrome associated with persistent pupillary membrane. J AAPOS. 2011;15(2):196–7.
4. Wilson ME Jr, Trivedi RH, Bartholomew LR, Pershing S. Comparison of anterior vitrectorhexis and continuous curvilinear capsulorhexis in pediatric cataract and intraocular lens implantation surgery: a 10-year analysis. J AAPOS. 2007;11(5):443–6.
5. Praveen MR, Vasavada AR, Koul A, Trivedi RH, Vasavada VA, Vasavada VA. Subtle signs of anterior vitreous face disturbance during posterior capsulorhexis in pediatric cataract surgery. J Cataract Refract Surg. 2008;34(1):163–7.
6. Hiles DA, Watson BA. Complications of implant surgery in children. J Am Intraocul Implant Soc. 1979;5(1):24–32.
7. Jackson CM, Bickford M, Trivedi RH, Wilson ME. Unplanned returns to the operating room within three months of pediatric cataract-related intraocular surgery: indications and risk factors. J AAPOS. 2019;23(4):224 e1–4.
8. Bothun ED, Wilson ME, Traboulsi EI, Diehl NN, Plager DA, Vanderveen DK, et al. Outcomes of unilateral cataracts in infants and toddlers 7 to 24 months of age: toddler Aphakia and Pseudophakia Study (TAPS). Ophthalmology. 2019;126(8):1189–95.
9. Medsinge A, Nischal K. Pediatric cataract: challenges and future directions. Clin Ophthalmol. 2015;9:77–90.
10. Plager DA, Lynn MJ, Buckley EG, Wilson ME, Lambert SR, Infant Aphakia Treatment Study G. Complications in the first 5 years following cataract surgery in infants with and without intraocular lens implantation in the Infant Aphakia Treatment Study. Am J Ophthalmol. 2014;158(5):892–8.
11. Bothun ED, Wilson ME, Vanderveen DK, Plager DA, Freedman SF, Trivedi RH, et al. Outcomes of bilateral cataracts removed in infants 1 to 7 months of age using the toddler Aphakia and Pseudophakia Treatment Study registry. Ophthalmology. 2020;127(4):501–10.
12. Bar-Sela S, Har-Noy N, Spierer A. Secondary membrane formation after cataract surgery with primary intraocular lens implantation in children. Int Ophthalmol. 2014;34(4):767–72.
13. Trivedi RH, Wilson ME. Posterior capsule opacification in pediatric eyes with and without traumatic cataract. J Cataract Refract Surg. 2015;41(7):1461–4.
14. Ruddle JB, Staffieri SE, Crowston JG, Sherwin JC, Mackey DA. Incidence and predictors of glaucoma following surgery for congenital cataract in the first year of life in Victoria, Australia. Clin Exp Ophthalmol. 2013;41:653–61.
15. Freedman SFLM, Beck AD, Bothun ED, Örge FH, Lambert SR, Infant Aphakia, Group TS. Glaucoma-related adverse events in the first 5 years after unilateral cataract removal in the Infant Aphakia Treatment Study. JAMA Ophthalmol. 2015;133(8):907–14.
16. Asrani S, Freedman S, Hasselblad V, Buckley EG, Egbert J, Dahan E, et al. Does primary intraocular lens implantation prevent "aphakic" glaucoma in children? J AAPOS. 2000;4(1):33–9.
17. Astle WF, Alewenah O, Ingram AD, Paszuk A. Surgical outcomes of primary foldable intraocular lens implantation in children: understanding posterior opacification and the absence of glaucoma. J Cataract Refract Surg. 2009;35(7):1216–22.
18. Mataftsi A, Haidich A, Kokkali S, Rabiah P, Birch E, Stager DJ, et al. Postoperative glaucoma following infantile cataract surgery: an individual patient data meta-analysis. JAMA Ophthalmol. 2014;132(9):1059–67.
19. Trivedi RH, Wilson ME Jr, Golub RL. Incidence and risk factors for glaucoma after pediatric cataract surgery with and without intraocular lens implantation. J AAPOS. 2006;10(2):117–23.
20. Muir KW, Duncan L, Enyedi LB, Wallace DK, Freedman SF. Central corneal thickness: congenital cataracts and aphakia. Am J Ophthalmol. 2007;144(4):502–6.
21. Simsek T, Mutluay AH, Elgin U, Gursel R, Batman A. Glaucoma and increased central corneal thickness

in aphakic and pseudophakic patients after congenital cataract surgery. Br J Ophthalmol. 2006;90(9):1103–6.
22. Wilson ME, Trivedi RH. Pediatric cataract surgery: techniques, complications and management. 2nd ed; 2014.
23. Kraus CL, Trivedi RH, Wilson ME. Intraocular pressure control with echothiophate iodide in children's eyes with glaucoma after cataract extraction. J AAPOS. 2015;19(2):116–8.e1.
24. CCPMOH SGo. Ocular hypertension after pediatric cataract surgery: baseline characteristics and first-year report. PLoS One. 2013;8(7):e69867.
25. Englert JA, Wilson ME. Postoperative intraocular pressure elevation after the use of Healon GV in pediatric cataract surgery. J AAPOS. 2000;4:60–1.
26. Latif K, Shakir M, Zafar S, Rizvi S, Naz S. Outcomes of congenital cataract surgery in a Tertiary Care Hospital. Pak J Ophthalmol. 2014;30(1):28–32.
27. Trivedi RH, Boden JH, Mickler C, Wilson ME. Intraocular pressure elevation during early postoperative period after secondary intraocular lens implantation in children and adolescents. J Cataract Refract Surg. 2012;38(9):1633–6.
28. Hellinger WC, Bacalis LP, Edelhauser HF, Mamalis N, Milstein B, Masket S, et al. Recommended practices for cleaning and sterilizing intraocular surgical instruments. J Cataract Refract Surg. 2007;33(6):1095–100.
29. Eydelman MB, Tarver ME, Calogero D, Buchen SY, Alexander KY. The Food and Drug Administration's proactive toxic anterior segment syndrome program. Ophthalmology. 2012;119(7):1297–302.
30. Mamalis N. Toxic anterior segment syndrome update. J Cataract Refract Surg. 2010;36(7):1067–8.
31. Cutler Peck CM, Brubaker J, Clouser S, Danford C, Edelhauser HE, Mamalis N. Toxic anterior segment syndrome: common causes. J Cataract Refract Surg. 2010;36(7):1073–80.
32. Ari S, Caca I, Sahin A, Cingu AK. Toxic anterior segment syndrome subsequent to pediatric cataract surgery. Cutan Ocul Toxicol. 2012;31(1):53–7.
33. Melo GB, Bispo PJ, Regatieri CV, Yu MC, Pignatari AC, Hofling-Lima AL. Incidence of endophthalmitis after cataract surgery (2002–2008) at a Brazilian University Hospital. Arq Bras Oftalmol. 2010;73:505–7.
34. Wheeler DT, Stager DR, Weakley DR Jr. Endophthalmitis following pediatric intraocular surgery for congenital cataracts and congenital glaucoma. J Pediatr Ophthalmol Strabismus. 1992;29(3):139–41.
35. Yao KZ, Zhu Y, Zhu Z, Wu J, Liu Y, Lu Y, Hao Y, Bao Y, Ye J, Huang Y, Li Z, Shentu X, Yu Y. The incidence of postoperative endophthalmitis after cataract surgery in China: a multicenter investigation of 2006–2011. Br J Ophthalmol. 2013;97(10):1312–7.
36. Packer M, Chang DF, Dewey SH, Little BC, Mamalis N, Oetting TA, et al. Prevention, diagnosis, and management of acute postoperative bacterial endophthalmitis. J Cataract Refract Surg. 2011;37(9):1699–714.
37. Umar M, Abubakar A, Achi I, Alhassan M, Hassan A. Pediatric cataract surgery in national eye Centre Kaduna, Nigeria: outcome and challenges. Middle East Afr J Ophthalmol. 2015;22(1):92–6.
38. Kurt E, Mayali H. Early post-operative complications in cataract surgery. Rijeka: InTech; 2013.
39. Carrasquillo AM, Gupta BK, Wilensky JT. Recurrent hyphema in an aphakic child: Swan syndrome. J AAPOS. 2001;5(1):55–7.
40. Trivedi RH, Wilson ME Jr, Bartholomew LR, Lal G, Peterseim MM. Opacification of the visual axis after cataract surgery and single acrylic intraocular lens implantation in the first year of life. J AAPOS. 2004;8(2):156–64.
41. Wilson ME, Elliott L, Johnson B, Peterseim MM, Rah S, Werner L, et al. AcrySof acrylic intraocular lens implantation in children: clinical indications of biocompatibility. J AAPOS. 2001;5(6):377–80.
42. Trivedi RH, Wilson ME Jr. Single-piece acrylic intraocular lens implantation in children. J Cataract Refract Surg. 2003;29(9):1738–43.
43. Vasavada AR, Trivedi RH, Nath VC. Visual axis opacification after AcrySof intraocular lens implantation in children. J Cataract Refract Surg. 2004;30(5):1073–81.
44. Summers CG, Letson RD. Is the phakic eye normal in monocular pediatric aphakia? J Pediatr Ophthalmol Strabismus. 1992;29(5):324–7.
45. Lenart TD, Drack AV, Tarnuzzer RW, Fernandes A, Lambert SR. Heterochromia after pediatric cataract surgery. J AAPOS. 2000;4(1):40–5.
46. Vasavada AR, Trivedi RH. Role of optic capture in congenital cataract and intraocular lens surgery in children. J Cataract Refract Surg. 2000;26(6):824–31.
47. Lim Z, Rubab S, Chan YH, Levin AV. Management and outcomes of cataract in children: the Toronto experience. J AAPOS. 2012;16(3):249–54.
48. Kleinmann G, Apple DJ, Werner L, Pandey SK, Neuhann IM, Assia EI, et al. Postoperative surface deposits on intraocular lenses in children. J Cataract Refract Surg. 2006;32(11):1932–7.
49. Pehere NK, Bojja S, Vemuganti GK, Vaddavalli PK, Samant M, Jalali S, et al. Opacification of intraocular lenses implanted during infancy: a clinicopathologic study of 4 explanted intraocular lenses. Ophthalmology. 2011;118(11):2128–32 e1.
50. Mullner-Eidenbock A, Amon M, Moser E, Kruger A, Abela C, Schlemmer Y, et al. Morphological and functional results of AcrySof intraocular lens implantation in children: prospective randomized study of age-related surgical management. J Cataract Refract Surg. 2003;29(2):285–93.
51. De la Huerta I, Williams GA. Rhegmatogenous retinal detachment after pediatric cataract surgery. Ophthalmology. 2018;125(1):4–5.
52. Rabiah PK, Du H, Hahn EA. Frequency and predictors of retinal detachment after pediatric cataract surgery without primary intraocular lens implantation. J AAPOS. 2005;9(2):152–9.

53. Haargaard B, Andersen EW, Oudin A, Poulsen G, Wohlfahrt J, la Cour M, et al. Risk of retinal detachment after pediatric cataract surgery. Invest Ophthalmol Vis Sci. 2014;55(5):2947–51.
54. Agarkar S, Gokhale VV, Raman R, Bhende M, Swaminathan G, Jain M. Incidence, risk factors, and outcomes of retinal detachment after pediatric cataract surgery. Ophthalmology. 2018;125(1):36–42.
55. Ahmadieh H, Javadi MA, Ahmady M, Karimian F, Einollahi B, Zare M, et al. Primary capsulectomy, anterior vitrectomy, lensectomy, and posterior chamber lens implantation in children: limbal versus pars plana. J Cataract Refract Surg. 1999;25(6):768–75.
56. Rao SK, Ravishankar K, Sitalakshmi G, Ng JS, Yu C, Lam DS. Cystoid macular edema after pediatric intraocular lens implantation: fluorescein angioscopy results and literature review. J Cataract Refract Surg. 2001;27(3):432–6.
57. Spierer A, Bar-Sela S. Changes in astigmatism after congenital cataract surgery and foldable intraocular lens implantation. J Pediatr Ophthalmol Strabismus. 2004;41(1):35–8.
58. Spierer A, Bar-Sela SM. Changes in astigmatism after congenital cataract surgery and intraocular lens implantation: a comparative study. Arch Ophthalmol. 2004;122(5):695–7.
59. Spierer A, Nahum A. Changes in astigmatism after congenital cataract surgery and intraocular lens implantation using scleral tunnel incision. Eye. 2002;16(4):466–8.
60. Spierer A, Shelah M. Changes in astigmatism after cataract extraction and intraocular lens implantation in children. Eye. 1999;13(Pt 3a):360–2.
61. Bar-Sela S, Glovinsky Y, Wygnanski-Jaffe T, Spierer A. The relationship between patient age and astigmatism magnitude after congenital cataract surgery. Eur J Ophthalmol. 2009;19(3):376–9.
62. Bar-Sela SM, Barequet IS, Spierer A. Vector analysis of high early postoperative astigmatism after congenital cataract surgery. Graefes Arch Clin Exp Ophthalmol. 2005;243(9):881–5.
63. Bar-Sela SM, Spierer A. Astigmatism outcomes of scleral tunnel and clear corneal incisions for congenital cataract surgery. Eye. 2006;20(9):1044–8.
64. Brown SM, Hodges MR, Corona J. Relaxation of postoperative astigmatism after lens implantation through a 6.25 mm scleral wound in children. J Cataract Refract Surg. 2001;27(12):2012–6.
65. Gupta A, Ramappa M, Kekunnaya R, Vaddavalli PK, Ray D, Chaurasia S, et al. Comparing the astigmatic outcome after paediatric cataract surgery with different incisions. Br J Ophthalmol. 2012;96(3):386–9.
66. Lifshitz T, Levy J. Secondary artisan phakic intraocular lens for correction of progressive high myopia in a pseudophakic child. J AAPOS. 2005;9(5):497–8.
67. Sharma N, Pushker N, Dada T, Vajpayee RB, Dada VK. Complications of pediatric cataract surgery and intraocular lens implantation. J Cataract Refract Surg. 1999;25(12):1585–8.

7 Visual Axis Opacification

Chirakshi Dhull and Sudarshan Kumar Khokhar

7.1 Introduction

Pediatric cataract surgery techniques have significantly improved over course of time with development of new microsurgical techniques. Despite this, pediatric eyes are more predisposed to development of media opacity following cataract surgery as compared to adult eyes. Visual axis opacification (VAO) includes any significant media opacity in the visual axis which hinders the transmission of light and thus, affect image formation. This defeats the purpose of early pediatric cataract surgery which is primarily to clear the media and prevent stimulus deprivation amblyopia.

There are various causes of media opacity, including early onset and late onset causes (Table 7.1). The most important and commonest cause is posterior capsular opacification (PCO) [1, 2]. It is the commonest complication requiring second surgical intervention following pediatric cataract [3]. Intraoperative and postoperative complications are discussed in the respective chapter. In this chapter, we will discuss VAO related to PCO and hyaloid face opacification. PCO is children is generally thicker than adults and most often would require surgical interven-

Table 7.1 Causes of visual axis opacification [4]

Early media opacification	Late media opacification
Corneal edema Hyphema Inflammatory or fibrinous membrane (Fig. 7.1) Cortical remnants Vitreous hemorrhage Vitreous exudates	Posterior capsular opacification (Fig. 7.2) Hyaloid face opacification IOL glistening (Fig. 7.3) IOL debris or pigments Late vitreous exudates

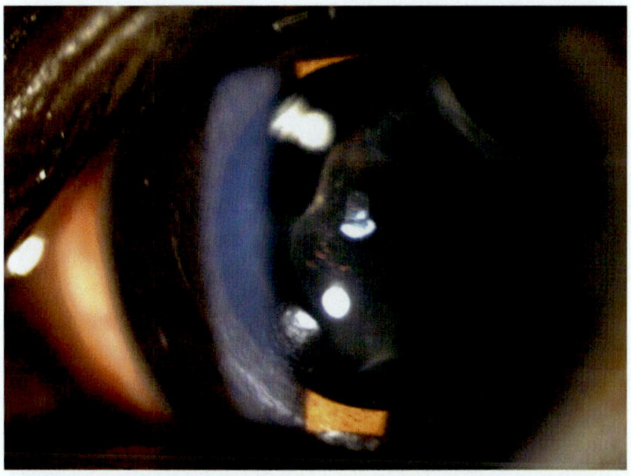

Fig. 7.1 Postoperative serial picture of 12-year-old boy with post traumatic cataract with fibrinous membrane in the anterior chamber on first postoperative day

Supplementary Information The online version of this chapter (https://doi.org/10.1007/978-981-16-0212-2_7) contains supplementary material, which is available to authorized users.

C. Dhull (✉)
Eye Q Hospital, Rohtak, Haryana, India

S. K. Khokhar
Professor Ophthalmology, Dr. RP Centre for Ophthalmic Sciences, All India Institute of Medical Sciences, New Delhi, India

S. K. Khokhar, C. Dhull (eds.), *Essentials of Pediatric Cataract Surgery*,
https://doi.org/10.1007/978-981-16-0212-2_7

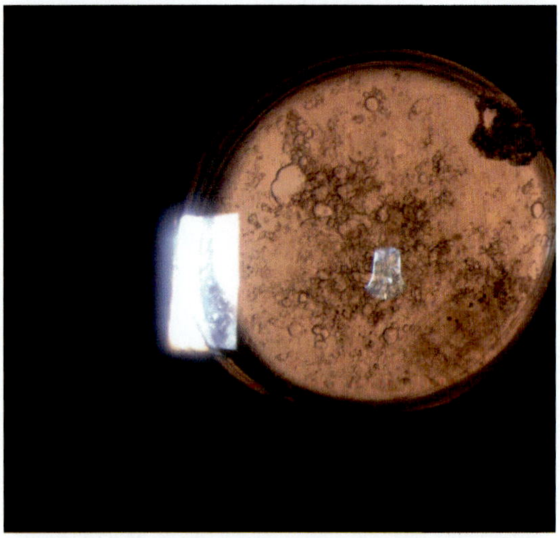

Fig. 7.2 Posterior capsular opacification seen 4 months post-surgery in 8-year-old child (Posterior capsule intact)

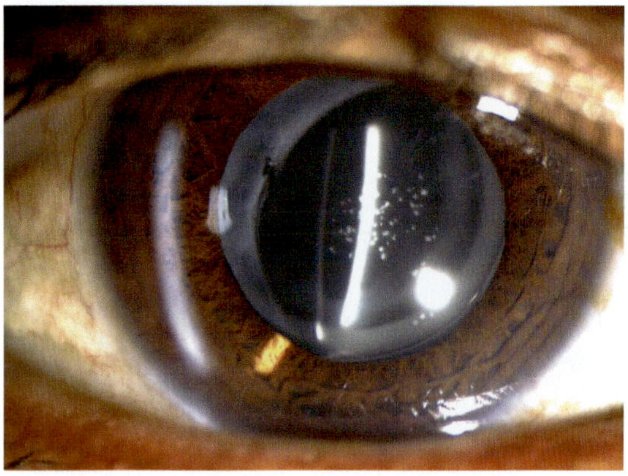

Fig. 7.3 IOL glistening seen with anterior capsular fibrosis 4 years after surgery

tion for removal. Understanding pathogenesis of PCO will help in understanding predisposing factors and prevention techniques for PCO formation. We would also discuss surgical approaches for successful PCO management.

7.2 Pathogenesis

After any extracapsular cataract surgery, lens epithelial cells (LECs) on the anterior capsule are invariably left behind. These LEC's are responsible for PCO formation [5]. The germinal equatorial E-type LECs show active mitosis and produce lens fibers throughout life. Some of the anterior or equatorial LECs left after surgery show the process of proliferation, migration and differentiation [6] as a healing response to surgery. There is epithelial to mesenchymal transition (EMT) along with collagen deposition and lens fiber [7–9].

There are two types of PCO: fibrotic and proliferative type. There may be contraction of fibroblasts deposited which may cause wrinkling and folds in the capsule. This leads to fibrotic variety of PCO [8, 9]. The lens fiber proliferation and regeneration from E-type LECs is responsible for proliferative type of PCO [6, 9]. Just like the posterior capsule, anterior hyaloid face can also act as the scaffold for this process of migration, proliferation and EMT.

Cytokines and growth factors such as transforming growth factor β (TGF-β), fibroblast growth factor 2 (FGF-2), Interleukins 1 and 6 also have a significant role in cellular response in PCO [10–12]. The inflammatory response in children following cataract surgery is significantly greater than adults. This explains thicker and more frequent PCO is younger children. Additionally, in conditions associated with more severe inflammatory response such as uveitis, trauma, etc., PCO may be more frequent.

7.3 Predisposing Factor

The incidence of PCO is variable and can be as high as 95% [13] without adequate protective measures. The incidence depends various predisposing factors: age at the time of surgery, etiology of cataract, surgical technique, IOL implantation and position, ocular comorbidities such as persistent fetal vasculature (PFV), systemic comorbidities such as juvenile idiopathic arthritis.

7.3.1 Age

Age is one of the most important factors in determining the predisposition to PCO. Younger age group is significantly more predisposed to PCO formation [14–19]. Peterseim et al. reported higher incidence of PCO in children <2 months of age when compared with older children [19].

Hosal and Biglan found the risk of secondary cataract formation to be 4.76-fold (odd's ratio) when operated at <1 year of age compared to children >1 year of age.

7.3.2 Etiology of Cataract

Traumatic cataracts may have higher risk of VAO formation compared to developmental or congenital cataract of non-infective origin [20]. This may be explained by higher inflammation in traumatic cases before and after surgery.

Systemic association such as JIA may significantly increase incidence of PCO. Incidence of PCO has been reported in as high as 70–80% eyes despite posterior capsulotomy with or without anterior vitrectomy [21, 22]. PCO formed may be very thick and vascularized (Fig. 7.4). In other cause of uveitis, there is increased incidence of PCO as well. Infective cataracts such as TORCH infections (Toxoplasma, others, rubella, cytomegalovirus, and herpes simplex virus) may also show more inflammation and hence greater risk of PCO.

Ocular association such as PFV has been associated with increased incidence of PCO [1, 2]. In addition to PCO, they may develop hyphema or more commonly vitreous hemorrhage which may be the cause of media opacity.

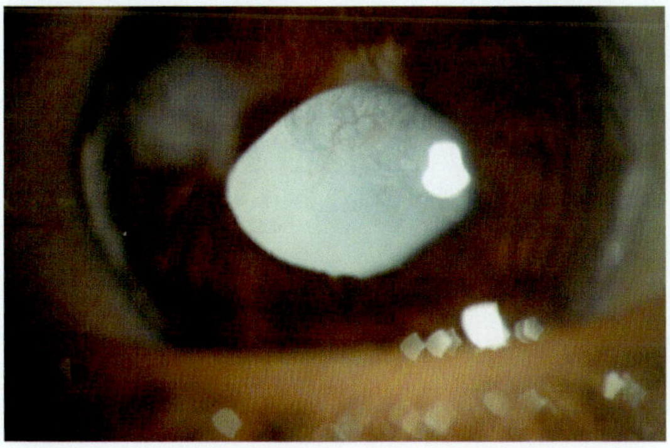

Fig. 7.4 8-year-old JIA patient with aphakia with vascularized visual axis opacification 1 year after surgery. Band shaped keratopathy is also seen

7.3.3 Surgical Technique

The importance of posterior capsulorhexis (PCCC) or capsulotomy with or without anterior vitrectomy (AV) in pediatric cataract surgery has been clearly established in the last 30 years. Incidence of PCO depend on the presence or absence of PCCC as well as AV. Posterior capsule or anterior hyaloid face act as a scaffold for PCO to form.

Hosal and Biglan clearly established the importance of PCCC and AV in their study of 152 patients with a mean follow of 6 years. PCO occurred 78.6% of eyes without PCCC, 42.9% with PCCC, and 22.5% with combined PCCC and AV [16].

7.3.4 Size of Capsulorhexis

A 5 mm opening in anterior capsulorhexis is considered as ideal. Smaller capsulorhexis may be associated with anterior capsular phimosis.

7.3.5 Aphakia or Pseudophakia

It has remained somewhat controversial over time whether the presence of IOL increases VAO formation. In our experience, we have not observed drastic difference between the two groups. However, a review of five studies including 597 eyes was published by J. Chen et al. where they found primary IOL implantation increased risk of VAO compared to contact lens fitted group [23]. There may be associated confounders such as surgical technique, surgeon's experience, and use of steroids which have been identified in the study.

7.3.6 IOL Position and Type

Incidence of VAO in the case of IOL in bag and IOL in sulcus in pediatric traumatic cataract was compared [24]. Complications including VAO and pupillary capture were observed more often in sulcus group. In other studies, no difference in

PCO was found based on IOL position [25]. IOL in sulcus with optic capture has been used to reduce PCO formation [26]. Besides these, poorly centered anterior capsulorhexis in the bag may also accelerate PCO formation if it does not cover all the edges of IOL.

Studies comparing the acylic material prove that hydrophilic acrylic material accelerates PCO formation more than hydrophobic material [27]. Heparin surface coating on polymethyl methacrylate (PMMA) i.e., heparin surface modified IOLs (HSM-IOLs) also cause less PCO formation and are used for uveitic cataracts [22]. (Hydrophilic acrylic IOL > PMMA IOL > hydrophobic IOL). A capsular bend with sharp and square optic edge induce contact inhibition to migrating LECs, thus reducing PCO formation [28].

7.4 Clinical Presentation

Detection of VAO is challenging in pediatric patients. Symptoms may be nonspecific and parents need to be counselled to look for anything out of the ordinary. In bilateral cataracts, if only one eye is affected, parents may not notice anything. Hence, the importance of regular follow ups and EUA needs to be explained beforehand. Sometimes, presence of whitish opacity or squint is observed by the caregivers. In unilateral cataracts, where patching is being followed with good compliance, the child may now be noted to resist occlusion of the good eye more than usual.

Most often, it is picked up on routine follow-up. Clinician may find poor visual acuity on Cardiff's tests and a poor glow (Bruckner reflex) through direct ophthalmoscope. A child presenting to clinic with a poor glow should be assessed through the corrective spectacles as high refractive error may show dull glow specially in aphakia.

VAO may be predominantly posterior to lens, anterior to lens or combination of both. It may be visual insignificant when central visual axis is clear. PCO is classified as:

- Fibrotic type: In fibrotic variety, capsule is thickened and fibrosed with folds and wrinkling in the capsule (Fig. 7.5).
- Proliferative type: Include both Elschnig pearls and Sommering ring. Elschnig pearls are round, clear pearl like clusters of residual LECs which are clearly demarcated on retroillumination (Fig. 7.6). Sommering ring forms in the periphery generally between anterior capsular edge and posterior capsule, it may

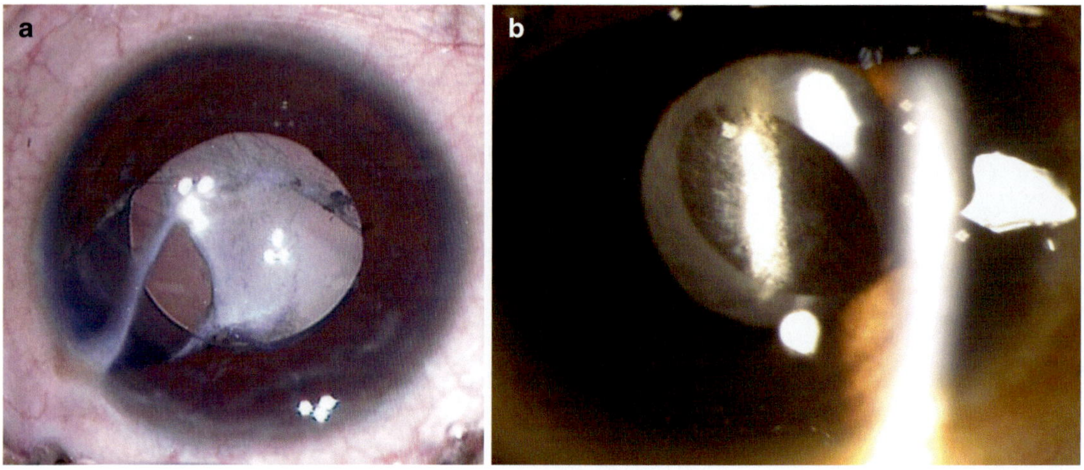

Fig. 7.5 Fibrotic type of VAO. (**a**) Anterior fibrotic VAO seen 4 months after surgery for post traumatic cataract. (**b**) Posterior fibrotic VAO seen 1 year after surgery for intermediate uveitis

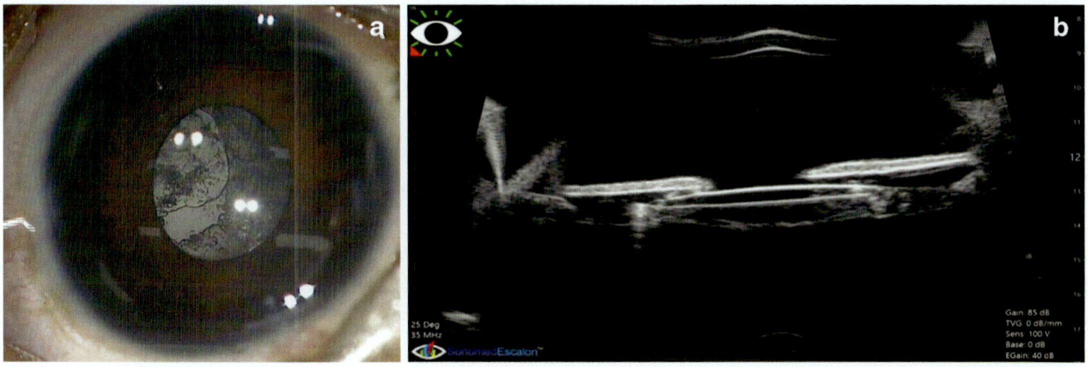

Fig. 7.6 Proliferative VAO with Elschnig pearl formation. (**a**) Clinical picture. (**b**) UBM of the same showing VAO posterior to IOL and intact posterior capsule

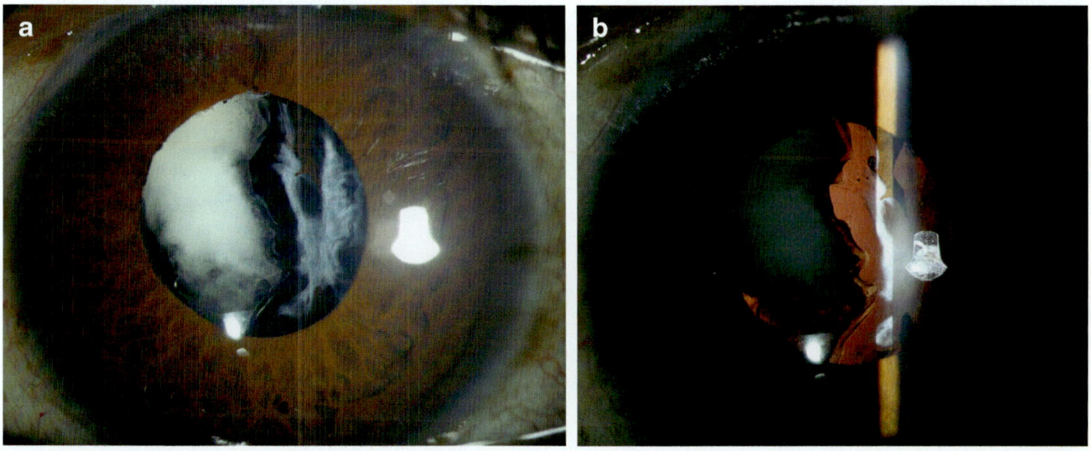

Fig. 7.7 Proliferative VAO with Soemmering ring seen in aphakic patient 20 months after surgery

proliferate further, contract and involve the visual axis (Fig. 7.7).

7.5 Investigations

Ultrasonography should be performed preoperatively to rule out posterior segment pathology such as retinal detachment. In uveitis cases, USG should be performed to evaluate activity in the posterior segment as well.

Ultrasound biomicroscopy (UBM) can be performed in cases of severe VAO or non-dilating pupil. It provides detailed information related to the location and severity of VAO. Anterior, posterior and mixed variety can be evaluated and surgery can be planned preoperatively (Fig. 7.8), it can also provide information regarding IOL position and associated pathology such as persistent fetal vasculature.

7.6 Prevention

7.6.1 Medical Preventive Measures

Use of topical steroids and cycloplegics post-surgery helps in control of inflammation and hence VAO formation. Slow taper of steroids is recommended.

In etiologies associated with excess inflammation such as uveitis, prophylactic use of systemic steroids or immunosuppressants is recommended.

7.6.2 Surgical Preventive Measures

ACCC: 5 mm circular central ACCC covering IOL 360° should be made as there are greater chances of PCO formation in eccentric IOLs (Fig. 7.9).

Hydrodissection and cortical clean up: We recommend performing good cortical clean up especially the equatorial fibers and cells. Residual cortical matter can promote VAO formation.

PCCC and AV: Studies have well established the role of primary PCCC with anterior vitrectomy to effectively delay the secondary cataract formation in infants and children [29].

Anterior vitrectomy breaks the scaffold for the LECs that are actively proliferating and prevents deposition of metaplastic cells, thus preventing PCO formation [30]. Posterior capsulotomy is must for all patients <6 years of age [18]. Vitrectomy can be deferred after 5 years of age [30].

The authors routinely perform PCCC with/without AV for all children operated for cataract at the age of less than 6 years and in special cases of older children with mental retardation, nystagmus or who are unable to follow-up frequently.

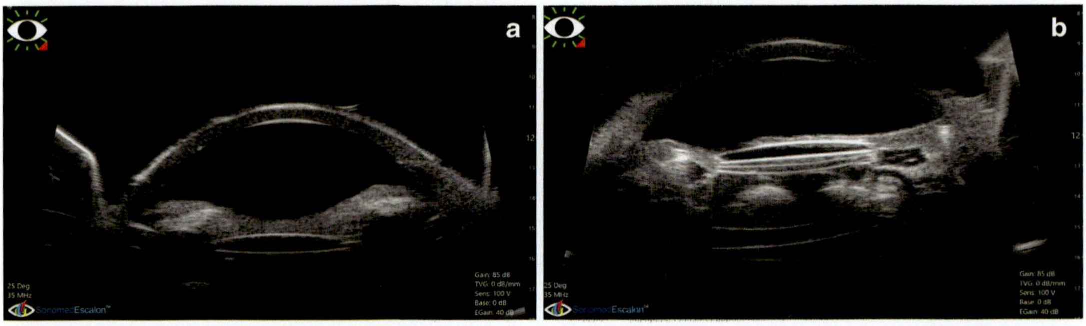

Fig. 7.8 UBM of dense VAO patients. (**a**) Anterior VAO seen, no VAO behind the lens. (**b**) Combined anterior and posterior VAO

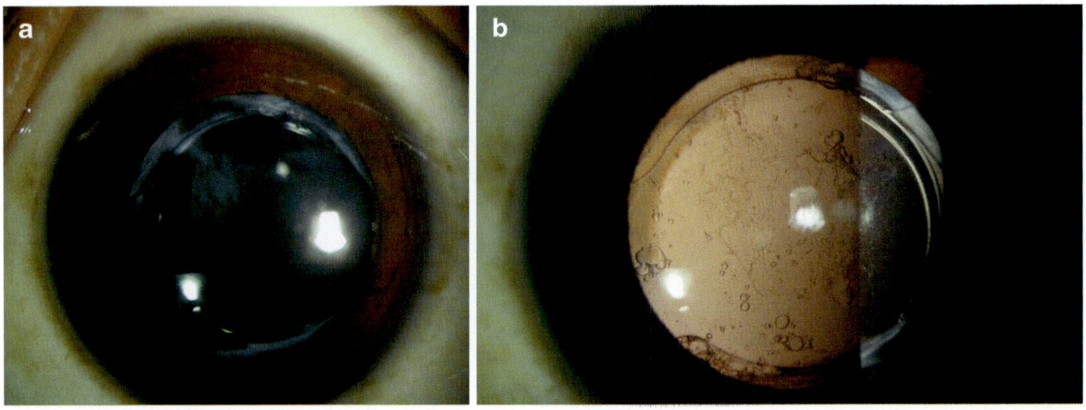

Fig. 7.9 PCO formation in case of larger capsulorhexis not covering IOL completely. (**a**) Diffuse illumination picture. (**b**) Retroillumination picture. Note both fibrotic and pearl like PCO formation

IOL: We recommend in the bag IOL implantation with square edge haptic IOL or in the sulcus IOL with optic capture with both anterior and posterior capsule depending on suitability, to reduce VAO.

7.7 Management

PCO is amblyogenic in the critical period of visual development and causes stimulus deprivation in a child, thereby interfering with the goal of a successful cataract surgery. If PCO is visually significant, it requires removal via laser or surgery.

7.7.1 Neodymium Yttrium Aluminum Garnet (Nd:YAG) Capsulotomy

Nd:YAG laser is a relatively noninvasive nonsurgical procedure to remove PCO in a day care setting. Since the procedure requires significant cooperation from the patient, it is used in older children with sufficient understanding.

The procedure is performed under topical anesthesia. An Abraham's Nd YAG laser lens is used. Energy requirement is generally low from 1–2 mJ/pulse. It can be titrated based on the thickness of PCO. Laser shots are directed at taut capsule to create a 4 to 5 mm circular opening [31]. Cruciate opening can also be used but generally not preferred due to risk of extension. A posterior offset may be required to avoid hitting the IOL. It is not preferred in cases of PMMA IOL.

However, with the use of Nd:YAG capsulotomy, few limitations remain: (1) the anterior hyaloid still remains intact, which may again act as scaffold for recurrent PCO formation; and (2) a very thick fibrous PCO may not be easily cut with laser. (3) Risks of treatment with Nd:YAG laser include: cystoid macular edema (CME) [32, 33] and low risk of retinal detachment [33]. IOL pitting can happen in uncooperative children especially with thick PCO.

7.7.2 Surgical Management

Most children especially under 6 years of age require surgical intervention for treatment of VAO. Surgical approach depends on the location of PCO, location of IOL and surgeon's experience. VAO must be managed promptly and child has to be taken up for resurgery under general anesthesia. An informed consent must be obtained from caretakers/parents in these cases, with clinician explaining them the risk of recurrent PCO and associated complications.

7.7.2.1 Limbal Route

Most anterior segment surgeons prefer membranectomy from anterior route or limbal route (Fig. 7.10). Two paracentesis incisions are made at the limbus nearly 180° apart. Anterior chamber is filled with viscoelastic and vitrectomy cutter and irrigator can be used for making an adequate opening in the PCO in aphakic eyes. If PCO is very thick intravitreal scissors and forceps may be required to cut and remove the membranes especially in cases such as uveitis, PFV, etc. Limited localized anterior vitrectomy is performed. If IOL is placed in the sulcus, a slight nudge can help to place the probe underneath it for membranectomy. If IOL is in the bag or fibrosed strongly with the capsule, excessive manipulation may weaken the zonules. We prefer a pars plana approach in such cases.

7.7.2.2 Pars Plana Route (Fig. 7.11)

A pars plana port is constructed first as described in chapter on surgical management. A limbal paracentesis is created for irrigation. Limited anterior vitrectomy is performed followed by membranectomy using vitrectomy cutter in Cut IA mode. Similar to limbal approach, in case of thick VAO, microincision (23 gauze) intravitreal

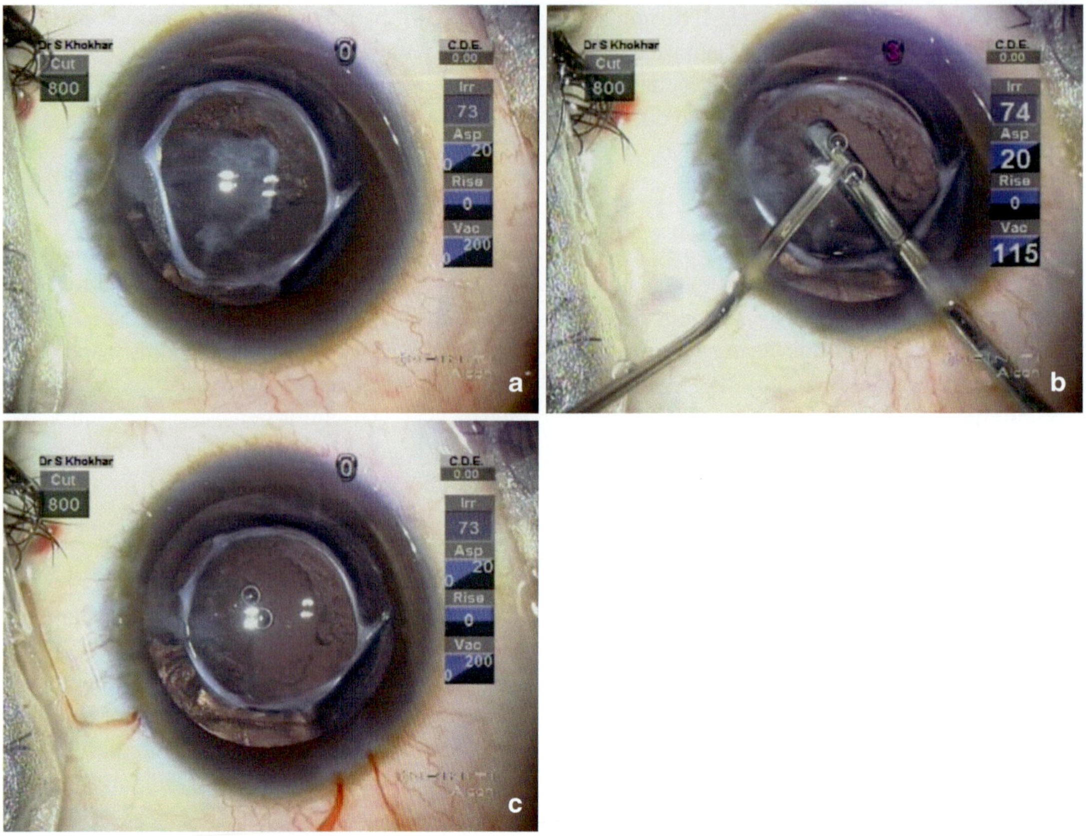

Fig. 7.10 Surgical management of PCO via anterior route. (**a**) Thick PCO behind IOL. (**b**) Membranectomy and anterior vitrectomy being performed by lifting the IOL slightly. (**c**) Surgery complete with clear 5 mm central zone

scissors and forceps can be used. There is minimal displacement of IOL and the irrigation probe can be used to support IOL throughout the procedure. Combined approach in cases of VAO both anterior and posterior to IOL can be used to achieve optimal outcome.

VAO associated with complicated surgery or mal-positioned IOL may require additional procedure to membranectomy and anterior vitrectomy. Pupilloplasty, IOL exchange, repositioning or explant may be required. This may be a surgical challenge due to extensive fibrosis and/or vascularization. Complications associated with membranectomy are similar to any intraocular procedure such as pediatric cataract surgery. Refractive correction after surgery is a must for early visual rehabilitation. Amblyopia therapy should be initiated as soon as media is rendered clear.

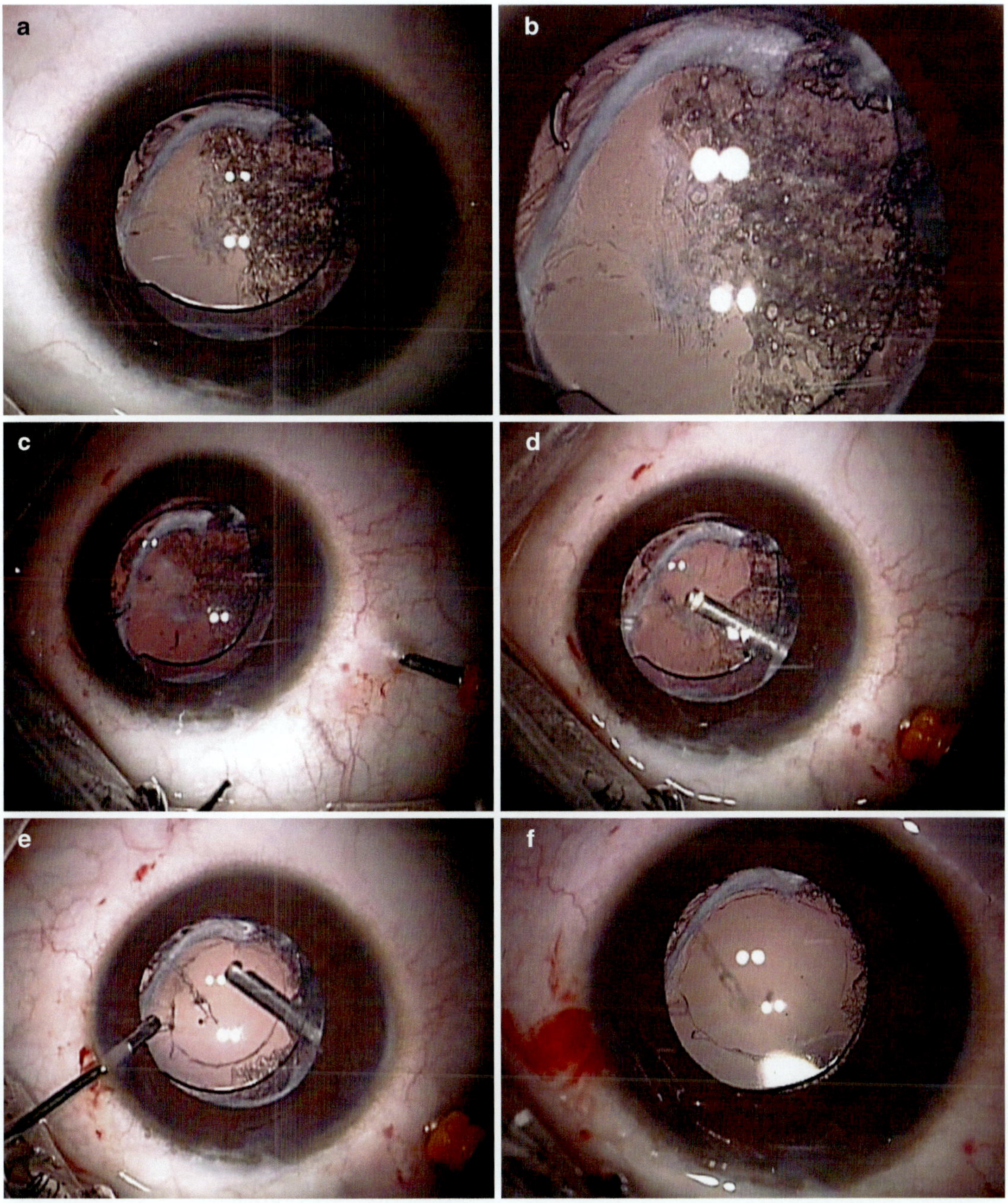

Fig. 7.11 Surgical management of PCO via pars plana route. (**a**) Clinical picture showing proliferative type of PCO. (**b**) Magnified view showing primarily posterior variety of VAO. (**c**) 23 g port being made. (**d**) Membranectomy is performed in cut IA mode. (**e**) Limited anterior vitrectomy done. (**f**) Post-surgery central 5 mm opening

7.8 Conclusion

VAO remains the commonest postoperative complication that requires surgical intervention. Since incidence of VAO is extremely high in younger children without posterior capsulotomy, primary surgery should include meticulous technique with PCCC and AV. Prevention of PCO formation can help in reducing the rate of secondary surgical intervention in children. However, if PCO form, early remedy by the most suitable method is warranted. Refractive correction and amblyopia therapy should be continued after treatment of PCO.

References

1. Apple DJ, Solomon KD, Tetz MR, et al. Posterior capsule opacification. Surv Ophthalmol. 1992;37:73–116.
2. Pandey SK, Apple DJ, Werner L, et al. Posterior capsule opacification: a review of the aetiopathogenesis, experimental and clinical studies and factors for prevention. Indian J Ophthalmol. 2004;52:99–112.
3. Sachdeva V, Katukuri S, Ali MH, Kekunnaya R. Second intraocular surgery after primary pediatric cataract surgery: indications and outcomes during long-term follow-up at a tertiary eye care center. Eye. 2016;30:1260–5.
4. Khokhar SK, Dhull C, editors. Atlas of pediatric cataract. Singapore: Springer Nature Singapore Pte Ltd; 2019. p. 145. https://doi.org/10.1007/978-981-13-6939-1_15.
5. Lambert SR, Drack AV. Infantile cataract. Surv Ophthalmol. 1996;40:427–8.
6. Marcantonio JM, Vrensen GF. Cell biology of posterior capsular opacification. Eye (Lond). 1999;13(Pt 3b):484–8.
7. McDonnell PJ, Zarbin MA, Green WR. Posterior capsule opacification in pseudophakic eyes. Ophthalmology. 1983;90(12):1548–53.
8. Cobo LM, Ohsawa E, Chandler D, et al. Pathogenesis of capsular opacification after extracapsular cataract extraction: an animal model. Ophthalmology. 1984;91(7):857–63.
9. Wormstone IM. Posterior capsule opacification: a cell biological perspective. Exp Eye Res. 2002;74(3):337–47.
10. Meacock WR, Spalton DJ, Stanford MR. Role of cytokines in the pathogenesis of posterior capsule opacification. Br J Ophthalmol. 2000;84(3):332–6.
11. Nishi O. Posterior capsule opacification, part 1: experimental investigations. J Cataract Refract Surg. 1999;25(1):106–17.
12. Wallentin N, Wickström K, Lundberg C. Effect of cataract surgery on aqueous TGF-β and lens epithelial cell proliferation. Invest Ophthalmol Vis Sci. 1998;39(8):1410–8.
13. Knight-Nanan D, O'Keefe M, Bowell R. Outcome and complications of intraocular lenses in children with cataract. J Cataract Refract Surg. 1996;22:730–6.
14. Morgan KS, Karcioglu ZA. Secondary cataracts in infants after lensectomies. J Pediatr Ophthalmol Strabismus. 1987;24:45–8.
15. Alexandrakis G, Peterseim MM, Wilson ME. Clinical outcomes of pars plana capsulotomy with anterior vitrectomy in pediatric cataract surgery. J AAPOS. 2002;6:163–7.
16. Hosal BM, Biglan AB. Risk factors for secondary membrane formation after removal. J Cataract Refract Surg. 2002;28:302–9.
17. Lambert SR, Buckley EG, Plager DA, et al. Unilateral intraocular lens implantation during the first six months of life. J AAPOS. 1999;3:344–9.
18. Trivedi RH, Wilson E, Vasavada AR, et al. Visual axis opacification after cataract surgery and hydrophobic acrylic intraocular lens implantation in the first year of life. J Cataract Refract Surg. 2011;37:83–7.
19. Peterseim MW, Wilson MW. Bilateral intraocular lens implantation in the pediatric population. Ophthalmology. 2000;107:1261–6.
20. Gimbel HV, Ferensowicz M, Raanan M, et al. Implantation in children. J Pediatr Ophthalmol Strabismus. 1993;30:69–79.
21. BenEzra B, Cohen E. Cataract surgery in children with chronic uveitis. Ophthalmology. 2000;107:1255–60.
22. Lundvall A, Zetterstrom C. Cataract extraction and intraocular lens implantation in children with uveitis. Br J Ophthalmol. 2000;84:791–3.
23. Chen J, Chen Y, Zhong Y, et al. Comparison of visual acuity and complications between primary IOL implantation and aphakia in patients with congenital cataract younger than 2 years: a meta-analysis. Cataract Refract Surg. 2020;46:465–73.
24. Pandey SK, Ram J, Werner L, et al. Visual results and postoperative complications of capsular bag and ciliary sulcus fixation of posterior chamber intraocular lenses in children with traumatic cataracts. J Cataract Refract Surg. 1999;25:1576–84.
25. Jensen AA, Basti S, Greenwald MJ, et al. When may the posterior capsule be preserved in pediatric intraocular. Ophthalmology. 2002;109:324–8.
26. Raina UK, Gupta V, Arora R, Mehta DK. Posterior continuous curvilinear capsulorhexis with and without optic capture of the posterior chamber intraocular lens in the absence of vitrectomy. J Pediatr Ophthalmol Strabismus. 2002;39(5):278–87.

27. Heatley CJ, Spalton DJ, Kumar A, Jose R, Boyce J, Bender LE. Comparison of posterior capsule opacification rates between hydrophilic and hydrophobic single-piece acrylic intraocular lenses. J Cataract Refract Surg. 2005;31(4):718–24.
28. Nishi O, Nishi K, Sakanishi K. Inhibition of migrating lens epithelial cells at the capsular bend created by the rectangular optic edge of a posterior chamber intraocular lens. Ophthalmic Surg Lasers. 1998;29(7):587–94.
29. Brady KM, Atkinson CS, Kilty LA, Hiles DA. Cataract surgery and intraocular lens implantation in children. Am J Ophthalmol. 1995;120(1):1–9.
30. Khokhar SK, Pillay G, Dhull C, Agarwal E, Mahabir M, Aggarwal P. Pediatric cataract. Indian J Ophthalmol. 2017;65(12):1340–9.
31. Atkinson CS, Hiles DA. Treatment of secondary posterior capsular membranes with the Nd:YAG laser in a pediatric population. Am J Ophthalmol. 1994;118(4):496–501.
32. Gilbard SM, Peyman GA, Goldberg MF. Evaluation for cystoid maculopathy after pars plicata lensectomy-vitrectomy for congenital cataracts. Ophthalmology. 1983;90:1201–6.
33. Hoyt CS, Nickel B. Aphakic cystoid macular edema; occurrence in infants and children after transpupillary lensectomy and anterior vitrectomy. Arch Ophthalmol. 1982;100:746–9.

Post-operative Management and Visual Rehabilitation in Pediatric Cataract

8

Seo Wei Leo

The difference between the paediatric eye and the adult eye is much more than the eye size. Children have ongoing visual development and nervous plasticity resulting in risk of amblyopia. In addition to effective surgery, meticulous operative care and visual rehabilitation is crucial for favourable outcome. The lack of compliance poses additional challenges.

Visual rehabilitation includes refraction correction and amblyopia management. In cases where the intraocular lens was not implanted, aphakic correction can be corrected by various modalities such as aphakic glasses, contact lenses, epikeratophakia. Situations where the intraocular lens was contraindicated and not implanted include the following:

- Very young child (minimum age for IOL implantation depends on laterality and surgeon preference).
- Ocular factors like uveitis, microphthalmia, persistent foetal vasculature.

Supplementary Information The online version of this chapter (https://doi.org/10.1007/978-981-16-0212-2_8) contains supplementary material, which is available to authorized users.

S. W. Leo (✉)
Dr Leo Adult & Paediatric Eye Specialist Pte Ltd, Singapore, Singapore

In cases of primary intraocular lens implantation, visual rehabilitation encompasses management of the residual refractive error.

8.1 Aphakia Correction

See Fig. 8.1.

8.2 Aphakic Glasses

Aphakic glasses are commonly used for the correction of bilateral aphakia in children. They are also useful in children who are contact lens intolerant or as back up. Disadvantages of aphakic glasses include restriction of visual field to approximately 30°, heavy weight, distortion of image and prismatic effect. It is not recom-

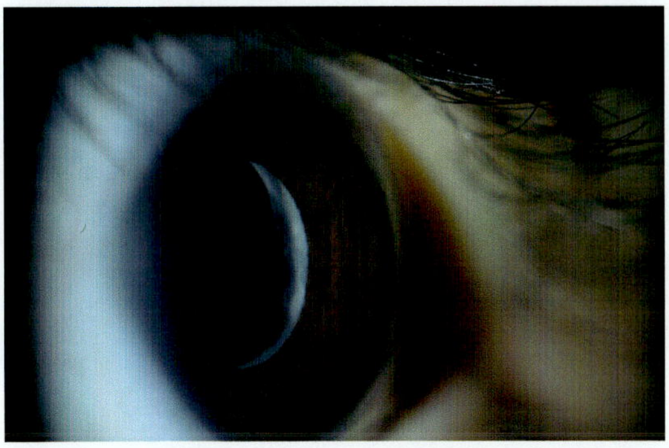

Fig. 8.1 Aphakia

S. K. Khokhar, C. Dhull (eds.), *Essentials of Pediatric Cataract Surgery*,
https://doi.org/10.1007/978-981-16-0212-2_8

mended for unilateral aphakia due to marked retinal image size disparity.

Due to increased trend towards primary IOL implantation and contact lens, the availability and advancement of technology for high power plus lens (>10 D) have declined. Primarily, three types of aphakic glasses are available [1]. Ultraviolet protection should be added to these lenses.

1. Lenticular lenses: These lenses have the prescribed power at the centre of lens surrounded by ring of little or no power. Although they are inferior to other lenses, they are the only option when requiring >20 D.
2. Aspheric lenticular lenses: They have aspherical central area lenses surrounded by ring of little or no power. Available 10–20 D, they are optically superior to lenticular lenses.
3. Multidrop lenses: They have spherical central zone that flattens into aspherical zone which further blends with ring of no power. The lens resembles the aspheric lenticular lenses without the noticeable ring. Far superior to other options, it is only available in the range of +10 to +16 D (Fig. 8.2).

Frame selection is very important in paediatric age group. Whenever possible the child should be included in decision making for the frame. The bridge of the frame should carefully conform in shape to that of the child. Cable temples (earpieces) which wrap around the back of the ear and spring hinges are recommended.

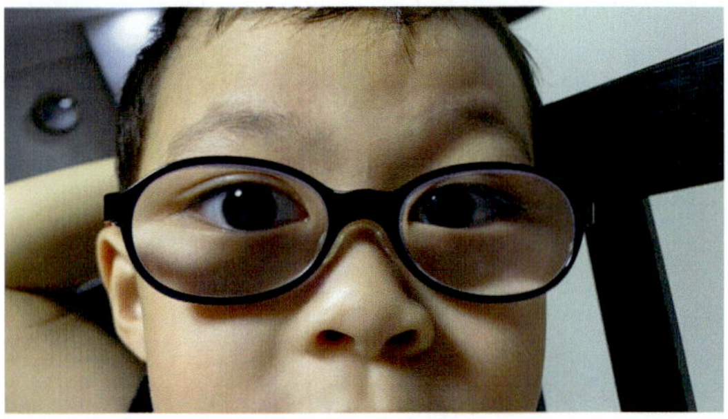

Fig. 8.2 Child with aphakic glasses

8.3 Contact Lenses

Studies have shown that better binocular vision and stereopsis can be obtained in patients who show excellent compliance with contact lens postoperatively [2]. In fact, aphakia with contact lens rehabilitation is the most common approach to the treatment of unilateral congenital cataract in infants less than 6 months [3]. The major advantage is the easy adjustability with the changing refractive error. Good lens fit, care, and hygiene compliance can prove to be an excellent alternative to primary IOL implantation, though inability to adhere these requirements can lead to hazardous consequences.

Contact lens in paediatric patients is demanding for adults/caregivers. Problems include difficult insertion and removal, poor compliance with long term use, loss of lenses, ocular irritation and infection. Compared to an adult, the paediatric conjunctival fornix is shallower, the globe is smaller, the sclera is steeper, the cornea is smaller and steeper. Coupled with changing refraction, increasing axial length, progressive corneal flattening, contact lens practice is much more challenging in paediatric patients.

Target refraction depends on the age of the patient:

- Less than 1 year of age: overcorrect by 2.0 D to get −2 D (which means near-point correction at 50 cm.)
- 1–2 years old: −1 to −1.5 D
- 3 years old and above: Bifocal glasses (near add +3).

There are three main type of contact lens to correct paediatric aphakia [4]:

1. Silicone elastomer (SE).
2. rigid gas permeable lens (RGP),
3. Hydrogel/Silicone hydrogel lenses.

In Singapore, the most commonly used contact lens to correct paediatric aphakia is an SE lens—the SilSoft (Bausch & Lomb). This was also used in the Infant Aphakia Treatment Study in the United States [5]. It has a high oxygen permeability (Dk = 340) and can be worn on an extended-wear basis. (The manufacturer recommends that the lens be removed for cleaning and disinfection at least once every 30 days and then left out of the eye overnight.) This wearing schedule is advantageous for young children, who often have a low tolerance for the insertion and removal of contact lenses. These SE lenses are limited for higher power (+23, +26, +29, +32 diopters [D]), 3 base curves (7.5, 7.7, 7.9 mm), and only 1 diameter (11.30 mm). Most aphakic infants are initially fitted with lenses that have a base curve of 7.5 mm. Lower-power SE contact lenses are available in 1 D increments (+11.50 D to +20.00 D), five base curves (7.5–8.3 mm), and 2 diameters (11.30, 12.50 mm). Some very young infants need higher power than what is available with the SE lenses. In addition, SE lenses have a limited capacity to correct corneal-induced astigmatism that exceeds 2 D in magnitude. The hydrophilic surface coating on SE lenses deteriorates over time, allowing its underlying hydrophobic surface to be exposed, which results in reduced wettability and accumulation of lipid-mucin deposits, thereby necessitating frequent lens replacement [6]. Silicon lenses are more costly, do not provide ultraviolet protection and can be uncomfortable initially (Fig. 8.3).

In contrast to SE lenses, RGP lenses can be customised to achieve virtually any power, base curve, or diameter. This means that they are more suitable for microphalmic eyes, small corneal diameters, 9.5 mm and those not within the power or base curve range of silicone lenses. For the high plus powers needed to correct paediatric aphakia, RGP lenses are commonly made from Menicon Z (Menicon, Nagoya, Japan) with a Dk = 189 or hexafocon B (Bausch & Lomb) with a Dk = 141.2, 7 The advantages of RGP lenses include availability in a wider range of powers, increased ability to correct corneal astigmatism (up to 6 D), better durability, and lower cost. RGP lens may be ordered with UV blockers. The primary disadvantage of RGP lenses is that for the high plus powers needed to correct paediatric aphakia, their effective oxygen permeability is not optimal for extended wear and hence they need to be removed daily. The lens replacement rate was approximately 50% higher for RGP lenses when compared to SE lenses [5].

There are many disadvantages associated with the use of soft lenses like hydrogel lenses for paediatric aphakia [7]. The major problem is corneal hypoxia. The combination of the low Dk and the large centre thickness in high plus power means that these lenses have very low oxygen transmissibility (Dk/t), leading to complications like corneal vascularisation, stromal oedema. Silicone hydrogel lenses provide a marked increase in oxygen supply to the cornea compared to hydrogel lenses. However, these lenses, especially if worn on an extended-wear basis, can accumulate high levels of lipid deposition and be associated with clinical complications such as superior epithelial arcuate lesions, mucin balls and contact lens related papillary conjunctivitis.

Contact lens fitting can be initiated during the cataract surgery by taking corneal measurements using handheld topography or keratometry. Postoperatively, the aphakic child should be fitted as soon as possible. Most infants require the

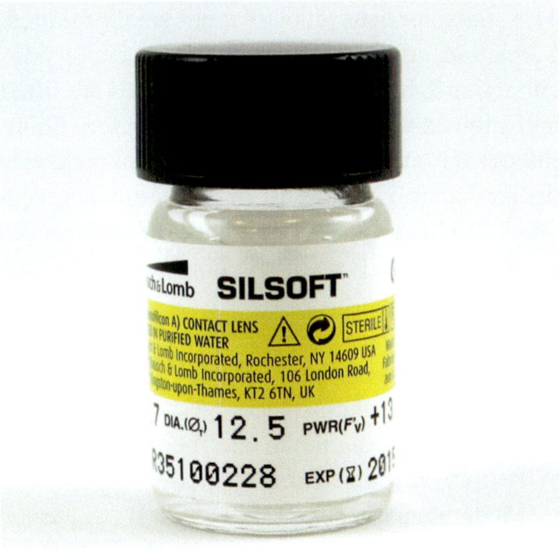

Fig. 8.3 Silsoft contact lens

11.3-diameter lens due to their small fissures. Premature infants may need much steeper base curves, such as 7.50 or 7.70. The lenses are fitted and allowed to settle for 15–20 min before doing fluorescein evaluation. A "steep" lens produces distinct central pooling of fluorescein whereas a "flat" lens results in an absence of fluorescein centrally. An ideal fit is obtained with the following:

- 1–2 mm movement on blink
- Minimal apical clearance
- Minimal bearing in the intermediate zone
- Peripheral edge clearance
- Moderate nasal edge lift
- There is no encroachment upon the limbus
- The optics are within the pupil

Preoperative biometry can also be used to estimate contact lens power for distance if an accurate refraction cannot be obtained initially [8]. These are the methods: (1) 30 D contact lens (32 D minus 2 D overcorrection for near vision based on IATS protocol); (2) regression-estimated contact lens power of 84.4–3.2 × axial length; and (3) IOL power calculated using the Sanders-Retzlaff-Kraff (SRK/T) regression formula with a modified A-constant (112.176) with mean prediction error of −4.0, −1.0, and −2.0 D respectively.

The compliance and success of contact lens treatment of aphakia depends on the caregiver/parents. They need to be educated and trained in lens insertion, lens removal, lens cleaning and care. It is crucial for them to understand and recognise complications such as infection, torn lenses, poorly fitting lens so that they can bring the child for requited medical care. Compliance to visits cannot be overemphasised.

8.4 Epikeratophakia

Epikeratophakia (or epikeratoplasty) is a surgical procedure in which a lamellar graft is sutured onto the surface of the recipient cornea to reproduce the effect of a highly positive contact lens [9]. This procedure has generally not been very successful for infantile aphakia due to graft failure. The only theoretical indication is unilateral aphakia where intraocular lens implantation is contraindicated and yet the patient is contact lens intolerant.

8.5 Management of Residual Refractive Errors After Intraocular Lens Implantation

Paediatric cataract surgery is associated with several sources of postoperative refractive error [10]. These include planned refractive error based on age or fellow eye status, loss of accommodation, and unexpected refractive errors due to inaccuracies in biometry technique, use of IOL power formulas based on adult normative values, and late refractive changes due to unpredictable eye growth (Fig. 8.4).

On average, the eye grows 4.5 mm in the first 2 years of life. From the age of 2–6 years, growth is slower but still substantial at 0.4 mm per year. We aim to correct the residual refractive errors with spectacle lenses or contact lenses. The target refraction is as follows:

1. in children less than 1 year: aim for mild myopia −2 D,
2. in children 1–2 year: aim for myopia −1 to −1.5 D,
3. Emmetropia for distance, Near add +3 for children 3 years and above (Fig. 8.5).

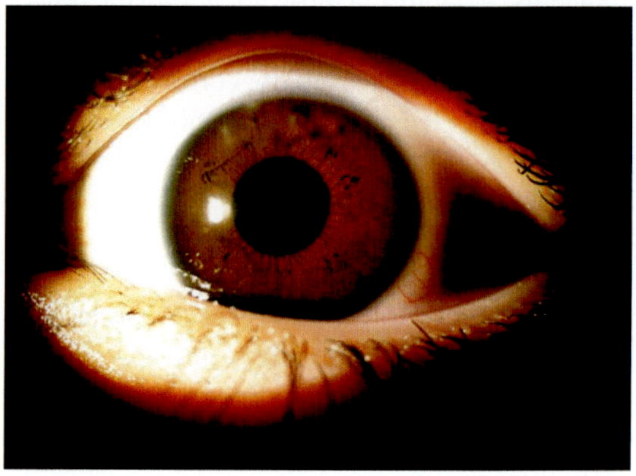

Fig. 8.4 Paediatric pseudophakia

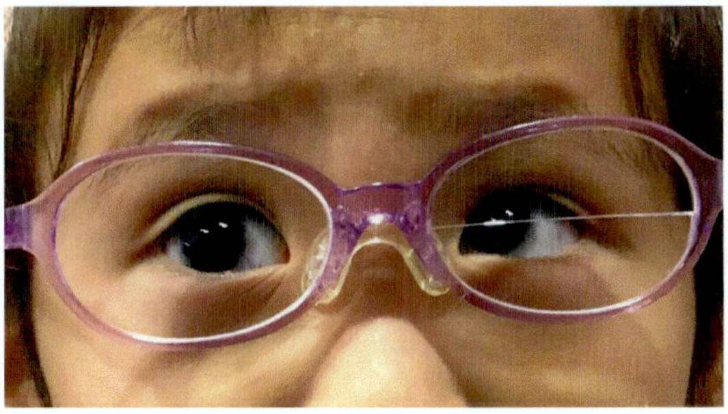

Fig. 8.5 Left IOL implantation with bifocal spectacle lens correction

In unilateral cases, the fellow eye must not be forgotten. Refractive errors like significant hyperopia, myopia and astigmatism need to be corrected with optical aids.

8.6 Amblyopia Treatment

In paediatric cataract, amblyopia is the result of preop deprivation and postop anisometropia. The treatment goal is to provide a clear retinal image as soon as possible and to correct ocular dominance by patching good eye. Timely treatment is critical. The amount of patching depends on the age when retinal image was cleared. Likewise, if an older child presents with a unilateral cataract, the prognosis for improvement depends on the age at which the opacity developed. If it has been present since early infancy, the prognosis is poor, because of amblyopia, even if the surgery is successful in itself [11].

The IATS regimen for patching is as follows:

- Patching of the good eye 1 h per day per month of age until the child is 8 months old starting the second week following cataract surgery.
- Patch all hours that the child is awake every other day or one-half the child's waking hours every day for children more than 8 months old.
- If compliance is poor and patching of less than 15 min for 3 months has been achieved, use occlusion contact lens (Fig. 8.6).

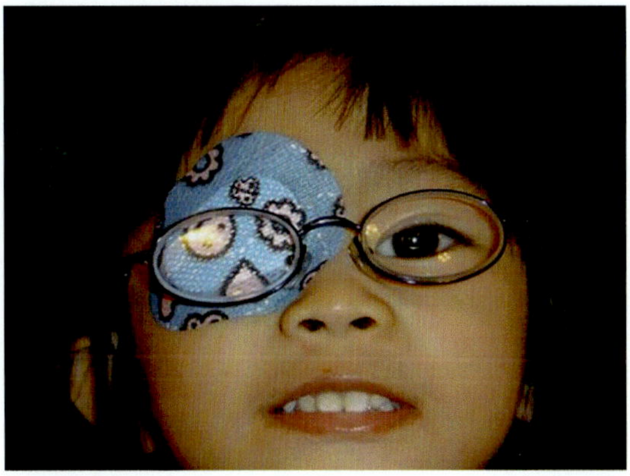

Fig. 8.6 Child with left amblyopia

8.7 Summary

Advancement in surgical techniques and methods of optical rehabilitation has substantially improved the functional and anatomic outcomes of paediatric cataract surgeries in recent years. In cases where primary IOL implantation is not done, contact lenses and aphakic glasses are viable options. In cases of primary IOL implantation, residual refractive errors need to be corrected. In all cases, amblyopia management is critical.

References

1. Trivedi R, Wilson ME. Correction of aphakia: glasses and contact lens. In: Pediatric cataract surgery: techniques, complication and management. Philadelphia: Lippincott; 2005. p. 306–7.
2. Ma JJ, Morad Y, Mau E, et al. Contact lens for the treatment of pediatric cataracts. Ophthalmology. 2003;110:299–305.
3. McAnena L, McCreery K, Brosnahan D. Migration to aphakia and contact lens treatment is the trend in the management of unilateral congenital cataract in Britain and Ireland. Ir J Med Sci. 2019;188(3):1021–4.
4. Lambert SR, Kraker RT, Pineles SL, Hutchinson AK, Wilson LB, Galvin JA, VanderVeen DK. Contact lens correction of aphakia in children: a report by the American Academy of Ophthalmology. Ophthalmology. 2018;125(9):1452–8.
5. Russell B, Ward MA, Infant Aphakia Treatment Study Group. Infant aphakia treatment study contact lens experience: one-year outcomes. Eye Contact Lens. 2012;38:234–9.

6. de Brabander J, Kok JH, Nuijts RM, Wenniger-Prick LJ. A practical approach to and long-term results of fitting silicone contact lenses in aphakic children after congenital cataract. CLAO J. 2002;28:31–5.
7. Lindsay RG, Chi JT. Contact lens management of infantile aphakia. Clin Exp Optom. 2010;93(1):3–14.
8. Trivedi RH, Lambert SR, Lynn MJ, Wilson ME, Infant Aphakia Treatment Study Group. The role of preoperative biometry in selecting initial contact lens power in the infant aphakia treatment study. J AAPOS. 2014;18(3):251–4.
9. Morgan KS, Somers M. Update on epikeratophakia in children. Int Ophthalmol Clin. 1989;29(1):37–42.
10. Indaram M, VanderVeen DK. Postoperative refractive errors following pediatric cataract extraction with intraocular lens implantation. Semin Ophthalmol. 2018;33(1):51–8.
11. Baradaran-Rafii A, Shirzadeh E, Eslani M, Akbari M. Optical correction of aphakia in children. J Ophthalmic Vis Res. 2014;9(1):71–82.

Part II

Pediatric Cataract Surgery in Challenging Situations

9 Surgery in Fibrotic Anterior and Posterior Capsule

Sudarshan Kumar Khokhar, Parmanand Kumar, and Chirakshi Dhull

In pediatric cataracts, the capsulorhexis decides the type and the site of IOL insertion. Even in normal capsule, the rhexis is difficult, presence of plaques or fibrosis makes it even more challenging.

Focal, multifocal or diffuse, dense, white opacity adherent to the internal surface of anterior and posterior lens capsule leads to the formation of capsule plaque. It appears as white opacity blocking the red glow of the fundus. Capsular fibrosis in immature cataract is visible as whitish plaque with striation or stretching of capsule (Fig. 9.1a). It is sometimes difficult to identify anterior capsular fibrosis (ACF) in white mature cataracts because of the lack of contrast. Posterior capsular fibrosis is also not visible in mature cataract due to lack of visualization. ACF is easily visible as wavy fibrotic lines intraoperatively after staining with Trypan blue dye (Fig. 9.1b). These could be located centrally or eccentrically and may be discrete or confluent covering almost the entire capsule. On ultrasound biomicroscopy (UBM), both anterior and posterior capsular plaque is easily visible as hyperreflective area (Fig. 9.1c, d).

Based on the area of anterior capsule involved, ACF is classified as [1]:

- Small (0.1 mm^2)
- Medium (0.1–0.3 mm^2)
- Large (>0.3 mm^2)

9.1 Incidence

Johar et al. found anterior capsular plaque in 11.5% of congenital cataracts [1]. Wilson reported 6% incidence of anterior capsular fibrosis in congenital cataracts [2]. The occurrence of anterior capsular plaque was more common in mature cataracts, three times more than other type of cataracts like nuclear, lamellar and mixed cataract [1].

Posterior capsular plaque was seen in 13.4% in congenital cataract [3] as compared to 10.1% in age related cataracts [4], mostly in total white cataracts [3, 4].

9.2 Pathophysiology

Human crystalline lens is highly organised structure. It consists of lens epithelial cells (LEC) and fibres secreted by these epithelial cells and cap-

Supplementary Information The online version of this chapter (https://doi.org/10.1007/978-981-16-0212-2_9) contains supplementary material, which is available to authorized users.

S. K. Khokhar (✉)
Professor Ophthalmology, Dr. RP Centre for Ophthalmic Sciences, All India Institute of Medical Sciences, New Delhi, India

P. Kumar
R P Center, AIIMS, New Delhi, India

C. Dhull
Eye Q Hospital, Rohtak, Haryana, India

S. K. Khokhar, C. Dhull (eds.), *Essentials of Pediatric Cataract Surgery*,
https://doi.org/10.1007/978-981-16-0212-2_9

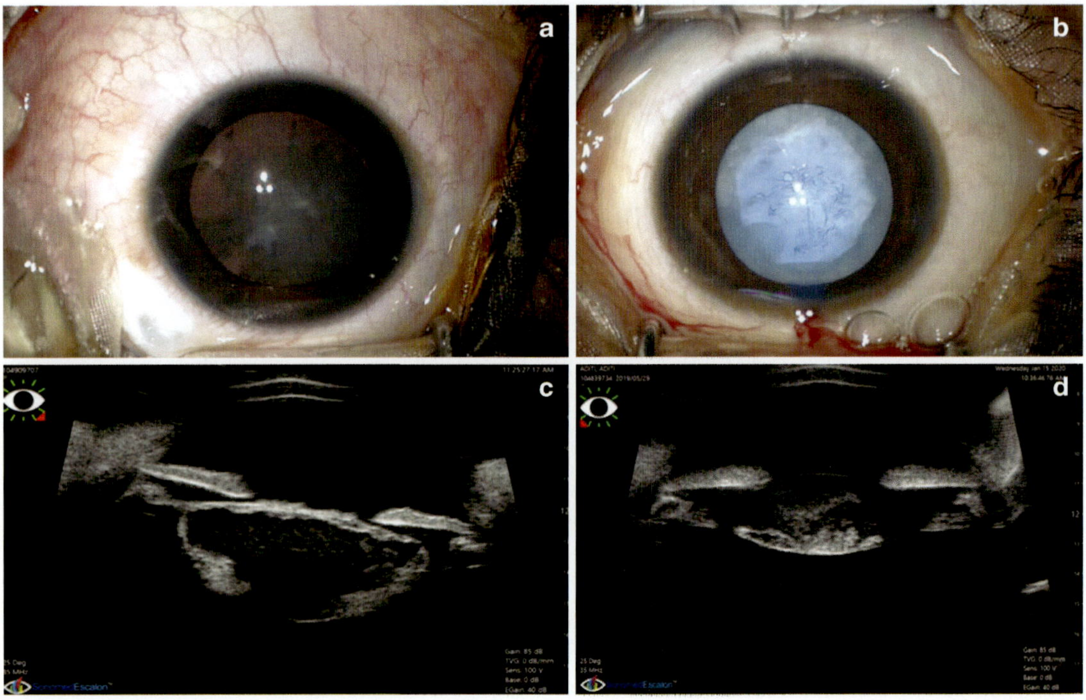

Fig. 9.1 (**a**) Congenital cataract with anterior capsular plaque. (**b**) Congenital cataract with anterior capsular fibrosis prominently visible after staining with Trypan Blue dye. (**c**) UBM showing hyperreflective anterior capsule suggestive of anterior capsular plaque. (**d**) UBM showing hyperreflective posterior capsule suggestive of posterior capsular plaque

sule. The capsule is formed by secretion of LEC. It is the basement membrane of LECs, which predominantly consists of type IV collagen with minor contributions of type I collagen, type III collagen, fibronectin, laminin, and sulfated glycosaminoglycans [5]. LECs are regularly arranged beneath the capsule and their nuclei were uniformly placed in the cells. LECs are cuboidal beneath anterior capsule and columnar in equatorial region. The LECs in the cataracts are having faintly stained cytoplasm. Their nuclei are heterogenous in the shape and size and are located unevenly [1].

The anterior lens epithelium obtained from eyes having cataract with ACF had two distinct regions: nonplaque and plaque region. The nonplaque region had LECs which were similar to the LECs of samples obtained from nonplaque cataract samples, such as faintly stained cytoplasm, heterogeneity in the shape and size of nuclei.

Plaque region shows lesser number of cells positive for α-SMA (smooth muscle actin) with abundance of collagen fiber particularly of type I collagen. This shows trans-differentiations of epithelial cells into myofibroblast called as epithelial mesenchymal trans-differentiation (EMT) [6–9]. Myofibroblast cells under the influence of TGF-β undergo mitotic proliferation with accumulation of fibroblastic material in extracellular matrix which leads to formation of distinct opaque region called plaque [6, 10–14].

Pathophysiology of plaque formation is same in both anterior and posterior capsule. Posterior capsular plaque formation more common because of association with anterior vitreo-lenticular interface dysgenesis [15].

9.3 Surgical Management

Continuous curvilinear capsulorhexis is mandatory for a successful cataract surgery with IOL implantation in pediatric cataracts [16].

The rhexis in pediatric cataract is tricky due to the increased elasticity of capsule in young age, positive vitreous pressure and also the lower scleral rigidity which adds to the surgeon's miseries [16, 17].

Now in cases with fibrosis of the capsule, it is difficult to perform rhexis and thus there is need to modify techniques which will be dealt in this chapter.

Anterior capsulorhexis—Staining with trypan blue dye is required in all cases of cataract with anterior capsular fibrosis. After staining, anterior chamber is filled with heavy molecular weight OVDs (Healon GV) to flatten the anterior capsule. Capsulorhexis is done according to the size, location and extent of anterior capsular plaque.

1. *Small capsular plaque* not extending in periphery (≤3 mm)—Capsulorhexis is done around the plaque, keeping the size of capsulorhexis at least 4–5 mm (Fig. 9.2).
2. *Central capsular plaque* (3–5 mm)—Capsulorhexis was done around the plaque, either continuous curvilinear as explained (Fig. 9.3) or by push–pull technique (Fig. 9.4).

   Push–pull technique of capsulorhexis—It was first performed by Nischal [18] in human and later by Hamada and colleagues [19]. It was two incisions push–pull technique. Later, Mohammadpour introduced four incisions push–pull technique.

   Two incisions push–pull technique—A stab incision is made on the capsule at the junction of the fibrous plaque and the clear capsule of lens with 26 G bent cystitome or MVR. The inner margin of flap is grasped with capsulorhexis microforceps and centripetal force is applied. When the anterior capsule has been folded almost halfway onto itself, the pulling is stopped and another incision is made at the diametrically opposite margin of the plaque. Again, the flap is pulled toward the center with the help of microforceps until the tear meets at both ends, resulting in a continuous capsulorhexis.

   Four incisions push–pull technique—Four stab incisions of 1–1.5 mm size is made at the junction of fibrotic and non-fibrotic area of anterior capsule with 26 G bent cystitome. The inner margin of flap is grasped with capsulorhexis microforceps and pulled centripetally. All the four flaps were joined together to complete the rhexis.

   According to authors, if the fibrosis is severe then more than four stab incisions can be made on anterior capsule. Oval capsulorhexis or extension of capsulorhexis is major drawback of this procedure. Authors do not recommend this technique if the plaque is irregular in shape and size of more than 6 mm and if any tail-like extension to the periphery is present.
3. *Anterior eccentric capsular plaque (<5 mm)*—In this scenario, authors recommend to complete the rhexis by opting partial rhexis and partial cutting. A stab incision is made with 26 G bent cystitome on anterior capsule away from the fibrotic part. Rhexis is done in non-fibrotic part with capsulorhexis forceps or microforceps. In fibrotic part, rhexis is done by cutting fibrotic anterior capsule with micro-scissors (Fig. 9.5).
4. *Anterior capsular plaque >6 mm or irregular plaque >5 mm*—In this case scenario, authors recommend to complete the rhexis by cutting the anterior capsule with micro-scissor all-around after stab incision with 26 G bent cystitome or MVR (Fig. 9.6). Vitreorhexis is another option in such cases.

Vitreorhexis—In this method, the rhexis is done using the vitrector with the slow cut rate and high infusion rate [20, 21]. The advantage of this

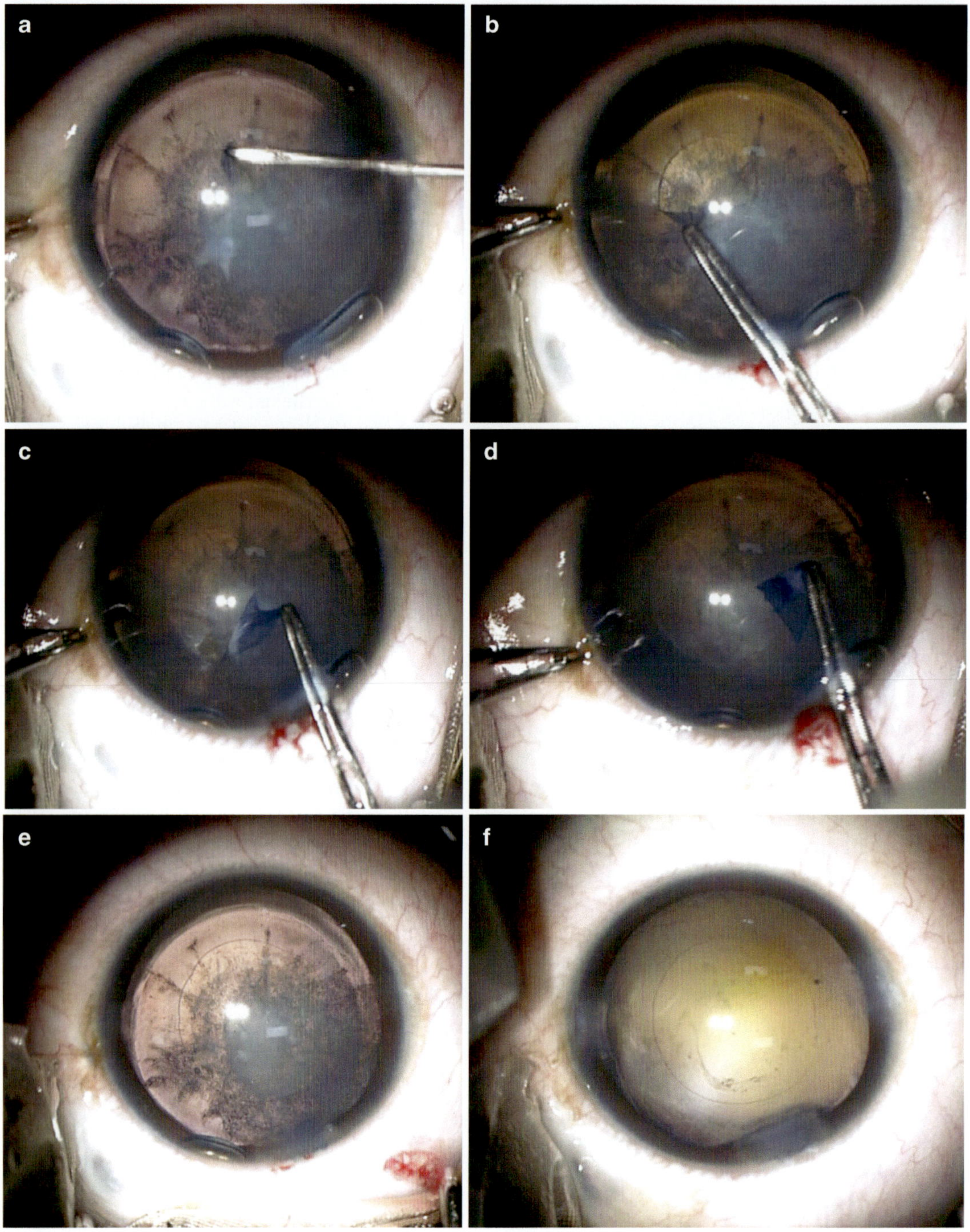

Fig 9.2 (**a**) Anterior capsule nick was given with 26 G bent cystitome. (**b**–**d**) Root of the capsular flap was grasped with utrata capsulorhexis forceps and rhexis was done covering the capsular plaque. (**e**, **f**) Figure showing final capsulorhexis size before and after lens aspiration

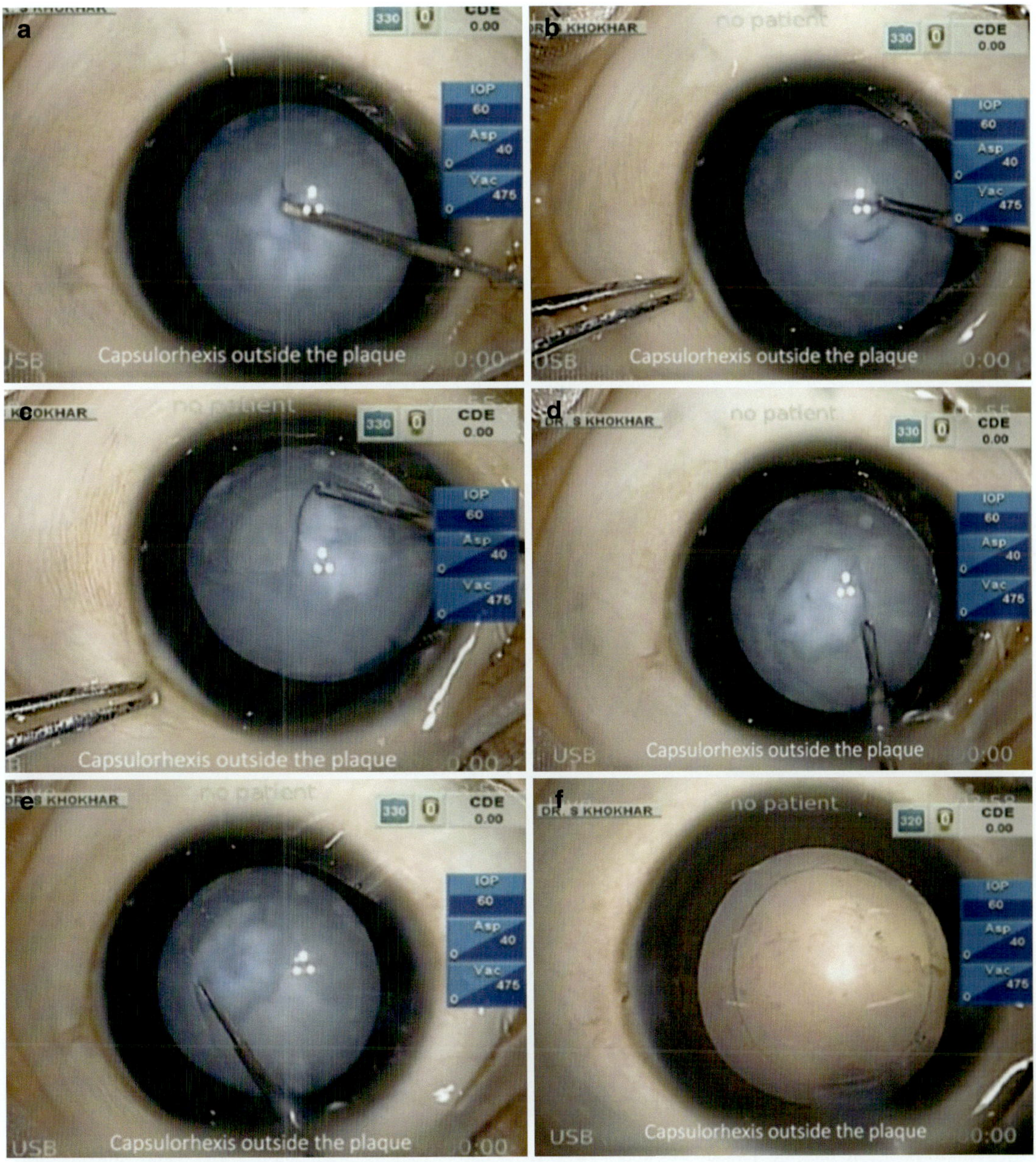

Fig. 9.3 Anterior capsular plaque of more than 3 mm but less than 5 mm rhexis around the plaque done with the help of 26 bent cystitome and 23 G Alcon forceps (**a**–**e**). (**f**) Final rhexis size visible clearly after lens aspiration

technique is that anterior capsulotomy, lens aspiration, posterior capsulotomy, and anterior vitrectomy can be done sequentially with the same instruments, avoiding repeated entries and exits of instrument into and out of the anterior chamber and thus minimizing the occurrence of mechanical injuries to the eye.

Plasma blade—Plasma blade also known as Fugo blade after the inventor, can also be used to do anterior capsulotomy. It is an electrosurgical device that uses pulses of plasma which are generated around its tip to cut and cauterize tissue in liquid medium (Fig. 9.7). The advantage of this technique is that it can be used to create an ante-

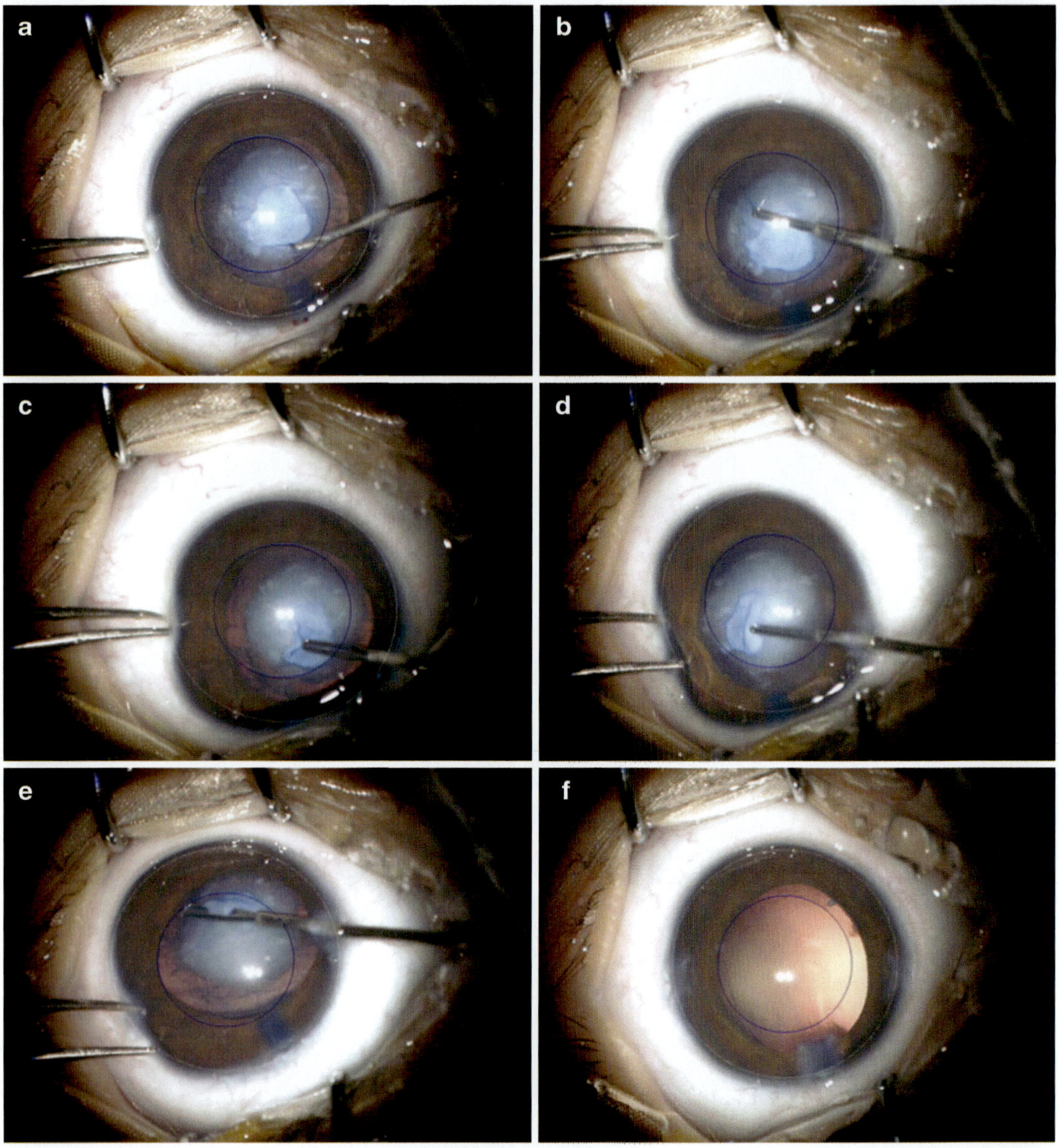

Fig. 9.4 (**a**) Four stab incision is made 90° apart. (**b–e**) Inner flap of each stab incision is grasped and pulled centripetally with 23 G Alcon forceps one by one till each flap joined to other flap. (**f**) Final rhexis size with nasal extension

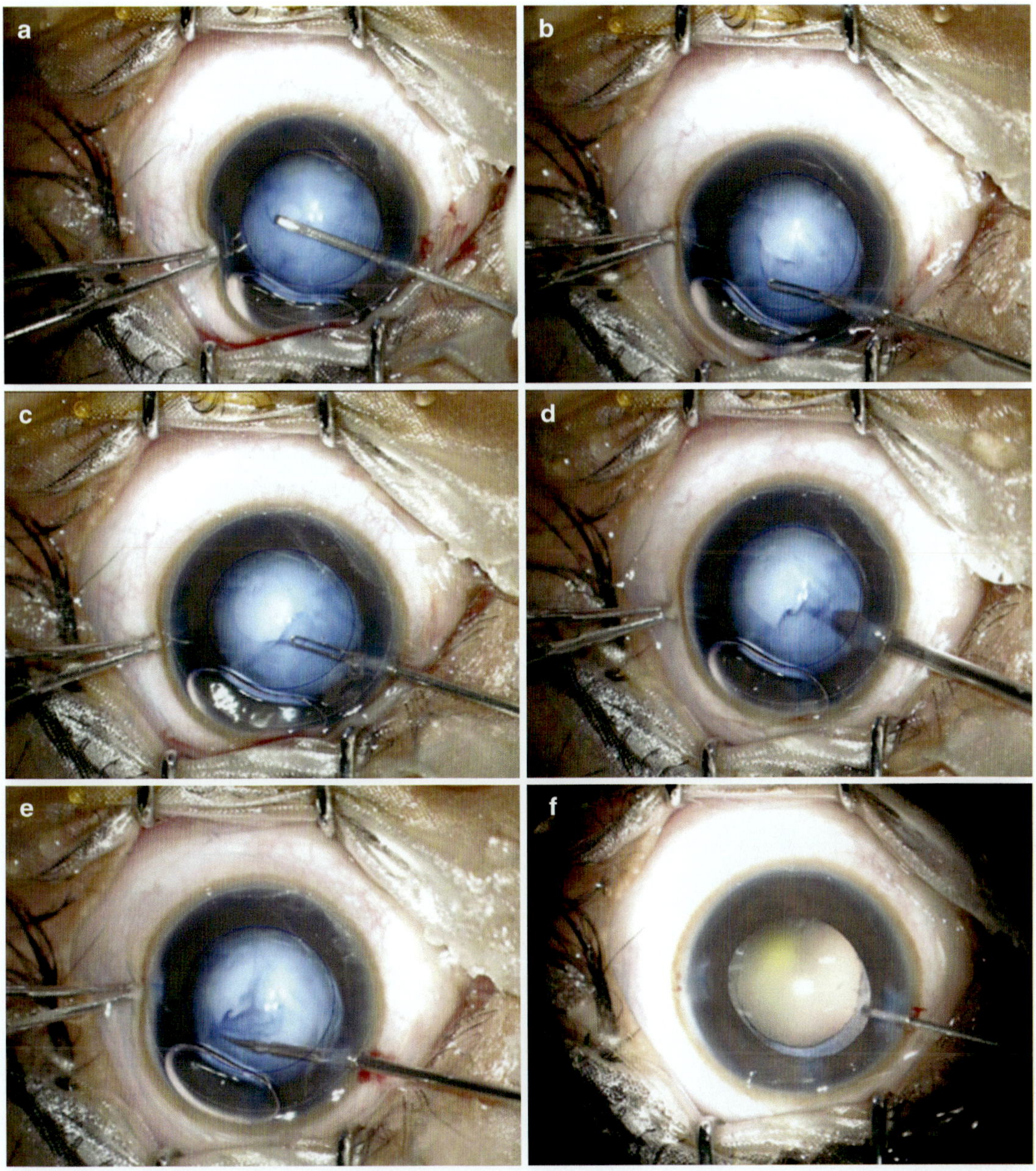

Fig. 9.5 (**a**) Anterior capsule stab incision is given with 26 G bent cystitome. (**b**, **c**) Rhexis is done with 23 G Alcon forceps in non-fibrotic part of anterior capsule. (**d**) Stab incision is made in fibrotic part of capsule. (**e**) Rhexis completed by cutting the fibrotic capsule with 23 G Alcon scissor. (**f**) Final capsulorhexis visible clearly after lens aspiration

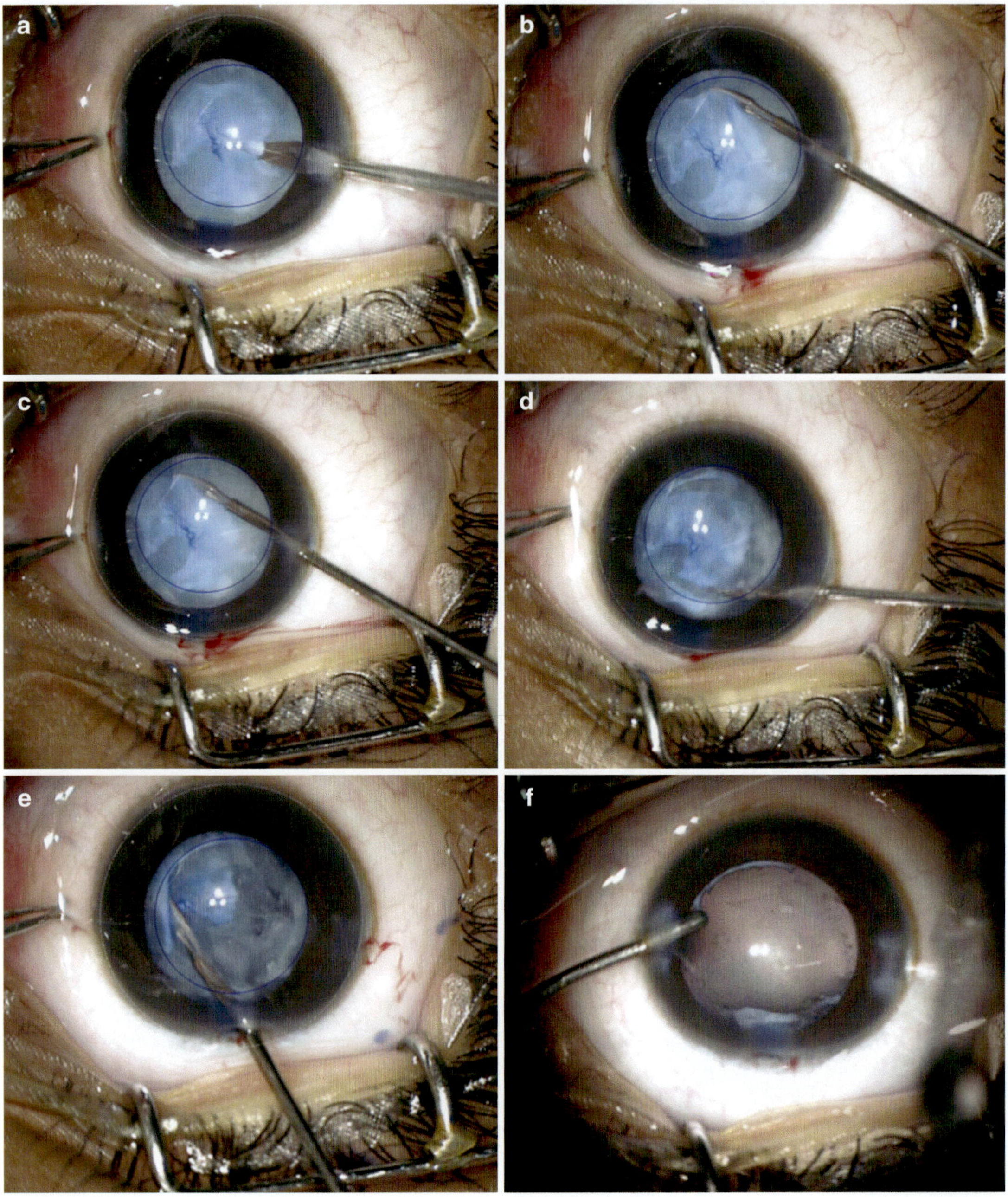

Fig 9.6 (**a**) Stab incision is made with MVR in anterior capsule. (**b–e**) Capsulorhexis is done by cutting the anterior capsule all-around with 23 G Alcon scissor. (**f**) Final capsulorhexis visible clearly after lens aspiration

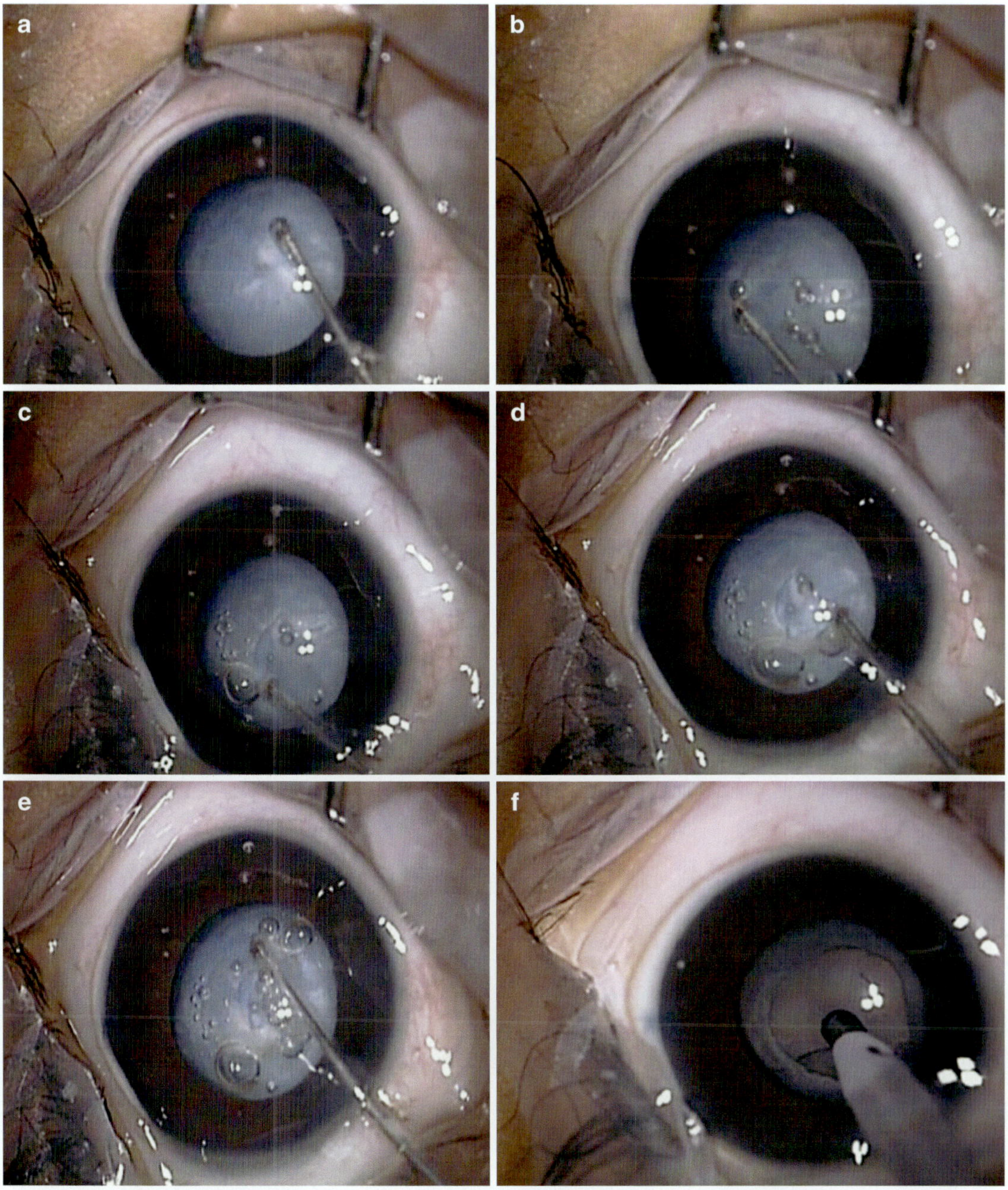

Fig 9.7 (**a**–**e**) Capsulorhexis is done with plasma blade. (**f**) Capsulorhexis clearly visible after lens aspiration

rior capsulotomy through plaque. The disadvantage of Fugo blade is formation of gas bubbles, impairing the surgeon's view [22].

9.4 Posterior Capsular Plaque Management

After lens aspiration anterior chamber and capsular bag is formed with viscoelastic substance. Always keep in mind that bag is not inflated so much, otherwise chances of posterior capsular tear increases. Posterior capsular plaque management varies according to size of plaque and whether plaque is tightly or loosely adherent to posterior capsule.

1. *Posterior capsule plaque <3mm—*
   Peeling of the plaque is done with the help of 26 G bent cystitome and microforceps (Fig. 9.8). After plaque removal, inspect the posterior capsular integrity. If intact make a stab incision, do

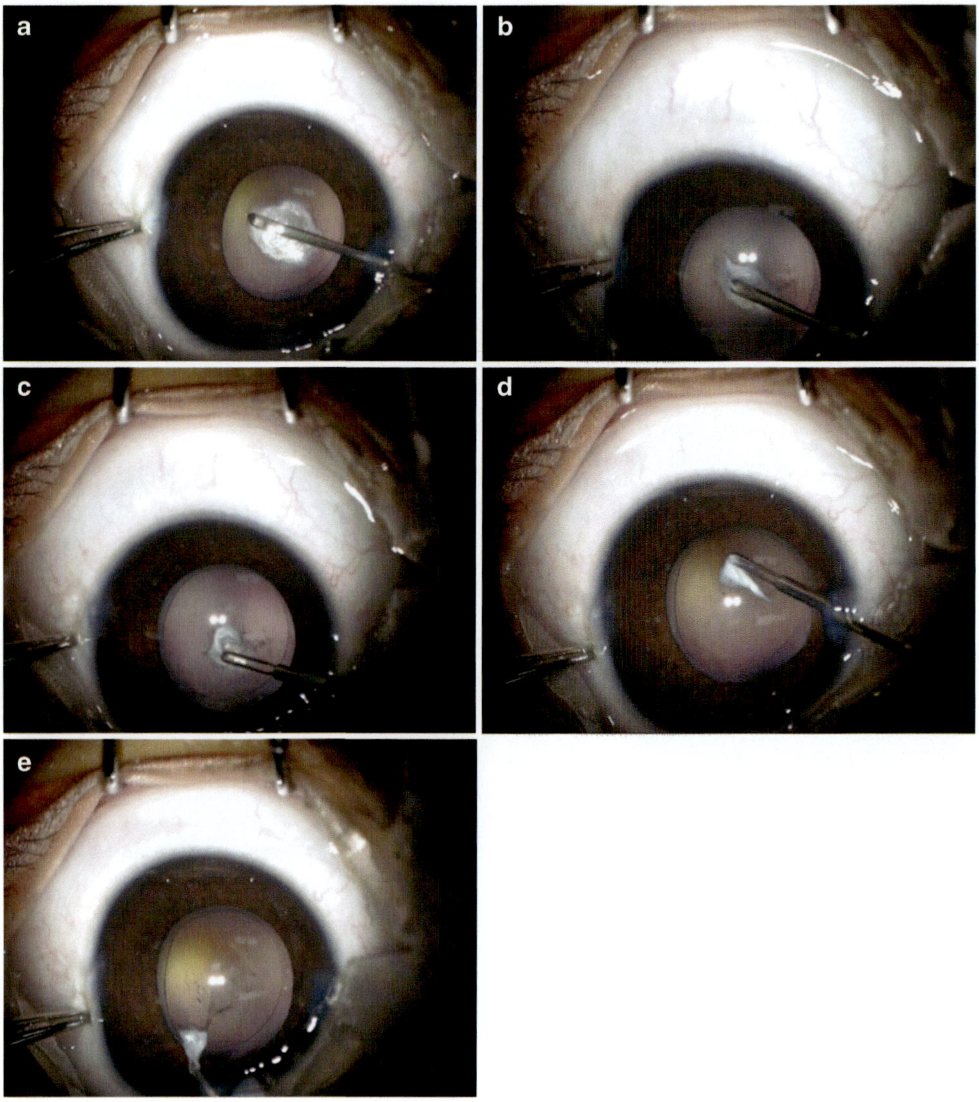

Fig. 9.8 (**a**) Scraping of edges of plaque is done with 26 G bent cystitome. (**b–d**) Edges of plaque grasped with 23 G Alcon forceps and pulled tangentially upwards. (**e**) Detached plaque from posterior capsule

capsulorhexis followed by anterior vitrectomy both according to age of the child.

If posterior capsule is ruptured and small in size, then one can proceed with capsulorhexis followed by anterior vitrectomy.

If the plaque is tightly adherent to the posterior capsule during peeling, make a stab incision in clear part of posterior capsule and do capsulorhexis covering the plaque.

2. *Posterior capsule plaque 3–5 mm*—If the plaque is loosely adherent, peeling of the plaque will be done in similar manner as explained above. If plaque is dense and tightly adherent, make a stab incision at margin of plaque with 26 G cystitome or MVR. Grasped the plaque with one hand with microforceps, complete the rhexis by cutting all around it by micro-scissor (Fig. 9.9).

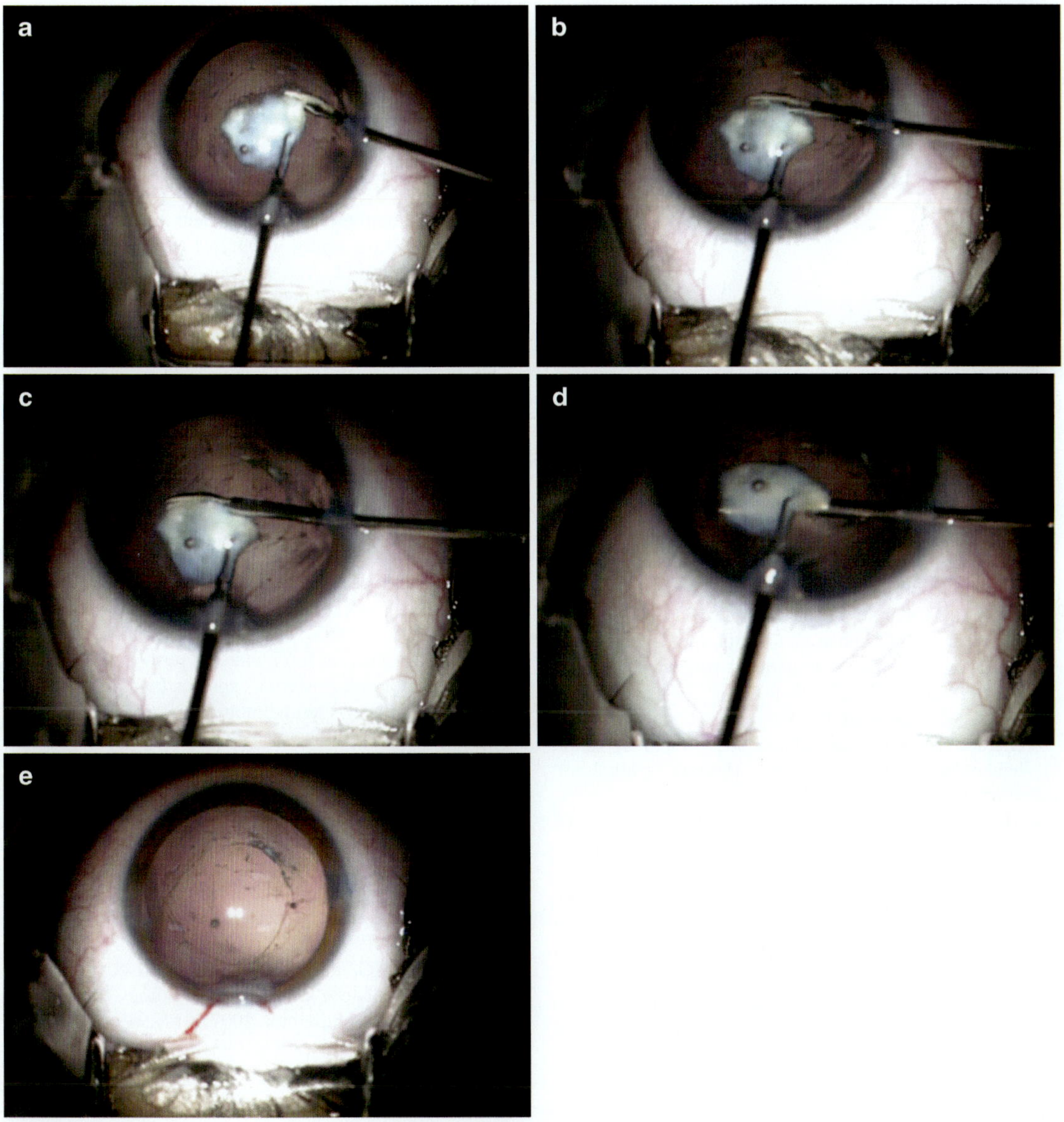

Fig 9.9 (**a**–**d**) Densely adherent plaque removed with the help and microforceps and micro-scissor. (**e**) Clear media with visible rhexis margin

3. *Posterior capsule plaque >5 mm*—Make central opening with MVR and use vitrector to create opening with a 0.5 mm rim left around the plaque

Surgical challenges

(a) You can use push–pull technique after making 4 nicks 90° apart and pull and push each to get a rhexis around the fibrotic area.
(b) Needs rhexis at normal rhexis area and cutting through fibrosis using intra vit scissors.
(c) Needs cutting with scissors after making a stab entry using MVR using all three ports.

These challenges are discussed and shown in detail in the videos of this chapter (Videos 9.1, 9.2, 9.3, 9.4, 9.5 and 9.6).

References

1. Johar K, Vasavada AR, Tatsumi K, et al. Anterior capsular plaque in congenital cataract: occurrence, morphology, immunofluorescence, and ultrastructure. Invest Ophthalmol Vis Sci. 2007;48:4209–14.
2. Wilson ME, Trivedi RH, Morrison DG, et al. The Infant Aphakia Treatment Study: evaluation of cataract morphology in eyes with monocular cataracts. J AAPOS. 2011;15(5):421–6.
3. Praveen MR, Shah SK, Vasavada AR, et al. Incidence, management, and postoperative outcomes in pediatric eyes with coexisting posterior capsule plaque and cataract. J Cataract Refract Surg. 2010;36:2094–9.
4. Vasavada AR, Chauhan H, Shah G. Incidence of posterior capsular plaque in cataract surgery. J Cataract Refract Surg. 1997;23:798–802.
5. Dische Z, Zelmenis G. The content and structural characteristics of the collagenous protein of rabbit lens capsules at different ages. Investig Ophthalmol. 1965;4:174–80.
6. Marcantonio JM, Syam PP, Liu CS, Duncan G. Epithelial transdifferentiation and cataract in the human lens. Exp Eye Res. 2003;77:339–46.
7. Rungger-Brandle E, Conti A, Leuenberger PM, Rungger D. Expression of alphasmooth muscle actin in lens epithelia from human donors and cataract patients. Exp Eye Res. 2005;81:539–50.
8. Nagamoto T, Eguchi G, Beebe DC. Alpha-smooth muscle actin expression in cultured lens epithelial cells. Invest Ophthalmol Vis Sci. 2000;41:1122–9.
9. Schmitt-Graff A, Pau H, Spahr R, Piper HM, Skalli O, Gabbiani G. Appearance of alpha-smooth muscle actin in human eye lens cells of anterior capsular cataract and in cultured bovine lens-forming cells. Differentiation. 1990;43:115–22.
10. Lovicu FJ, Ang S, Chorazyczewska M, McAvoy JW. Deregulation of lens epithelial cell proliferation and differentiation during the development of TGFbeta-induced anterior subcapsular cataract. Dev Neurosci. 2004;26:446–55.
11. Saika S, Kono-Saika S, Ohnishi Y, et al. Smad3 signaling is required for epithelial-mesenchymal transition of lens epithelium after injury. Am J Pathol. 2004;164:651–63.
12. Shirai K, Saika S, Tanaka T, et al. A new model of anterior subcapsular cataract: involvement of TGFbeta/Smad signaling. Mol Vis. 2006;12:681–91.
13. Peng Q, Hennig A, Vasavada AR, Apple DJ. Posterior capsular plaque: a common feature of cataract surgery in the developing world. Am J Ophthalmol. 1998;125:621–6.
14. Vasavada AR, Thampi P, Bhatt DS. Degeneration and transdifferentiation of human lens epithelial cells. J Cataract Refract Surg. 1999;25:1312–3.
15. Van Looveren J, Van Gerwen V, Schildermans K, Laukens K, Baggerman G, Tassignon MJ. Proteomic analysis of posterior capsular plaques in congenital unilateral cataract. Acta Ophthalmol. 2018;96(8):e963–9. https://doi.org/10.1111/aos.13782.
16. Wilson ME. Anterior capsule management for pediatric intraocular lens implantation. J Pediatr Ophthalmol Strabismus. 1999;36(6):314–43.
17. Wilson ME Jr. Anterior lens capsule management in pediatric cataract surgery. Trans Am Ophthalmol Soc. 2004;102:391–422.
18. Nischal KK. Two-incision push-pull capsulorhexis for pediatric cataract surgery. J Cataract Refract Surg. 2002;28:593–5.
19. Hamada S, Low S, Walters BC, Nischal KK. Five-year experience of the 2-incision push-pull technique for anterior and posterior capsulorrhexis in pediatric cataract surgery. Ophthalmology. 2006;113:1309–14.
20. Wilson ME, Bluestein EC, Wang XH, et al. Comparison of mechanized anterior capsulectomy and manual continuous capsulorrhexis in pediatric eyes. J Cataract Refract Surg. 1994;20:602–6.
21. Wilson ME, Saunders RA, Roberts EL, et al. Mechanized anterior capsulectomy as an alternative to manual capsulorhexis in children undergoing intraocular lens implantation. J Pediatr Ophthalmol Strabismus. 1996;33:237–40.
22. Priglinger SG, Palanker D, Alge CS, et al. Pulsed electron avalanche knife: new technology for cataract surgery. Br J Ophthalmol. 2007;91(7):949–54. https://doi.org/10.1136/bjo.2006.109546.

Preexisting Posterior Capsular Defect

10

Chirakshi Dhull and Sudarshan Kumar Khokhar

10.1 Introduction

Preexisting posterior capsular defect (PCD) is a rare entity associated with congenital cataracts. This unique condition requires special surgical considerations for satisfactory outcomes. The incidence varies from 2% to 6.7% [1, 2] and it is more commonly reported in developing world. Preexisting PCD includes congenital cataract associated with a defect in posterior capsule which may or may not be associated with fibrosis [3]. Trauma is excluded from this terminology and in this chapter PCD refers to congenital PCD. This entity was first published by Vajpayee et al. in 1992 [4]. PCD may be associated with posterior capsular plaque, dense posterior, nuclear or total cataract [2, 3]. Posterior polar cataracts is a unique morphology which may be associated with localized posterior capsular defect; but they generally present in adulthood [5, 6].

Supplementary Information The online version of this chapter (https://doi.org/10.1007/978-981-16-0212-2_10) contains supplementary material, which is available to authorized users.

C. Dhull (✉)
Eye Q Hospital, Rohtak, Haryana, India

S. K. Khokhar
Professor Ophthalmology, Dr. RP Centre for Ophthalmic Sciences, All India Institute of Medical Sciences, New Delhi, India

10.2 Pathogenesis

The pathogenesis of PCD is not completely understood. Various theories have been put forward. It has been hypothesized that PCD starts as posterior lenticonus/lentiglobus, which may later progress to a full thickness defect [7]. Posterior lenticonus may result secondary to traction caused by remnants of hyaloid vasculature. This has been supported by reports of association of posterior lenticonus with persistent fetal vasculature (PFV) in both unilateral and bilateral cases [8, 9]. Other theory for formation of posterior lenticonus include thinning of the posterior capsule which has been supported by histopathological evidence [10]. Role of genetics has been identified in bilateral cases [11]. Overall, there is a defect or weakness in the posterior capsular wall and this breach is the primary defect leading to cataract formation.

Once the integrity of posterior capsule is compromised, clear crystalline lens fibers come in contact with the fluid in Berger's space. This leads to hydration of lens proteins and opacification of lens ensues. The cataract may range from only posterior localized area to the whole lens. Afterwards, the lens absorption and posterior migration starts. In early stage, there may be only slight decrease in lens volume with localized cataract. In late stages, the lens may be partially or full absorbed.

S. K. Khokhar, C. Dhull (eds.), *Essentials of Pediatric Cataract Surgery*,
https://doi.org/10.1007/978-981-16-0212-2_10

In some cases of PCD, there may be a healing response seen which may try to close the defect. According to the theory of cicatrization, hyalocytes, and equitorial lens epithelial cells (LECs) migrate and proliferate leading to formation of posterior capsular plaque [12, 13]. This may be incomplete or complete, which determines the type of PCD as discussed in the subsequent section.

10.3 Clinical Presentation

The presentation in pediatric cataract associated with PCD is similar to any other congenital cataract. It is easy to miss by the caregivers at an early stage due to its posterior location. A history of rapid progression of whitish opacity by the mother or caregiver may provide a hint toward the diagnosis.

It may be difficult to diagnose PCD in undilated pupil with a torch examination in a small child. A dilated slit lamp examination may help in picking subtle but key signs for diagnosis. A similar examination can be performed using direct ophthalmoscope for a small baby and further details may be elicited during examination under anesthesia using microscope. The step wise examination in a fully dilated pupil should include the following:

- **Anterior chamber depth (ACD):** *Unusually deep* anterior chamber should raise a suspicion of posterior capsular opening or partially absorbed cataract.
- **Anterior capsule curvature:** *Flat or concave* anterior capsule is generally observed with PCD. There may be wrinkling of anterior capsule in cases with more severe cicatricial response.
- **Morphology of cataract:** Variable morphology of cataract has been noted with PCD. It may be localized posterior, posterior cortical, posterior polar, dumbbell shaped, total, or membranous cataract.
- Presence of vacuoles in the vicinity of cataract may be suggestive. In addition, *lens thickness* is generally reduced.
- **Posterior capsular assessment:** Well-defined defect in posterior capsule may be seen, could be any shape but **spindle shape** is the commonest in our experience. In rare cases, there may be association of persistent fetal vasculature.
- **Assessment of anterior vitreous:** Two specific signs may be seen and are regarded as highly indicative of PCD.
  - **Fish tail Sign:** As seen in cases of Posterior polar cataract and PCD is indicative of breach in posterior capsule. It is exaggerated by eye movements [1].
  - **White dot sign:** Presence of white dots on the posterior capsule and/or in the anterior vitreous [1] is highly suggestive of PCD (Fig. 10.1).

10.4 Classifications

Zhangliang Li [3] et al. have classified PCD after removal of cataract in three types. In type I, a large defect with cortex sinking in the anterior vitreous is seen, as observed in 38.1% in their study. In type II, a cluster of fibrotic spots are

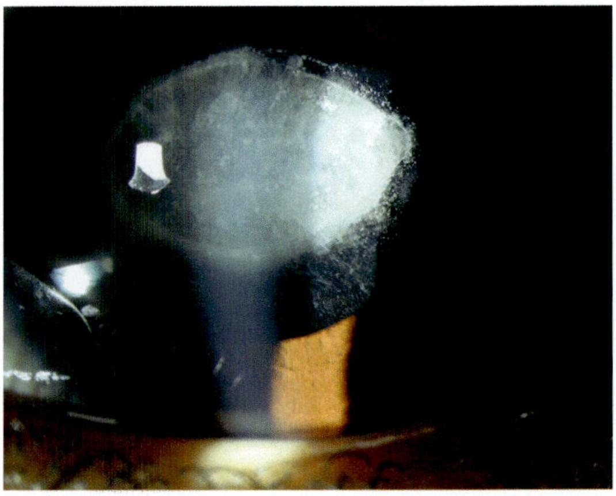

Fig. 10.1 Congenital cataract with tell-tale signs of PCD. Deep AC, white dot sign is seen along with well-defined spindle shaped PCD

seen in posterior capsule, as observed in 47.6% in their study. Type III has concurrent PFV (14.3%) [3]. This classification system is based on the theory of cicatrization.

10.4.1 Surgical Classification

We have proposed an alternate classification of PCD [14] which is based on the surgical approach required for appropriate management. Classification of PCD is shown in Table 10.1.

We will discuss in detail, the surgical approach for type 1 and type 2. Type 3 is discussed in detail with management of fibrotic plaques (Chap. 9).

10.5 Investigations

10.5.1 Ultrasonography

Ultrasonography (USG) should be performed to rule out PFV which is a known association with PCD [3]. Tabatabaei et al. have described the role of 20 MHz USG for evaluation of posterior capsule in traumatic cases [15]. There are isolated reports of using 10 MHz probe USG in lateral longitudinal axis for detection of posterior capsular defect [16]. Although not as precise, USG probe can detect large defects especially in cases of posterior displacement of lens matter in anterior vitreous.

10.5.2 Ultrasound Biomicroscopy

In cases of diagnostic difficulty, ultrasound bimicroscopy (UBM) with 35 MHz should be performed for confirmation. Signs of PCD are enhanced and discontinuity in posterior capsule is generally visible (Fig. 10.5). Lens thickness is significantly reduced. It can be helpful in subtle presentations where partially absorbed cataract is visible but other clinical signs are absent. Very small PCD can also be visualized with UBM (Fig. 10.6). Other than that, biometric parameters such as lens thickness, vitreous

Table 10.1 Classification of preexisting PCD [14]

Type 1	Well-defined defect, with sharp edges and minimal fibrosis (Fig. 10.2)
Type 2	Circular or regular defect with fibrosis (Fig. 10.3)
Type 3	Posterior capsular plaque where the defect is sealed (Fig. 10.4)

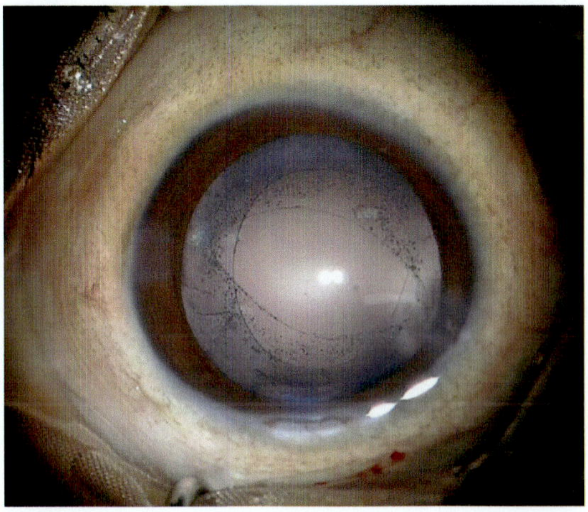

Fig. 10.2 Intraoperative picture of Type 1 PCD, notice the spindle shape, sharp edges and lack of fibrosis

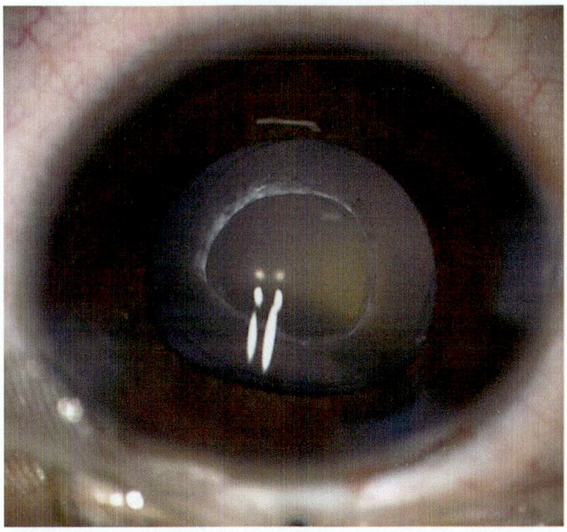

Fig. 10.3 Type 2 PCD with fibrosed margins

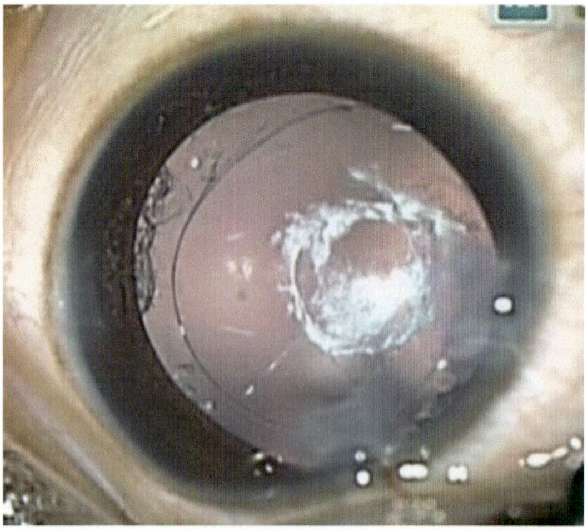

Fig. 10.4 Type 3 PCD with posterior capsular plaque

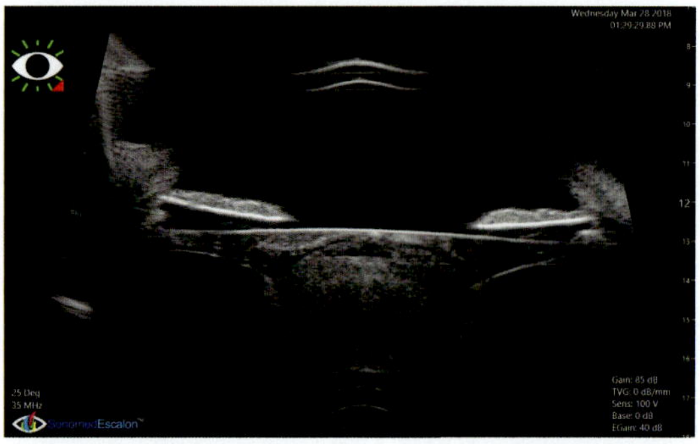

Fig. 10.5 UBM of a 2 month baby with congenital cataract showing large PCD and lens matter in anterior vitreous cavity

chamber depth and corneal diameter may help in prediction of PCD [3].

10.5.3 Anterior Segment Optical Coherence Tomography

Anterior Segment Optical Coherence tomography (ASOCT) can be useful in older children especially in cases of posterior polar cataract where defects may be minute. Due to higher resolution, in such cases, ASOCT can detect these defects preoperatively [17].

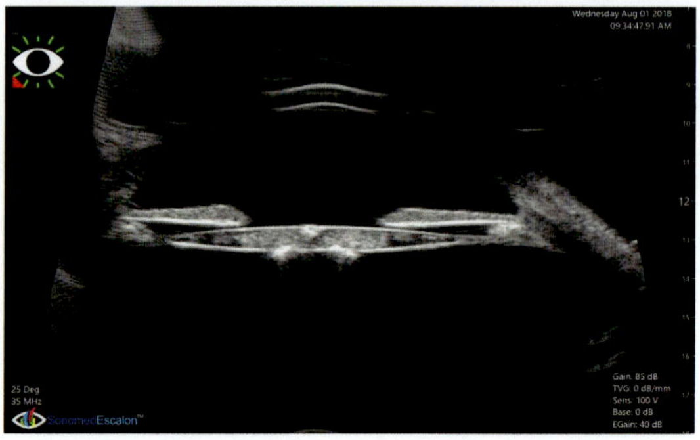

Fig. 10.6 UBM of a child with partially absorbed cataract showing anterior and posterior capsular plaque with small defects and lens matter in Berger's space. Also notice the increase in anterior chamber depth and decrease in lens thickness

10.6 Management

Most cases with PCD are rapidly progressive and associated with significant cataract. They require early cataract surgery to prevent amblyopia from setting in. In some cases such as posterior polar cataract, visually insignificant cataract may be seen. These children can be followed up regular with adequate refractive correction.

10.6.1 Surgical Management

Apart from the usual standard surgical steps for pediatric cataract surgery, certain precautions should be taken. Figures 10.7 and 10.8 will aid in better understanding of the below mentioned points. We would highlight step wise care to ensure successful surgical outcome:

10.6.2 Incisions

Small paracentesis should be made. Main incision can be avoided in the beginning. This provides tighter chamber and prevents wound leak which can potentially extend pre-existing PCD.

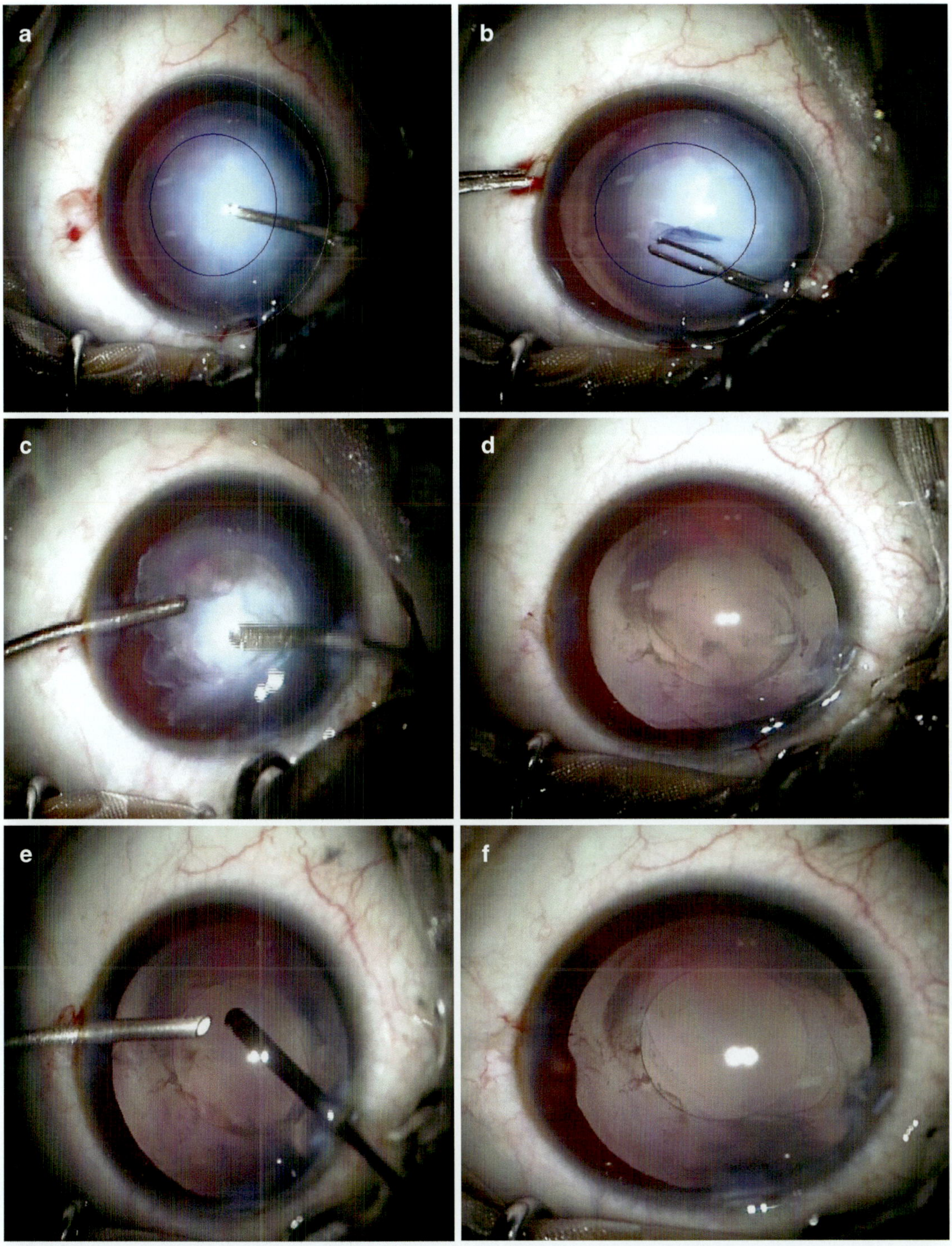

Fig. 10.7 Surgical steps in a case of total cataract preexisting PCD. (**a**) Callisto ring of 5 mm size is used to ensure capsulorhexis size. (**b**) ACCC is performed using microincision forceps. (**c**) Lens aspiration is performed with bimanual irrigator and aspirator. (**d**) PCD is visible following lens aspiration, notice a faint PFV stalk in the superior field. (**e**) Anterior vitrectomy is performed. (**f**) PCCC margins are more clearly visible. (**g**) PCIOL is places in bag using safe technique. (**h**) Final lens stability during viscoelastic removal

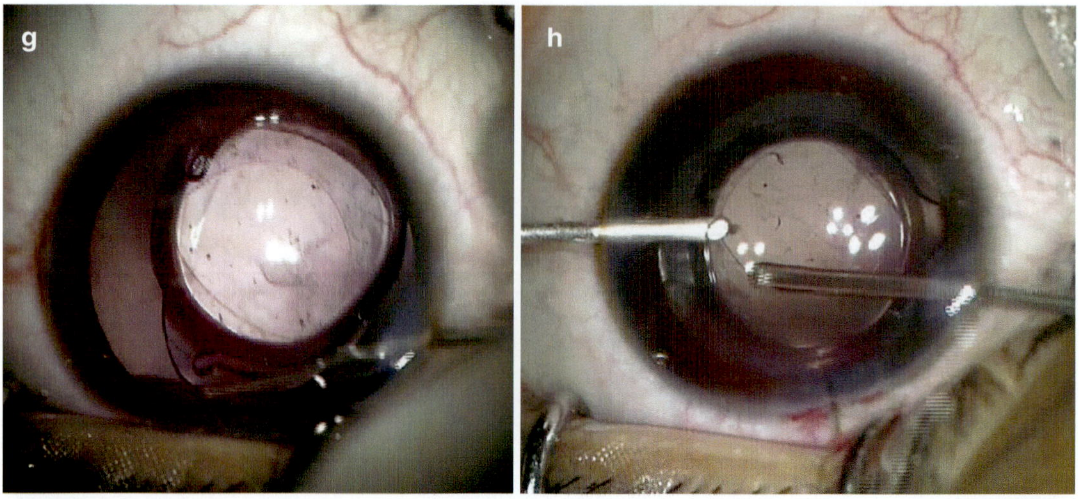

Fig. 10.7 (continued)

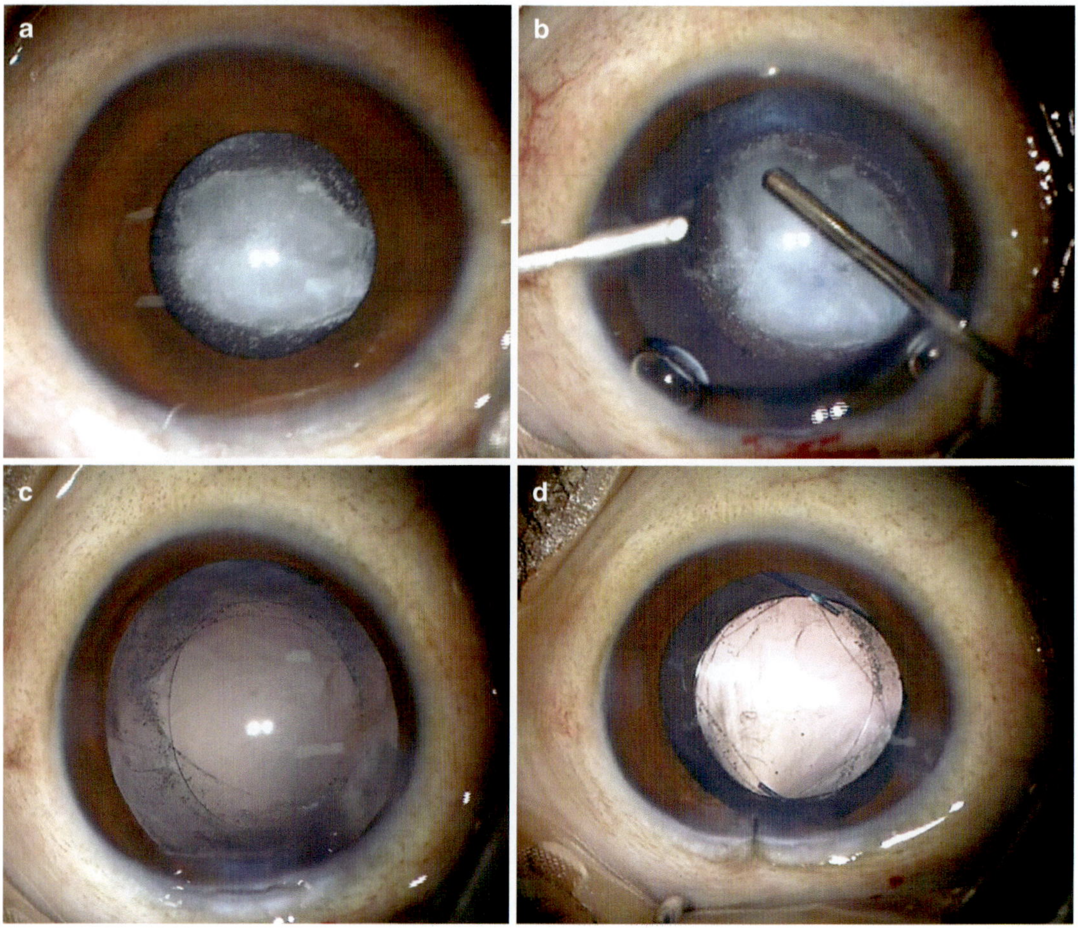

Fig. 10.8 Surgical steps in partially absorbed cataract with large PCD. (**a**) Preoperative image showing absorbed cataract and white dot sign. (**b**) Following ACCC, Lens aspiration is performed in IA cut mode followed by anterior vitrectomy in cut IA mode with same vitrectomy probe. (**c**) PCD visible following vitrectomy. (**d**) PCIOL is placed in sulcus with optic capture due to large PCD

10.6.3 Anterior Chamber (AC)

AC has to be maintained throughout the surgery. Heavy ophthalmic viscosurgical devices (OVDs) can be used to maintain the chamber.

10.6.4 Anterior Capsulorhexis

We prefer to perform anterior capsulorhexis (ACCC) from microincision forceps in such cases. It has a twofold advantage. First, it can be used via a small incision has provides greater chamber stability. Also, anterior chamber is usually deep in cases of PCD. Microincision forceps, being longer compared to Utrata's forceps, helps in easier access to anterior capsule; without distorting the surgical wounds.

10.6.5 Hydro Maneuvers

Hydrodissection is avoided to prevent PCD extension and lens matter drop in vitreous cavity.

10.6.6 Lens Matter Removal

During lens matter removal, lower flow rate and IOP settings are used. A bimanual technique is preferred due to better control and small incision size. Slow removal can be performed. Generally vitreous is well formed in children and whole lens matter can be removed with ease.

We use 23 gauge vitrectomy cutter for irrigation and aspiration (IA) instead of the convention bimanual probes. This can be used in IA cut mode for lens matter removal and switched to cut IA mode for anterior vitrectomy. This reduces manipulation and chamber fluctuation while insertion and removal of instruments. Localized anterior vitrectomy can be completed.

10.6.7 Posterior Capsule Management

Posterior capsule management depends on type of PCD.

In type 1, margins of PCD are sharp and not fibrosed. If PCD is small, attempt can be made to convert the defect into posterior capsulorhexis (PCCC). Care has to be taken to not overfill the chamber and avoid filling the bag. IOL can be implanted in the bag in such cases with safe technique [18]. In larger defects, this may not be possible and hence IOL can be placed in the such cases with or without capture.

In type 2, PCD capsular margins are fibrosed and hence IOL can be placed in the bag with similar technique. We should ensure central 3 mm opening in these cases.

In type 3, where there is capsular plaque, various techniques are available. They are discussed in depth in the respective chapter.

10.6.8 Anterior Vitrectomy

After initially performing vitrectomy, it is generally not required after posterior capsular maneuvering. If required, it can be performed before IOL implantation. Triamcinolone can be used to improve visualization.

10.6.9 IOL Implantation

IOL need to be implanted with caution either in the bag or sulcus depending on the suitability. A circular, 5 mm anterior capsulorhexis is the key in these cases for successful IOL implantation. Most cases achieve good surgical outcomes [1, 2].

10.7 Visual Rehabilitation

Visual rehabilitation in such cases is similar to congenital cataract cases. Additional inflammation is not expected in such cases unless associated with PFV. Refractive correction along with amblyopia therapy as per requirement can performed for these children.

10.8 Conclusion

We would like to conclude preexisting PCD as a unique association with congenitial cataract. Diagnosis is essential as these present with surgical challenges. Clinical signs can provide hint to the diagnosis in most cases while additional investigation such as UBM may be required in some subtle cases. Careful surgery can help in preventing inadvertent complications and attain good outcomes.

References

1. Vasavada AR, Praveen MR, Nath V, Dave K. Diagnosis and management of congenital cataract with preexisting posterior capsule defect. J Cataract Refract Surg. 2004;30:403–8.
2. Wilson ME, Trivedi RH. Intraocular lens implantation in pediatric eyes with posterior lentiglobus. Trans Am Ophthalmol Soc. 2006;104:176–82.
3. Li Z, et al. Morphological and biometric features of preexisting posterior capsule defect in congenital cataract. J Cataract Refract Surg. 2018;44(7):871–7.
4. Vajpayee RB, Sandramouli S. Bilateral congenital posterior-capsular defects: a case report. Ophthalmic Surg. 1992;23:295–6.
5. Kalantan H. Posterior polar cataracts: a review. Saudi J Ophthalmol. 2012;26(1):41–9. https://doi.org/10.1016/j.sjopt.2011.05.001.
6. Vasavada AR, Vasavada VA. Managing the posterior polar cataract: an update. Indian J Ophthalmol. 2017;65(12):1350. https://doi.org/10.4103/ijo.IJO_707_17.
7. Wilson ME, Trivedi RH, Pandey SK. Pediatric cataract surgery: techniques, complications, and management. Philadelphia: Lippincott Williams & Wilkins; 2005.
8. Kilty LA, Hiles DA. Unilateral posterior lenticonus with persistent hyaloid artery remnant [letter]. Am J Ophthalmol. 1993;116:104–5.
9. Khokhar S, Dhull C, Mahalingam K, Agarwal P. Posterior lenticonus with persistent fetal vasculature. Indian J Ophthalmol. 2018;66(9):1335–6.
10. Khalil M, Saheb N. Posterior lenticonus. Ophthalmology. 1984;91:1429–30.
11. Vivian AJ, Lloyd C, Russel-Eggit I, Taylor D. Familial posterior lenticonus. Eye. 1995;9:119–23.
12. Van Looveren J, Van Gerwen V, Timmermans J-P, Tassignon M-J. Immunohistochemical characteristics of the vitreolenticular interface in congenital unilateral posterior cataract. J Cataract Refract Surg. 2016;42:1037–45.
13. Peng Q, Hennig A, Vasavada AR, Apple DJ. Posterior capsular plaque: a common feature of cataract surgery in the developing world. Am J Ophthalmol. 1998;125:621–6.
14. Khokhar SK, Dhull C, editors. Atlas of pediatric cataract. Singapore: Springer Nature. https://doi.org/10.1007/978-981-13-6939-1_5.
15. Tabatabaei A, Kiarudi MY, Ghassemi F, et al. Evaluation of posterior lens capsule by 20-MHz ultrasound probe in traumatic cataract. Am J Ophthalmol. 2012;153(1):51–4. https://doi.org/10.1016/j.ajo.2011.05.038.
16. Bergaal SK, Gagrani M, Pujari A, et al. Ultrasonographic assessment of the lens. Case Rep. 2018;2018:bcr-2018-226205.
17. Pujari A, Selvam H, Yadav S, et al. Preoperative assessment of posterior capsular integrity using posterior segment OCT with a +20 D intraocular lens: conical sign to suggest capsular deficiency. J Cataract Refract Surg. 2020;46(6):844–8. https://doi.org/10.1097/j.jcrs.0000000000000197.
18. Khokhar S, Sharma R, Patil B, Sinha G, Nayak B, Kinkhabwala RA. A safe technique for in-the-bag intraocular lens implantation in pediatric cataract surgery. Eur J Ophthalmol. 2015;25(1):57–9.

Persistent Fetal Vasculature

11

Chirakshi Dhull and Sudarshan Kumar Khokhar

11.1 Introduction

Persistent Fetal Vasculature (PFV) is a congenital anomaly of the eye resulting from failure of the embryological, primary vitreous, and hyaloid vasculature to regress [1, 2]. Cloquet reported it for the first time as early as 1818 [3]. It was named persistent hyperplastic primary vitreous (PHPV) based on the embryology and origin and described in detail by Reese in 1955 [1]. This term was used for a long time till Goldberg introduced the term persistent fetal vasculature or PFV combining the anterior, posterior, and mixed presentation to the terminology [3]. This is a more inclusive term and is currently the most accepted terminology for the condition.

PFV may be present as congenital cataract or leukocoria. It may involve some or all the component of hyaloid and fetal vasculature. Based on the structures involved, it can be classified as anterior, posterior, or combined variety. The surgical management and prognosis depend on the structures involved by this anomaly. It is usually unilateral but may be bilateral in rare cases [4].

11.2 Pathogenesis

During intrauterine life, the fetal vasculature is important for development of iris, lens, vitreous and retina. The vascular system comprises of three parts: vasa hyaloidea propria (VHP) or hyaloid vessels in vitreous, tunica vasculosa lentis (TVL), or hyaloid vessels covering posterior surface of lens and anterior pupillary vessels covering anterior surface of the lens which anastomose with TVL. These vessels start to grow in first month of gestation and begin to involute by 5 months of gestation via the process of apoptosis [5, 6]. These vessels usually disappear completely by birth leaving behind an acellular hyaloid canal called Cloquet's canal [2, 3, 5]. Any abnormality in the involutional process can result in partial or complete failure of vascular regression. This causes different clinical presentations ranging from mild to severe; anterior, posterior or combined variety.

Cause for the abnormality in regression of fetal vasculature is not completely understood [7]. Most cases are sporadic in nature [1, 2, 7]. Some have been reported to be associated with genetic abnormalities, but no specific locus has been identified in humans [8]. In animal models, gene mutations have been documented in bilateral

Supplementary Information The online version of this chapter (https://doi.org/10.1007/978-981-16-0212-2_11) contains supplementary material, which is available to authorized users.

C. Dhull (✉)
Eye Q Hospital, Rohtak, Haryana, India

S. K. Khokhar
Professor Ophthalmology, Dr. RP Centre for Ophthalmic Sciences, All India Institute of Medical Sciences, New Delhi, India

S. K. Khokhar, C. Dhull (eds.), *Essentials of Pediatric Cataract Surgery*,
https://doi.org/10.1007/978-981-16-0212-2_11

PFV [9, 10]. In the current literature, various animal models have been used to study the role of angiogenic and antiangiogenic factors [6, 11–13]. Vascular endothelial growth factor (VEGF) and placental growth factor (PGF) have been reported to have a regulatory role in involution of hyaloid vessels [13]. An association of PFV has been reported in p53-deficient and Bax/Bak proapoptotic Bcl-2-deficient mice [14]. This suggests a disturbance in proapoptotic, and antiapoptotic factors may have an influence in pathogenesis of PFV.

11.3 Clinical Presentation

PFV presents with a wide spectrum of presentation [15, 16] (Table 11.1). Anterior presentation may involve presence of pupillary membrane, Mittendorf dot, cataract, vessels over lens, enlarged ciliary processes, glaucoma, and/or retrolental membranes. Posterior presentation may contain Bergmeister papilla, stalk of PFV, falciform fold and/or retinal detachment. Combined variety, which contains the combination of the two, is the commonest presentation (Fig. 11.1).

Following are the important clinical presentation of PFV:

11.3.1 Anterior Presentation

11.3.1.1 Persistent Pupillary Membrane (PPM)

PPM is considered a mild presentation of anterior PFV where anterior TVL fails to regress. Most cases have a small PPM with no visual implications. In some cases, it may be vascularized and associated with other abnormalities such as anterior pyramidal cataract [17] or capsular plaque,

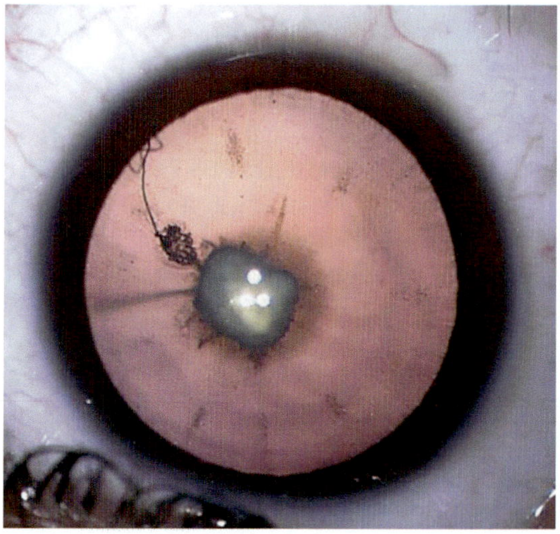

Fig. 11.1 Mixed variety of PFV with PPM, central cataract and stalk of PFV seen on the left

Table 11.1 Classification of PFV on the basis of clinical presentation [15, 16]

	Anterior PFV	Posterior PFV	Combined PFV
Clinical presentation	• Microphthalmia • Leucocoria • Shallow anterior chamber • Persistent pupillary membrane • Cataract • Elongated ciliary processes • Retrolental fibrovascular membrane • Intralenticular hemorrhage • Chronic inflammation • Glaucoma • Strabismus • Ectropion uvea • Coloboma Iridis	• Microphthalmia • Leucocoria • Mittendorf Dot • Vitreous membranes and stalk • Bergmeister papilla • Retinal fold • Tractional retinal detachment of posterior pole • Hypoplastic optic nerve • Dysplastic optic nerve • Pigment maculopathy • Hypoplastic macula • Clear lens • Strabismus	Clinical features from both anterior and posterior PFV

aniridia [17] or posterior stalk of PFV. If cataract is visually significant, surgery may be required.

In severe cases of PFV (Fig. 11.2), visual acuity may be affected. It can cause changes in the capsular curvature and lead to lenticular myopia. If visual acuity is significantly affected, surgery may be required. Lim et al. [18] reported surgical intervention in five eyes with PPM. They recommended the use of vitrectomy scissors instead of Vannas scissors for removal of PPM. After 22.6 months of follow up, no complication was reported, and visual acuity improved in 60% cases [18].

11.3.1.2 Cataract

PFV is considered one of the most important cause for unilateral cataract across the world, although it may cause bilateral cataract as well. The incidence of PFV in unilateral cataract varies. We detected PFV in 27.6% cases of unilateral cataract and it was the most common identifiable cause [19]. *Unilateral cataract* associated with ***microphthalmos*** should raise suspicion of PFV [20].

Morphology of cataract may vary from posterior capsular plaque, partially absorbed cataract or total cataract. Posterior capsular plaques have been hypothesized to develop from regressing hyaloid vasculature which may or may not be associated with stalk of PFV [21]. Posterior capsular plaque may be the remnant of the strong adhesions formed by capsule and hyaloid vessels which regress later [21]. Posterior lenticonus has also been hypothesized to have causal association with PFV [22].

Associated features of PFV should be looked for in all cases of unilateral cataract. Significant cataract associated with combined or anterior PFV requires surgical intervention [23]. Since surgical intervention is more difficult and requires additional instrumentation, timely clinical diagnosis is important.

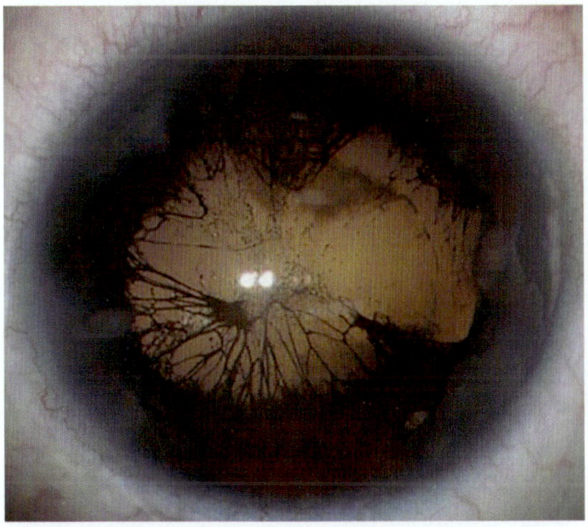

Fig. 11.2 PPM seen in association with minimal lamellar cataract

11.3.1.3 Enlarged Ciliary Processes

Prominent and elongated ciliary processes may be associated with cataractous lens or retrolental membrane. They may result from traction caused by contraction of the fibrovascular membrane. Prominent ciliary processes can be visualized following pupillary dilatation. They are considered a telltale sign of PFV (Fig. 11.3).

11.3.2 Posterior Presentation

11.3.2.1 Mittendorf Dot

This is also a mild presentation of PFV where there is near completer regression hyaloid artery, only a small white dot or cone is left on posterior capsule or just behind it. It is generally slightly nasal to the visual axis and is visually insignificant. It may be seen in 0.7–2% of the normal population [5, 23].

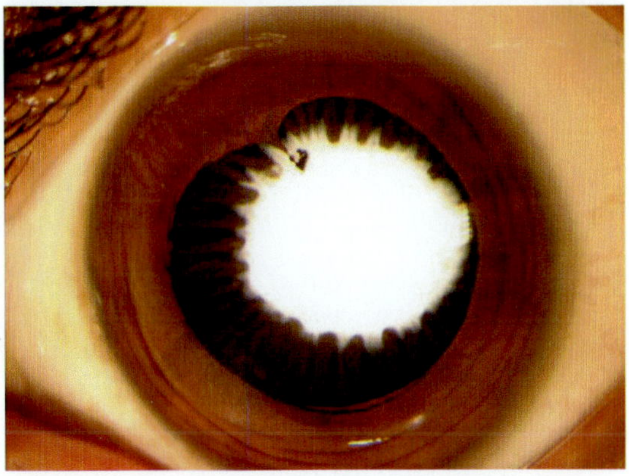

Fig. 11.3 Anterior variety of PFV with enlarged ciliary processes

11.3.2.2 Fibrovascular Membrane

Retrolental fibrovascular membrane has been described in literature as an important sign of PFV by Reese in 1955 [1]. It is considered the remnant of posterior TVL and may vary from small thin membrane to complete membrane covering posterior surface of the lens. The lens may be clear and this membrane may be the cause of leukocoria in children. This is not pathognomic of PFV and may be seen in retinopathy of prematurity or retinal detachment [24].

11.3.2.3 Persistent Hyaloid Artery

The fetal hyaloid artery lies within the Cloquet canal and regresses around the seventh month of gestation. If it persists, a stalk may be seen arising from the disc to behind the lens (Fig. 11.4).

11.3.2.4 Bergmeister Papilla

Refers to remnant of hyaloid artery to disc and can be seen as fibrovascular tuft at disc. It may be associated with other disc or macular abnormalities.

11.3.2.5 Tractional Detachment

PFV may be associated with congenital tent shaped detachment of retina where it may adhere to lens or ciliary body. If the detachment is severe, visual prognosis is poor.

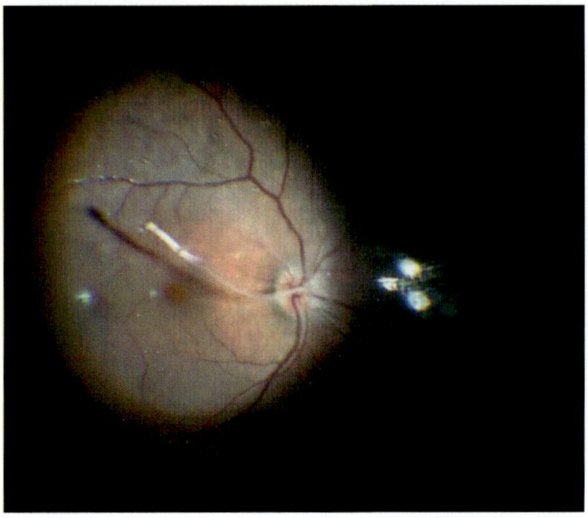

Fig. 11.4 Stalk of hyaloid artery remnant seen intraoperatively using wide angle viewing system

11.3.3 Associations

PFV may be associated with retinal folds, optic disc hypoplasia, macular hypoplasia, anterior segment dysgenesis, lens subluxation, ocular coloboma, etc. [25–30] These are relatively rare as compared to the other features of PFV. Systemic association include cleft palate and lip, polydactyly, and microcephaly [31]; and trisomy 13 [2].

11.3.4 Complications

PFV is associated with arrest in the normal of growth of eye ball and is usually associated with microphthalmia [15, 16]. Secondary glaucoma is a common sequalae to untreated PFV. This may be associated vitreous hemorrhage, hyphema, corneal edema and/or buphthalmos [32, 33]. These complications can occur suddenly and may result in eventual phthisis bulbi or painful blind eye. In the past, even in eyes with very poor prognosis, surgery has been recommended to avoid these complications [34].

11.4 Investigations

Diagnosis of PFV solely bases on clinical findings, may be challenging. A high suspicion of PFV should be kept in all cases with unilateral cataract. A differential diagnosis of leukocoria should be kept in mind when differentiating PFV from other entities (Table 11.2).

The following investigations are useful in confirming the diagnosis of PFV:

11.4.1 Ultrasonography (USG)

Ultrasonography needs to be performed in all cases of leukocoria where fundus is not visible. It is a noninvasive and inexpensive tool which can be useful in diagnosis of PFV. USG has been useful in diagnosis PFV and ruling out mass lesions such as retinoblastoma [35, 36]. Depending on the presentation, USG may show a thin stalk of remnant hyaloid vessel in the vitreous cavity between the disc and posterior lens capsule

Table 11.2 Differential diagnosis of leukocoria [15, 20, 23]

- Retinoblastoma
- Coat's disease
- Familial exudative vitreoretinopathy
- Retinopathy of prematurity
- Norrie's disease
- Ocular toxocariasis
- Retinal dysplasia
- Incontinentia pigmenti
- Uveitis
- Congenital cataract
- Fundal coloboma
- Juvenile xanthogranuloma
- Myelinated nerve fibers
- Endopthalmitis

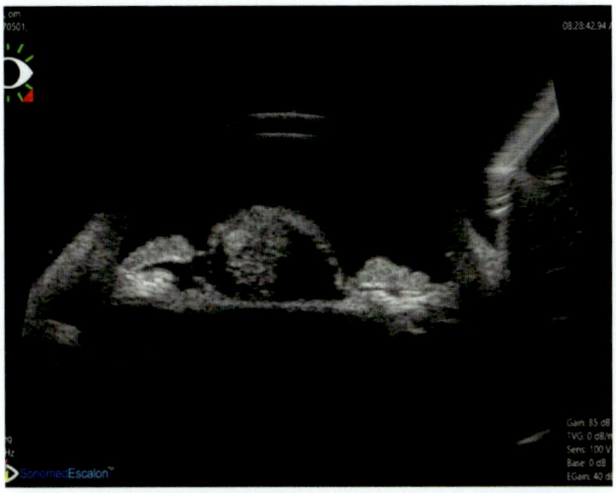

Fig. 11.6 UBM showing swollen anterior lens with posterior capsular plaque and enlarged and centrally displaced ciliary processes

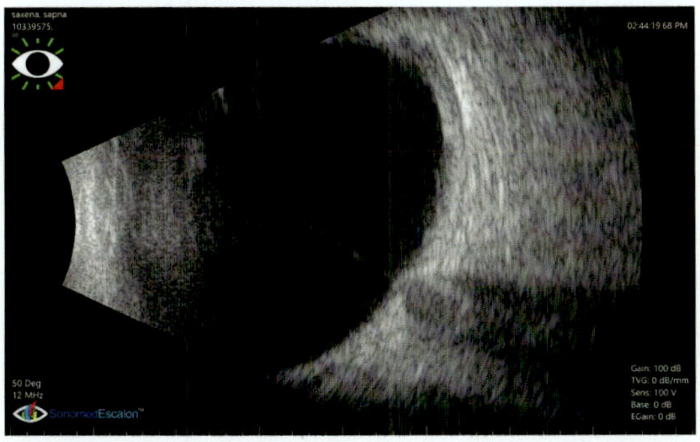

Fig. 11.5 USG picture showing hyperechoic stalk seen attached from disc to posterior surface of lens

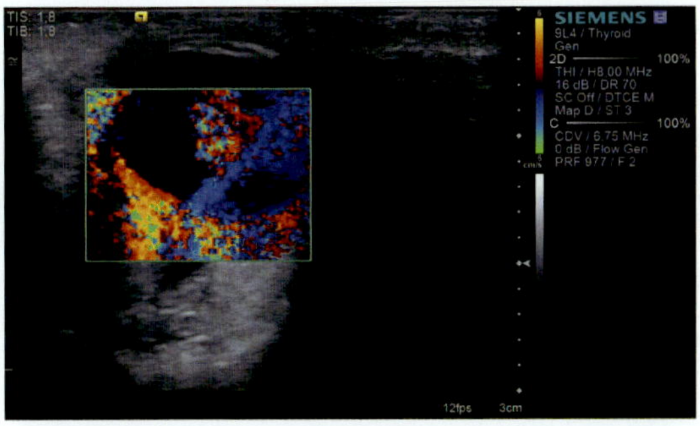

Fig. 11.7 Color Doppler of a 1 year old child suggestive of arterial blood flow in the stalk

(Fig. 11.5). USG may reveal presence or absence of retinal detachment. Although effective, sensitivity ranges from 70 to 80% [20].

11.4.2 Ultrasound Biomicroscopy (UBM)

UBM is particularly useful in cases of anterior presentation or combined presentation. Lens may be swollen or partially absorbed with prominent and enlarged ciliary processes (Fig. 11.6). In some cases, a stalk attached to posterior capsule may also be visible.

11.4.3 Color Doppler Imaging

It can detect a stalk of PFV based on the flow [37]. It can also differentiate between arterial or venous flow (Fig. 11.7). It is not useful in avascular cases or cases with no flow.

11.4.4 Magnetic Resonance Imaging (MRI)

MRI is considered highly sensitive and specific for diagnosis for PFV [38–40]. It is more expensive and may require anesthesia or sedation for the child to be performed accurately. Sensitivity is almost 100% (Fig. 11.8).

Computerized Tomography (CT scan) have also been reported as diagnostic tool [39]. It helps in ruling out more severe differential diagnosis such as retinoblastoma.

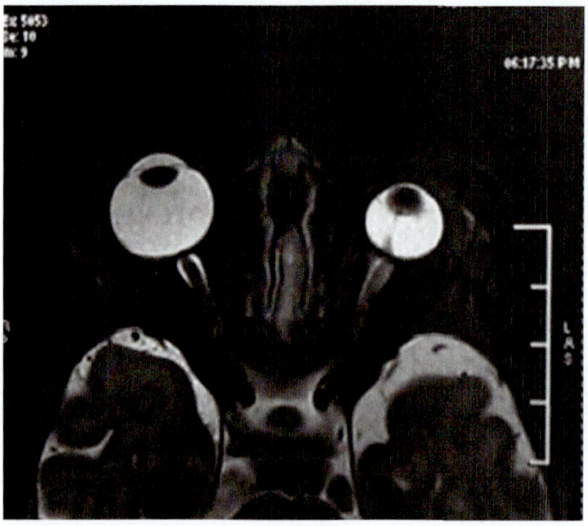

Fig. 11.8 T-2W image of MRI of a 3 month old baby showing left eye smaller in size with hypointense stalk attached from disc to lens confirm PFV

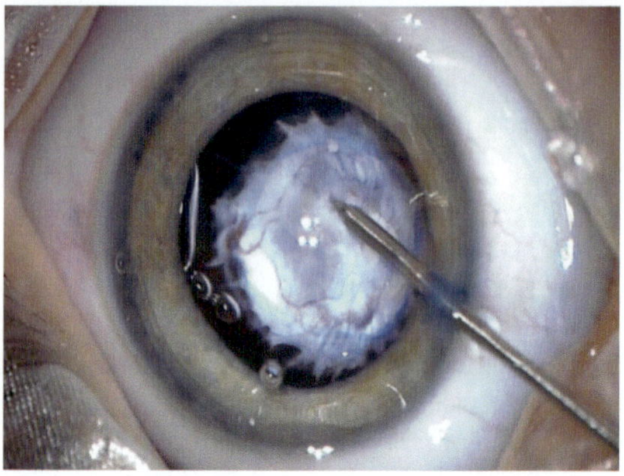

Fig. 11.9 Intraoperative image of anterior PFV where vessels are being cauterized using diathermy

11.5 Management

Historically, surgery was indicated to primarily avoid severe complications such as secondary glaucoma, buphthalmias, painful blind eye or phthisis bulbi with guarded to nil visual prognosis [1, 2, 31, 41, 42]. With time there have been advances in the surgical technique which has improved the anatomical and functional outcomes to a certain extent [43–46]. Surgery can be performed via anterior or posterior approach. Each has its merits and demerits.

11.5.1 Anterior Approach

Anterior approach has been commonly utilized by congenital cataract surgeon for management of PFV [31, 43]. It has certain advantages over posterior approach. IOL implantation can be performed with this method in the same surgery allowing better visual rehabilitation and cosmetic results [43]. This technique provides better visualization of small bleeders on the posterior capsule which can be tackled better. ***Salmon patch sign*** has been described to identify PFV in cases of posterior capsular plaque [47]. Intraoperatively, appearance pink hue on the plaque suggests leaking vessels, which can help in diagnosis of a previously missed PFV.

The principle of PFV surgery, in addition to providing clear media, is achieving *hemostasis*. In addition to the usual steps performed for congenital cataract surgery including lensectomy with anterior vitrectomy, additional steps are required to avoid intraoperative bleeding.

After making 2 MVR entry, 180° apart, ACCC and lens aspiration are performed as usual in cases with posterior capsular plaque. In absorbed cataract, there may be a vascularized membrane. Hemostasis is achieved by a variety of maneuvers before cutting the plaque or vascularized membrane. Heavy viscosity OVD is used and IOP is maintained/increased throughout surgery.

Additional instruments may be required to manage vascular component. **Diathermy** is an easily available instrument which can be used to coagulate the blood vessels (Fig. 11.9). Following this, a microincision scissors and forceps can be used for removal of plaque. Caution is required while cutting plaque as stalk of PFV may be present underneath. If stalk is present, it needs to be cauterized before cutting the anterior end. Following hemostasis, stalk is allowed to fall back and anterior vitrectomy can be performed.

Plasma knife or Fugo blade is an ingenious alternate to diathermy [48]. The plasma knife (Fugo blade) is a radiofrequency electrosurgical incising instrument that uses electromagnetic energy to perform cutting and provides non-cauterizing hemostasis called "autostasis" [48, 49]. The advantage of this technique is no heat production and minimal damage to adjacent tissue. Figure 11.10a–d shows the steps of surgery where after lensectomy, vascular stalk is visible. The posterior capsular plaque with attached stalk is cut using plasma knife (Fugo blade) avoiding inadvertent bleed. Afterward, the stalk is cut with microincision forceps. We can see finally we are left with intact rim of sulcus for placement of IOL.

11.5.2 Posterior Approach

It is commonly employed by retinal surgeons. The advantage of this technique is if associated vitreous hemorrhage, vitreous membranes, retinal folds or retinal detachment is present, it can

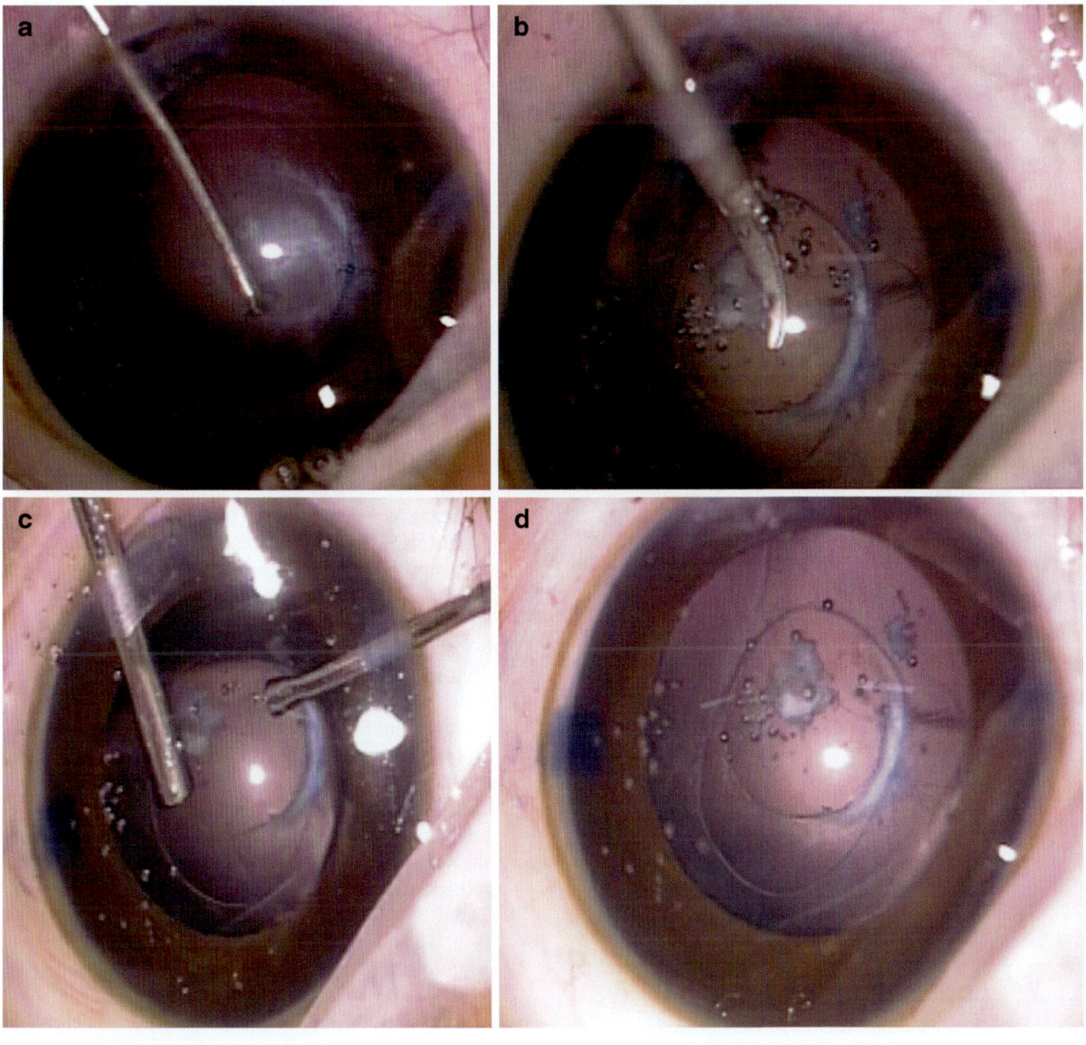

Fig. 11.10 (**a**) Fugo blade is used to cut the posterior capsule along with PFV stalk. (**b**) After hemostasis, stalk is cut with microincision forceps. (**c**) Stalk seen falling back. (**d**) After anterior vitrectomy, rim of sulcus is intact, IOL can be placed

be managed simultaneously. The disadvantage includes reduced feasibility for IOL implantation and requirement of vitreoretinal setup.

Two pars plana ports are made and lensectomy is performed starting from a stab in the posterior capsule. Following lensectomy, opening can be made of adequate size in anterior and posterior capsule. If bleeders are encountered, diathermy can be performed [50]. If thick plaque or membranes are encountered, intravitreal scissors can be used to cut the membranes [50]. A third port for illumination can be placed for associated retinal pathology. Prognosis is usually poor in cases of extensive retinal abnormalities.

11.6 Prognosis

Favorable outcomes may be achieved in children with PFV by early intervention followed by aggressive amblyopic treatment [43–46, 51]. Hunt et al. [34] found visual acuity of 6/60 or better in 18% of eyes with PFV in a long-term follow-up. Early surgery before 77 day was identified as good prognostic marker. Anteby et al. [43] found visual acuity of 20/200 (6/60) or better in 25% of the eyes. They implanted IOL in 30 eyes for better visual rehabilitation and found visual acuity of 20/50 or better in 20% and 20/200 or better in 33.3% eyes. Sisk et al. [52] found posterior manifestations of PFV, bilaterality, and microphthalmos were associated with poorer visual outcomes. They also compared the outcomes of limbal and pars plana approach and found similar visual and anatomical outcomes.

Outcomes remain inferior compared to other children with unilateral cataract without PFV. It may be due to higher percentage of complications including glaucoma, visual axis opacification, vitreous hemorrhage, and retinal detachment [43, 44, 53, 54].

11.7 Conclusion

PFV is a congenital anomaly caused by partial or complete failure of fetal vasculature to regress. It commonly presents as unilateral cataract. It has anterior, posterior or combined presentation. Diagnosis using clinical findings and USG (MRI if needed and available) is important as surgical approach is different than normal congenital cataract. Vascular hemostasis is required throughout surgery, diathermy, or plasma blade can be used for the same. Despite best efforts, visual outcomes remain lower than most pediatric cataracts. Nevertheless, a good surgical technique followed by refractive correction and amblyopia therapy provides hope for useful visual and cosmetic outcome.

References

1. Reese AB. Persistent hyperplastic primary vitreous. Am J Ophthalmol. 1955;40:317–31.
2. Goldberg M. Persistent fetal vasculature (PFV): an integrated interpretation of signs and symptoms associated with persistent hyperplastic primary vitreous (PHPV). LIV Edward Jackson Memorial Lecture. Am J Ophthalmol. 1997;124:587–626.
3. Cloquet, J. Mémoire sur la membrane pupillaire, et sur la formation du petit cercle artérial de l'iris. Paris, 1818. Cited by: Gulati N, Eagle RC Jr, Tasman W. Unoperated eyes with persistent fetal vasculature. Trans Am Ophthalmol Soc. 2003;101:59–64; discussion, 64–65.
4. Sanghvi DA, Sanghvi CA, Purandare NC. Bilateral persistent hyperplastic primary vitreous. Australas Radiol. 2005;49:72–4.
5. Wright KW. Embryology. In: Cook CS, Sulik KK, Wright KW, editors. Pediatric ophthalmology and strabismus. St. Louis: Mosby; 1995. p. 1–43.
6. Balazs EA, Toth LZ, Ozanics V. Cytological studies on the developing vitreous as related to the hyaloid vessel system. Albrecht Von Graefes Arch Klin Exp Ophthalmol. 1980;213(2):71–85.
7. Mullner-Eidenbock A, Amon M, Moser E, Klebermass N. Persistent fetal vasculature and minimal fetal remnants: a frequent cause of unilateral congenital cataracts. Ophthalmology. 2004;111:906–13.
8. Khaliq S, Hameed A, Ismail M, et al. Locus for autosomal recessive nonsyndromic persistent hyperplastic primary vitreous. Invest Ophthalmol Vis Sci. 2001;42:2225–8.
9. Grahn BH, Storey ES, McMillan C. Inherited retinal dysplasia and persistent hyperplastic primary vitreous in miniature Schnauzer dogs. Vet Ophthalmol. 2004;7:151–8.
10. Allgoewer I, Pfefferkorn B. Persistent hyperplastic tunica vasculosa lentis and persistent hyperplastic primary vitreous (PHTVL/PHPV) in two cats. Vet Ophthalmol. 2001;4:161–4.

11. Khokhar S, Dhull C. Commentary: understanding angiogenic factors in pathogenesis of persistent fetal vasculature. Indian J Ophthalmol. 2019;67:1622–3.
12. Gajjar DU, Vasavada AR, Patel P, Praveen MR, Shah SR. Evaluation of collagen derived antiangiogenic factors and matrix metalloproteinases in anterior lens epithelial cells of pediatric eyes with persistent fetal vasculature. Indian J Ophthalmol. 2019;67:1618–22.
13. Feeney SA, Simpson DA, Gardiner TA, Boyle C, Jamison P, Stitt AW. Role of vascular endothelial growth factor and placental growth factors during retinal vascular development and hyaloid regression. Invest Ophthalmol Vis Sci. 2003;44:839–47.
14. Hahn P, Lindsten T, Tolentino M, Thompson CB, Bennett J, Dunaief JL. Persistent fetal ocular vasculature in mice deficient in bax and bak. Arch Ophthalmol. 2005;123:797–802.
15. Pollard ZF. Persistent hyperplastic primary vitreous: diagnosis, treatment and results. Trans Am Ophthalmol Soc. 1997;95:487–549.
16. Saint-Geniex M, D'Amore P. Development and pathology of the hyaloid, choroidal and retinal vasculature. Int J Dev Biol. 2004;48:1045–58.
17. Khokhar S, Sinha G, Sharma R, Patil B, Mahabir M, Nayak B. Anterior pyramidal cataract: a rare association. JAMA Ophthalmol. 2015;133(4):e144626. https://doi.org/10.1001/jamaophthalmol.2014.4626.
18. Lim KH, Yu YS. Surgical management for persistent pupillary membrane with vitreous scissors. Korean J Ophthalmol. 1996;10(2):124–6. https://doi.org/10.3341/kjo.1996.10.2.124.
19. Khokhar S, Jose CP, Sihota R, Midha N. Unilateral congenital cataract: clinical profile and presentation. J Pediatr Ophthalmol Strabismus. 2018;55(2):107–12. https://doi.org/10.3928/01913913-20170703-11.
20. Khokhar SK, Pillay G, Dhull C, Agarwal E, Mahabir M, Aggarwal P. Pediatric cataract. Indian J Ophthalmol. 2017;65(12):1340–9. https://doi.org/10.4103/ijo.IJO_1023_17.
21. Mullner-Eidenbock A, Amon M, Moser E, et al. Persistent fetal vasculature and minimal fetal remnants: a frequent cause of unilateral congenital cataracts. Ophthalmology. 2004;111:906–13.
22. Khokhar S, Dhull C, Mahalingam K, Agarwal P. Posterior lenticonus with persistent fetal vasculature. Indian J Ophthalmol. 2018;66(9):1335–6. https://doi.org/10.4103/ijo.IJO_276_18.
23. Wilson E, Trivedi R. Pediatric cataract surgery: techniques, complications and management. Wolters Kluwer Health. 2014;34:226–32.
24. Appelbaum A. Retrolental fibroplasia; blindness in infants of low weight at birth. Calif Med. 1952;77(4):259–65.
25. Khokhar S, Takkar B, Pillay G, Venkatesh P. Three cases of associated persistent fetal vasculature and ocular coloboma: posterior segment dysgenesis. J Pediatr Ophthalmol Strabismus. 2017;54:e77–80. https://doi.org/10.3928/01913913-20170907-06.
26. Lasky JB, Sandu M, Balashanmugan A. PHACE syndrome: association with persistent fetal vasculature and coloboma–like iris defect. J AAPOS. 2004;8(5):495–8. https://doi.org/10.1016/S1091853104001272.
27. Khokhar S, Gupta Y, Raj N, Vardhan Azad S, Kashyap S, Dhull C. Persistent fetal vasculature with subluxated lens, posterior segment pathology, and bifid fibrous membrane: an atypical presentation. J Pediatr Ophthalmol Strabismus. 2020;57:e38–40. https://doi.org/10.3928/01913913-20200512-02. Published 2020 Jun 23.
28. Cennamo G, Liguori G, Pezone A, et al. Morning glory syndrome associated with marked persistent hyperplastic primary vitreous and lens coloboma. Br J Ophthalmol. 1989;73:684–6.
29. Matsubara A, Ozeki H, Matsunaga N, et al. Histopathological examination of two cases of anterior staphyloma associated with Peters' anomaly and persistent hyperplastic vitreous. Br J Ophthalmol. 2001;85:1421–5.
30. Khokhar S, Gupta S, Arora T, Gogia V, Dada T. Unilateral persistent fetal vasculature coexisting with anterior segment dysgenesis. Int Ophthalmol. 2013;33(4):399–401. https://doi.org/10.1007/s10792-013-9757-z.
31. Haddad R, Font RL, Reeser F. Persistent hyperplastic primary vitreous. A clinicopathologic study of 62 cases and review of the literature. Surv Ophthalmol. 1978;23:123–34.
32. Alward WL, Krasnow MA, Keech RV, et al. Persistent hyperplastic primary vitreous with glaucoma presenting in infancy. Arch Ophthalmol. 1991;109:1063–4.
33. Wieckowska A, Napierala A, Pytlarz E, et al. Persistent hyperplastic primary vitreous—diagnosis and differentiation [in Polish]. Klin Ocz. 1995;97:234–8.
34. Hunt A, Rowe N, Lam A, Martin F. Outcomes in persistent hyperplastic primary vitreous. Br J Ophthalmol. 2005;89(7):859–63. https://doi.org/10.1136/bjo.2004.053595.
35. MacKeen LD, Nischal KK, Lam WC, et al. High-frequency ultrasonography findings in persistent hyperplastic primary vitreous. J AAPOS. 2000;4:217–24.
36. Frazier Byrne S, Green RL. Intraocular tumors. In: Fraziet Byrne S, Green RL, editors. Ultrasound of the eye and orbit. St. Louis: Mosby; 1992. p. 201–4.
37. Hu A, Pei X, Ding X, et al. Combined persistent fetal vasculature: a classification based on high-resolution B-mode ultrasound and color doppler imaging. Ophthalmology. 2016;123(1):19–25. https://doi.org/10.1016/j.ophtha.2015.09.001.
38. Jain TP. Bilateral persistent hyperplastic primary vitreous. Indian J Ophthalmol. 2009;57(1):53–4. https://doi.org/10.4103/0301-4738.44487.
39. Mafee MF, Goldberg MF. Persistent hyperplastic primary vitreous (PHPV): role of computed tomography and magnetic resonance. Radiol Clin N Am. 1987;25:683–92.
40. Potter PD, Shields CL, Shields JA, et al. The role of magnetic resonance imaging in children with intraocular tumors and simulating lesions. Ophthalmology. 1996;103:1774–83.

41. Jensen OA. Persistent hyperplastic primary vitreous. Cases in Denmark. Acta Ophthalmol (Copenh). 1968;46:418–29.
42. Olsen J, Moller PM. Persistent primary hyperplastic vitreous. Acta Ophthalmol. 1968;46:412–7.
43. Anteby I, Cohen E, Karshai I, et al. Unilateral persistent hyperplastic primary vitreous: course and outcome. J AAPOS. 2002;6:92–9.
44. Alexandrakis G, Scott IU, Flynn HW Jr, et al. Visual acuity outcomes with and without surgery in patients with persistent fetal vasculature. Ophthalmology. 2000;107:1068–72.
45. Dass AB, Trese MT. Surgical results of persistent hyperplastic primary vitreous. Ophthalmology. 1999;106:280–4.
46. Mittra RA, Huynh LT, Ruttum MS, et al. Visual outcomes following lensectomy and vitrectomy for combined anterior and posterior persistent hyperplastic primary vitreous. Arch Ophthalmol. 1998;116:1190–4.
47. Khokhar S, Gupta S, Gogia V, Nayak B. Salmon pink patch sign: Diagnosing persistent fetal vasculature. Oman J Ophthalmol. 2016;9(1):68–9.
48. Khokhar S, Tejwani LK, Kumar G, Kushmesh R. Approach to cataract with persistent hyperplastic primary vitreous. J Cataract Refract Surg. 2011;37:1382–5.
49. Fugo RJ, Delcampo DM. The Fugo Blade: the next step after capsulorhexis. Ann Ophthalmol. 2001;33:13–20.
50. Paysse EA, McCreery KM, Coats DK. Surgical management of the lens and retrolental fibrotic membranes associated with persistent fetal vasculature. J Cataract Refract Surg. 2002;28:816–20.
51. Lambert SR, Buckley EG, Drews-Botsch C, et al. A randomized clinical trial comparing contact lens with intraocular lens correction of monocular aphakia during infancy: grating acuity and adverse events at age 1 year. Arch Ophthalmol. 2010;128:810–8.
52. Sisk RA, Berrocal AM, Feuer WJ, Murray TG. Visual and anatomic outcomes with or without surgery in persistent fetal vasculature. Ophthalmology. 2010;117(11):2178–83.e832. https://doi.org/10.1016/j.ophtha.2010.03.062.
53. BenEzra D. The surgical approaches to pediatric cataract. Eur J Implant Refract Surg. 1990;2:241–4.
54. BenEzra D, Cohen E. Posterior capsulectomy in pediatric cataract surgery: the necessity of a choice. Ophthalmology. 1997;104:2168–74.

12 Pediatric Traumatic Cataract

Mehul A. Shah and Shreya M. Shah

12.1 Introduction

Trauma is a cause of monocular blindness in the developed world, although few studies have addressed the problem of trauma in rural areas. The etiology of ocular injury likely differs from that in urban areas and is worthy of investigation. Any prevention strategy requires knowledge of the cause of injury, which may enable more appropriate targeting of resources toward preventing such injuries [1, 2]. Both eye trauma victims and society bear a large, potentially preventable burden, as ocular injury in children has a poor prognosis [3, 4]. After introduction of BETTS traumatic blindness understood well [5].

Children are highly vulnerable to ocular injury, especially sports-related ocular injury Traumatic cataracts can be an immediate, early, or late sequel of any ocular trauma. Management of traumatic cataract remains a challenge, in part because each case is unique. Surgical techniques need to be customized case by case based on associated ocular injuries. Pediatric cataract surgery is challenging and a traumatic etiology simply adds mere challenges. Such surgery in children should draw from both the principles of pediatric nontraumatic cataract removal techniques and the advancements in adult traumatic cataract removal techniques. Optimum timing of cataract surgery (duration between development of cataract and removal of cataract) is debatable. The timing of lens removal surgery is important in children—not only to achieve better anatomical outcome but also to achieve better visual outcome. Surgery too early may result in excessive postoperative inflammation and many cell deposits on the intraocular lens (IOL). Surgery too late may result in deprivational amblyopia [6–8].

12.2 Epidemiology

Cataract formation after traumatic injury is a common cause of ocular morbidity and visual loss. While no segment of society escapes the risk of eye injury, the victims primarily at risk are the young (median age 9.7 years). The majority of all eye injuries occur in persons under 30 years of age (57%).The toll of injury in terms of human suffering, as well as long-term disabilities, loss of productivity, and economic impact, can only be imagined [9–11].

Shah et al. reported has reported to be responsible for up to 29% of all childhood cataracts. At the Drashti Netralaya, our database includes 671 eyes with traumatic cataract in children (ophthalmology, wjo). Boys are more frequently affected

Supplementary Information The online version of this chapter (https://doi.org/10.1007/978-981-16-0212-2_12) contains supplementary material, which is available to authorized users.

M. A. Shah (✉) · S. M. Shah
Drashti Netralaya, Dahod, Gujarat, India

S. K. Khokhar, C. Dhull (eds.), *Essentials of Pediatric Cataract Surgery*,
https://doi.org/10.1007/978-981-16-0212-2_12

than girls (66% versus 35%). The majority of traumatic cataract cases occur in children while playing or when they are involved in sport-related activities. Commonly implicated objects include knives, BB guns, firecrackers, sticks thorns, rocks, pencils, arrows, wooden sticks, thorns and toys. Prevention of eye injuries is of utmost importance and is the team responsibility of parents, teachers, coaches, ophthalmologists, pediatricians, and optometrists. The American Academy of Pediatrics and the American Academy of Ophthalmology published a statement recommending types of protective lenses and frames for specific sports [4, 12, 13].

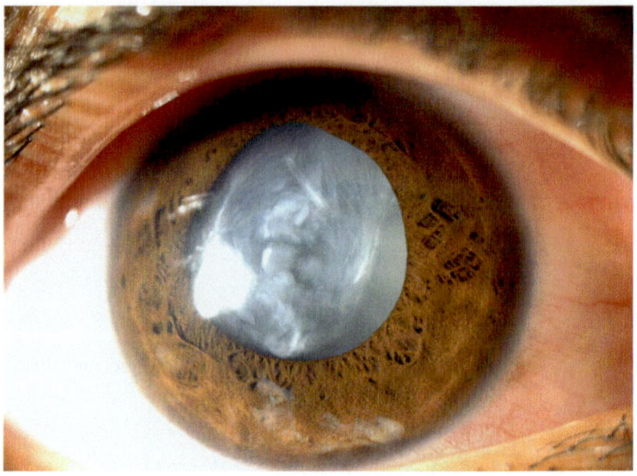

Fig. 12.2 Penetrating injury cap rupture

12.3 Pathophysiology

1. Blunt trauma is responsible for coup and countercoup ocular injury. Coup is the mechanism of direct impact. It is responsible for the Vossius ring (Fig. 12.1) (imprinted iris pigment) sometimes found on the anterior lens capsule following blunt injury. Countercoup refers to distant injury caused by Shockwaves traveling along the line of concussion. When the anterior surface of the eye is struck bluntly, there is a rapid anterior posterior shortening accompanied by equatorial expansion. This equatorial stretching can disrupt the lens capsule, zonules, or both. Combinations of coup, countercoup and equatorial expansion are responsible for the formation of traumatic cataract following blunt ocular injury.
2. Penetrating trauma that directly compromises the lens capsule often leads to cortical opacification at the site of injury. If the rent is sufficiently large, the entire lens rapidly opacifies (Fig. 12.2) When the capsular rent is small, however, the capsule may seal and the cortical cataract may remain localized.

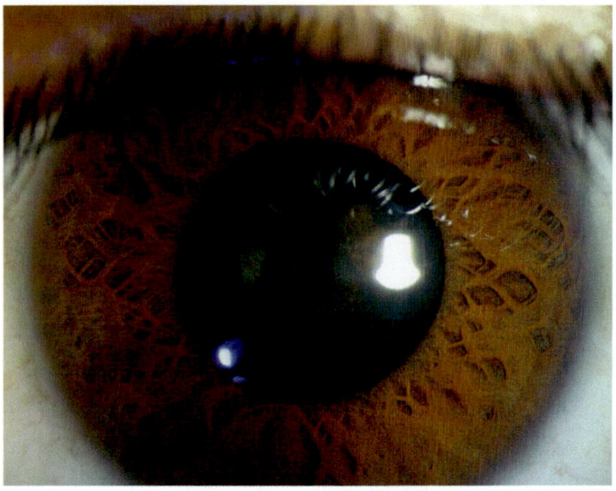

Fig. 12.1 Vossius ring because of blunt trauma and impression on lens (picture credits Dr Sudarshan Khokhar)

12.3.1 Preoperative Evaluation

12.3.1.1 Morphological Consideration

In the setting of traumatic cataract, the ophthalmologist must first "take a step back" and examine other ocular injuries in detail. The surgeon doing cataract surgery should be suspicious of injury to other ocular structures. Management depends on the degree and type of injury. Localized traumatic cataracts (especially if not in the visual axis) may be managed conservatively, while more significant lens opacities generally require cataract extraction. Similarly, capsular perforation may be managed with observation if small and not centrally located. Frequently, such injuries will develop only very localized opacification of the underlying cortex without progression to generalized cataract. Morphology of traumatic cataract may be classified into soft cataract with ruptured anterior capsule (Fig. 12.3a–c), Total cataract

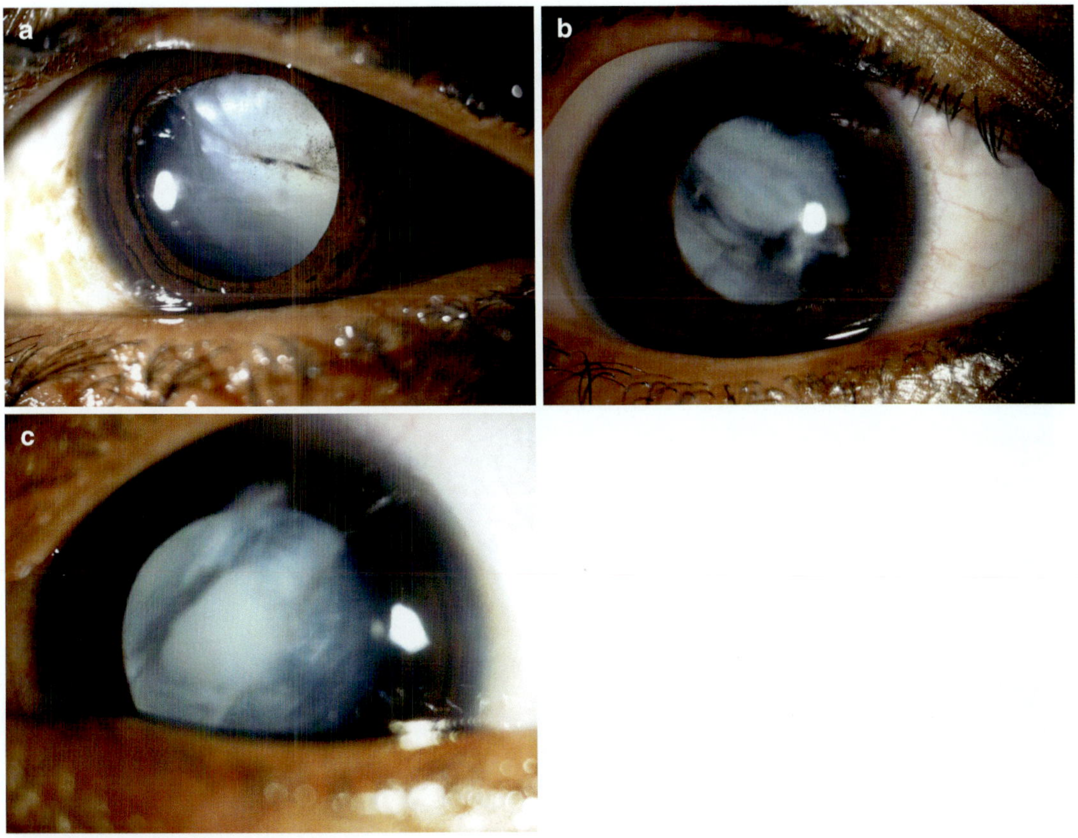

Fig. 12.3 (**a**) Soft cataract-1. (**b**) Soft cataract-2. (**c**) Soft cataract-3

(Fig. 12.4a–c), Membranous cataract with fusion of anterior and posterior capsule (Fig. 12.5a–c), and Rossette cataract (Fig. 12.6a–c). Surgical technique may be decided by the same [9]. Special type of morphology is also to be considered (Figs. 12.7, 12.8, and 12.9).

The initial patient evaluation is one of the most important critical steps in the management of any traumatic cataract. Data gathered during this examination, to a large extent, direct further investigations and establish immediate priorities. One of the most important aspects of this first examination is the description of the exact circumstances of the injury. This facilitates the development of risk estimates for occult injuries, such as intraocular foreign body (IOFB), chemical exposure, and posterior rupture of the globe (Fig. 12.10).

12.3.2 Examination

Before Dilation

1. Best-corrected visual acuity (BCVA).
2. Fixation preference.
3. Pupillary reflex: Presence of afferent pupillary defect may be indicative of traumatic optic neuropathy.
4. Intraocular pressure (if there is no evidence of ocular rupture).
5. Iris: Multiple small ruptures of the pupillary sphincters are common and result in a permanent traumatic mydriasis (Fig. 12.10). The clinical evaluation should also including a careful predilatation examination of the iris form trans-illumination defects. If present, it should be documented and following dilatation, the underlying lens surface should also

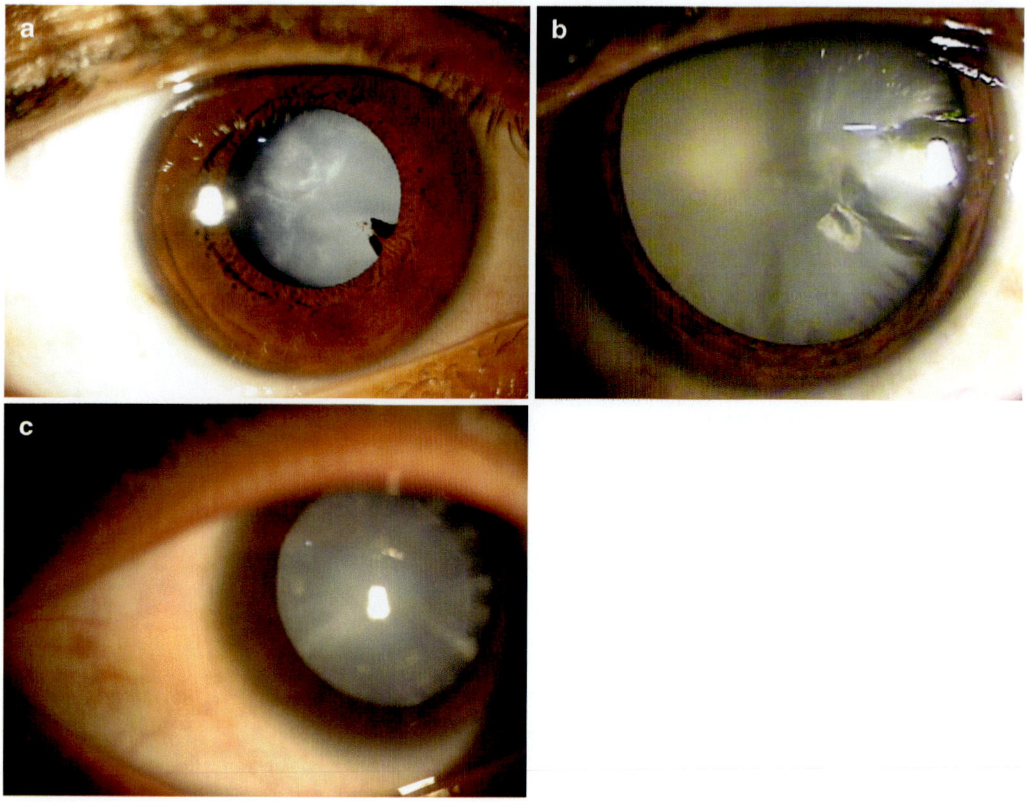

Fig. 12.4 (**a**) Total cataract-1. (**b**) Total cataract-2. (**c**) Total cataract-3

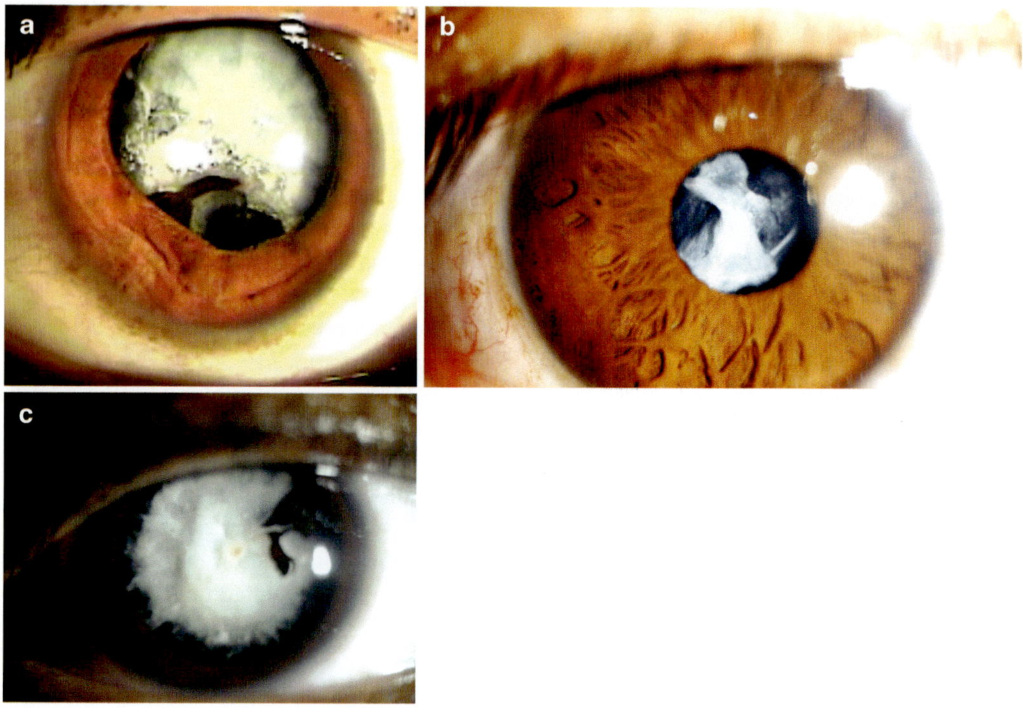

Fig. 12.5 (**a**) Membranous cataract-1. (**b**) Membranous cataract-2

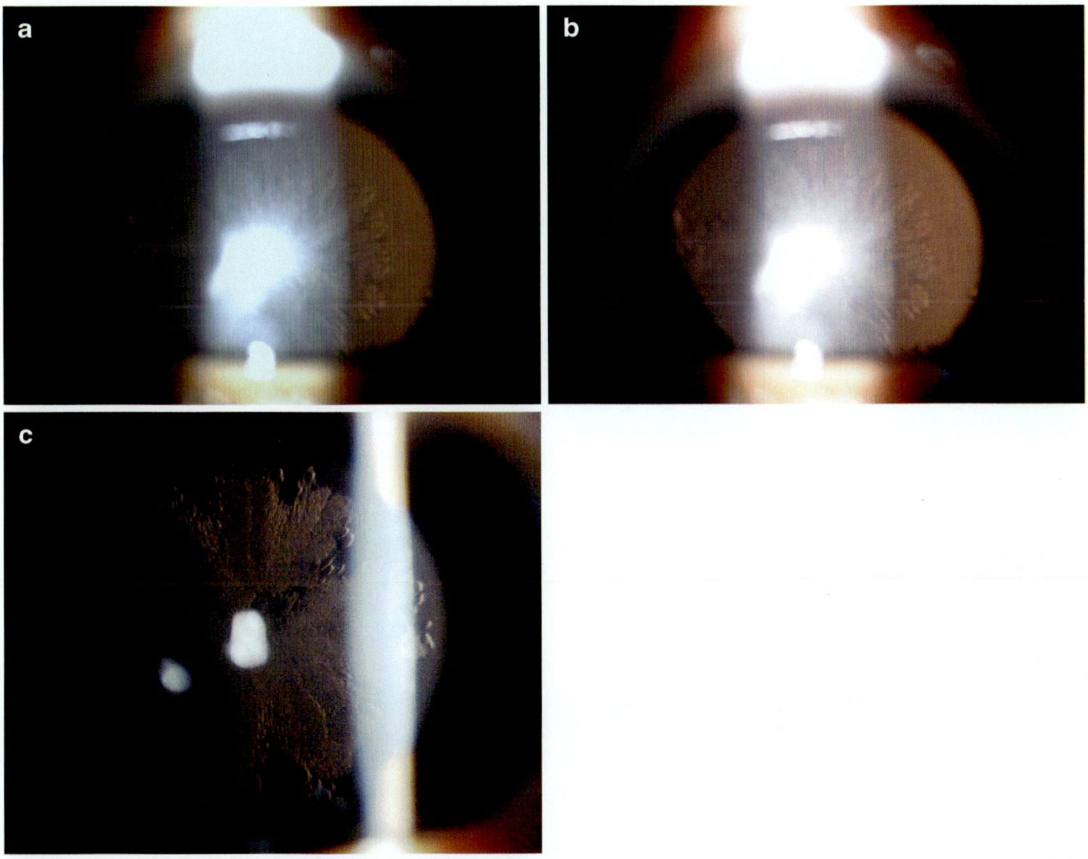

Fig. 12.6 (**a**) Rossette cataract-1. (**b**) Rossette cataract-2, Rossette cataract-3

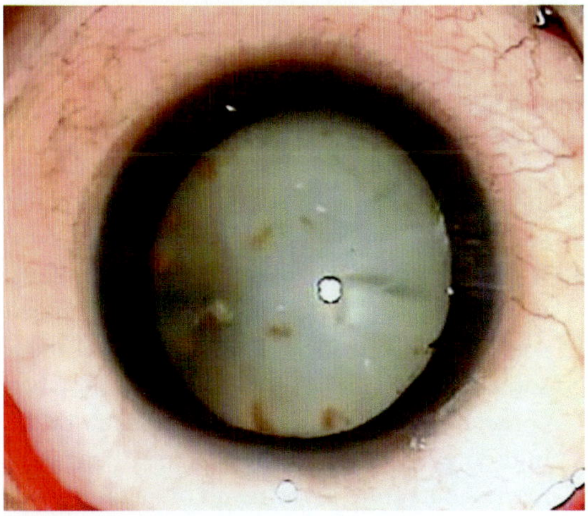

Fig. 12.7 Siderosis bulbi

be inspected for anterior capsular defect that indicate a penetrating injury or IOFB.

6. Zonules: Although detect on of zonular loss is not always possible prior to pupil dilation, suggestive findings include phacodonesis, an increase in myopic refractive error, abnormal peripheral lens curvature in one or more quadrants, an abnormal light reflex on retinoscopy, a visible lens equator, or vitreous in the anterior chamber (Fig. 12.11).

After Dilation

1. Slitlamp examination (after pupillary dilation) is recommended if feasible. This helps identify and document the type of cataract, the position and stability of the lens, integrity of the lens capsule and the overall status of the anterior segment. When slitlamp examination is not possible in the awake state, it can be done using a portable instrument in the oper-

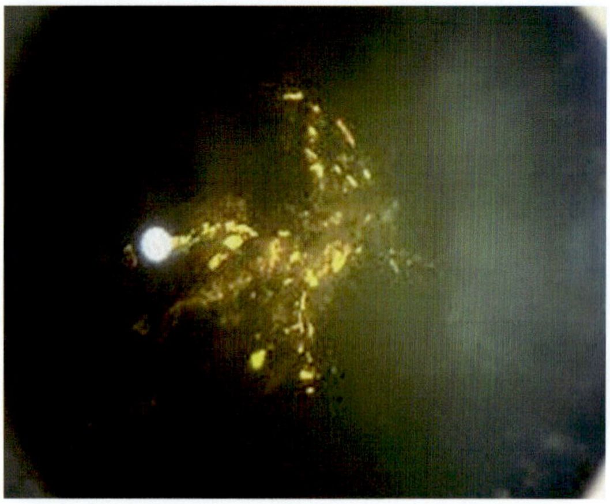

Fig. 12.8 Chalcosis lentis

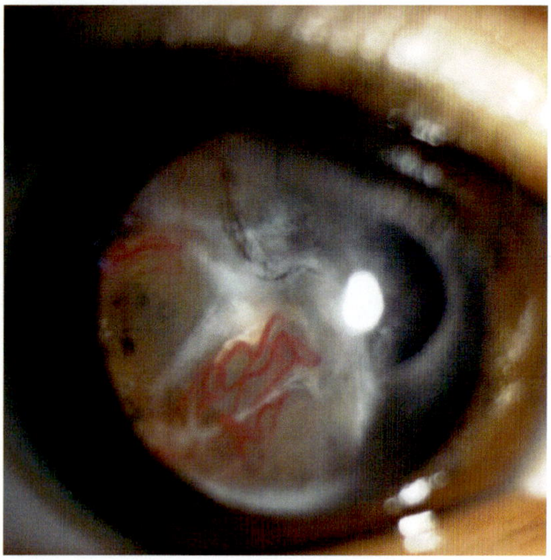

Fig. 12.9 Traumatic cataract following penetrating injury resulting in vascularized pupillary membrane

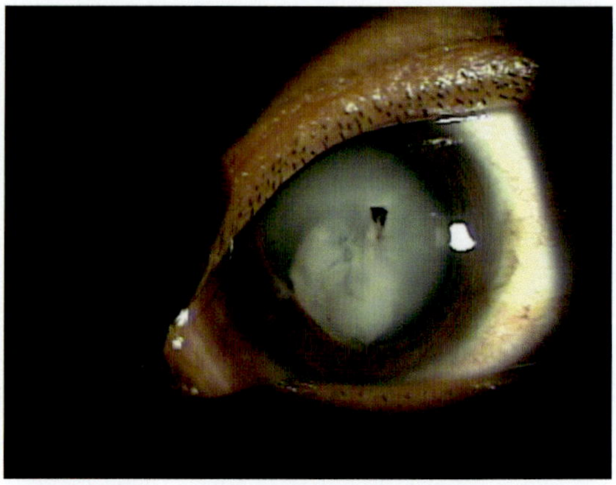

Fig. 12.10 Intra lenticular foreign body

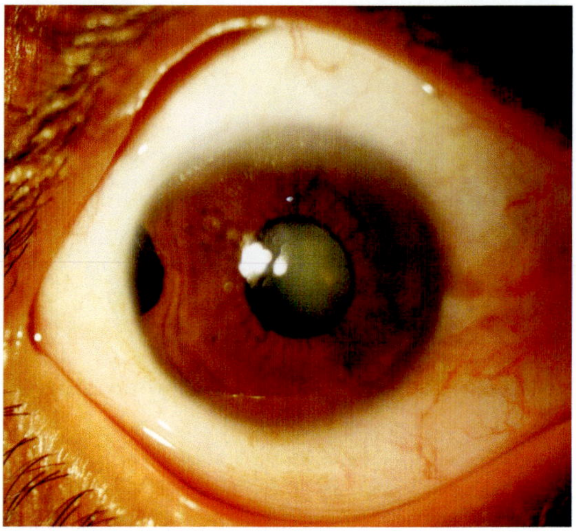

Fig. 12.11 Iridodialyses

ating room in conjunction with the examination using the operating microscope.

2. A posterior segment examination, including examination of the retinal periphery, should be carried out in detail if the view through the lens allows. Posterior segment examination is to be done using indirect ophthalmoscopy if media is opaque. B-scan is essential for evaluation.
3. Gonioscopy may be helpful to evaluate the angle structures and for recognizing vitreous at the lens equator or areas of loss of zonular support.
4. If planning for IOL implantation, keratometry using hand held keratometer and A-scan ultrasound or optical for globe axial length measurement should be attempted. Even when corneal scarring is present, keratometry of the injured eye should be attempted. Changes in corneal curvature as the result of an injury will change the IOL power needed to achieve the refractive goal. At times the keratometry readings of the fellow eye need to be used but this will further compromise the accuracy of the

postoperative refraction in relation to the postoperative goal.

A guarded prognosis for anatomical and functional outcome is to be thoroughly explained to the patient and patient's relatives. The full extent of the eye injuries are not always known prior to cataract surgery. It is also important to explain about the possible need for additional surgeries depending on the type of injury (retinal detachment, keratoplasty for dense corneal scar obstructing visual axis, etc.).

Documentation: During the examination, data should be entered in format designed by the International Society of Ocular Trauma (initial and follow-up forms) [14].

Ocular trauma score is calculated for each eye and visual outcome is compared with predicted value. Pediatric Ocular Trauma Score is other predictive model specifically designed for consideration of amblyopia [7, 8, 15–20].

12.3.3 Timing of Surgery

The timing of traumatic cataract surgery in children is important. Some authors have reported cataract surgery at the time of primary repair. While the development of amblyopia in children necessitates prompt removal of a cataract when it develops, cataract surgery is not necessarily required at the time of initial repair even when anterior capsular rupture is present. Cataract surgery can be deferred while the inflammatory response is treated with topical steroids. Advantages of secondary cataract removal are better visibility, better IOL power calculation, anterior segment reconstruction, and stabilization of a hemato-ocular barrier. Shah et al. reported visual outcome is significantly better in case of traumatic cataract if intervention done between 2 and 4 weeks of injury [11].

All patients with injuries and without an infection were treated with topical and systemic corticosteroids and cycloplegics. The duration of medical treatment depended on the degree of inflammation in the anterior and posterior segments of the operated eye. The operated patients were re-examined after 24 h, 3 days, and 1, 2, and 6 weeks to enable refractive correction. Follow-up was scheduled for day 3, weekly for 6 weeks, monthly for 3 months, and every 3 months for 1 year.

At every follow-up examination, visual acuity was tested according to age using the AAO guidelines. The anterior segment was examined with a slit lamp and the posterior segment with an indirect ophthalmoscope.

12.3.4 Surgical Details

General principles of pediatric cataract surgery should be followed. Specific differences have been described herein.

- Anesthesia: In anticipation of difficult surgery, general anesthesia is preferable even in older children who might otherwise be cooperative for local anesthesia. Combination of general and regional anesthesia is very useful technique [21].
- Morphological consideration may be considered for surgical technique, soft cataract may be removed by unimanual or bimanual aspiration. Membranous cataract may be dealt with pars plana lensectomy.
- Anterior capsule management: Performing the capsulorhexis may be difficult in pediatric traumatic cataract. Besides higher elasticity of pediatric anterior capsule, traumatic cataracts are often associated with ruptured anterior lens capsule or fibrosis of the anterior capsule.
  - Preexisting opening may be used for cortical clean up.
  - Long-standing thick capsule may be removed using wannas' scissors or vitrectomy hand piece. Synechiolysis may be done if required.
  - Small opening preexisting may be converted in capsulorhexis using 23 G forceps.

- Posterior capsule and vitreous management: Management of the posterior capsule depends on the age of the patient and the status of the posterior capsule (intact v/s torn) [8, 15, 22].
  - In young patients with complex trauma, after lens insertion primary posterior capsulotomy and vitrectomy using pars plana approach may be used.
  - Staged approach (leaving behind intact posterior capsule at the time of initial cataract surgery and planning a same sitting or secondary surgery to remove the center of the posterior capsule after the 10 L is properly fixed into the lens capsule) may help proper placement of the IOL. This staged approach may not be necessary for the surgeon who operates on children frequently. However, it may be better for surgeons unaccustomed to operating on children. Posterior capsule opacification occurs quickly in most cases of complex traumatic cataract surgery. Therefore, prepare the family that the best vision will likely come after this planned second surgery. Repair of iris defects or other more elective surgical maneuvers can also be done during this secondary procedure, which is often done 4–8 weeks after the initial cataract removal.
  - In case of posterior capsular defect vitrectomy performed using existing opening and anterior vitreous with blood debris and pigments should be removed using vitrector either before or after lens insertion.

12.3.5 The Surgical Technique

The surgical technique was selected according to morphology and the condition of tissues other than the lens. Phacoemulsification may be used to operate on cataracts with hard, large nuclei. With a lens that had either a white soft or rosette type cataract, unimanual or bimanual aspiration was used. Membranectomy and anterior vitrectomy, via either an anterior or a pars plana route, were performed when the cataract was membranous [9].

- In all patients undergoing corneal wound repair in cases of globe rupture, the traumatic cataract may be managed in first or second procedure. Recurrent inflammation was more prominent in patients who had undergone previous surgery for trauma [7, 8]. In such cases, when the ocular medium was hazy due to inflammation of the anterior vitreous, we performed a capsulectomy and vitrectomy via an anterior/pars plana route [23].
- In children younger than 2 years of age, both a lensectomy and vitrectomy via a pars plana route were performed, leaving the rim of the anterior capsule available for secondary lens implantation, and the same surgical procedures were used to manage the traumatic cataracts. Lens implantation as part of the primary procedure was avoided in all children younger than 2 years of age; these children were rehabilitated with optical correction, and secondary implantation was done after their second birthday.
- All children received supportive amblyopia therapy from a pediatric orthoptist, and a pediatric ophthalmologist treated strabismus for improvement in stereopsis.
- In young children, it is generally best to undercorrect an eye in anticipation of a myopic shift as the child becomes older.
- In-the-bag fixation is believed to be most preferred site by most to be the surgeons.
- If bag is destroyed during trauma capsular remnant may be used for implantation.
- If capsular bag is subluxated capsular tension ring may be used and sutured using 10/0 prolene if beg is very unstable.
- The use of multifocal capsular bag IOLs following removal of a traumatic cataract has also been explored. In comparison with capsular bag IOLs, the clinical lenses resulted in improved uncorrected near visual acuity and stereopsis, as well as decreased spectacle dependency. However, multifocal IOLs reply on centration of the IOL and the pupil. Neither are achievable in all cases of trauma. Since traumatic cataracts are most often unilateral, the child will rely mostly on the natural accommodation of the uninjured eye for near viewing.

Multifocal IOLs are best when used bilaterally. For these reasons, the use of multifocal IOLs in pediatric trauma has remained low.

- Several reports on groups of patients with angle-supported anterior chamber IOLs in traumatic pediatric aphakia have been published. Due to the high incidence of secondary glaucoma, progressive pupil distortion, endothelial loss, and the limited experience with these IOLs in children, angle-supported IOLs have not gained wide spread acceptance.
- Scleral-fixated IOLs are consider a more acceptable alternative for the bag or ciliary sulcus implantation of posterior chamber IOLs, in the absence of capsular support in children. However, concerns have been raised about the risk of conjunctival and scleral erosion of scleral sutures leading to Infection, IOL tilt, dislocation of the lens in the vitreous cavity, vitreous or ciliary body hemorrhage, and secondary glaucoma (Fig. 12.12).

12.3.6 Postoperative Medication

All patients if not infected are treated with systemic and local steroids.

Depending on the case, we may sometimes increase the frequency of steroid drops. Also, a short course of systemic steroids may be indicated. If IOP control had been a problem after the original trauma, perhaps during hyphema resolution, it is likely that elevated IOP will be seen transiently after cataract surgery. Prophylactic oral acetazolamide is recommended during the early healing phase in such cases.

12.3.6.1 Follow-up

The operated patients were re-examined after 24 h, 3 days, and 1, 2, and 6 weeks to enable refractive correction. Follow-up was scheduled for day 3, weekly for 6 weeks, monthly for 3 months, and every 3 months for 1 year.

At every follow-up examination, visual acuity was tested according to age using the AAO guidelines. The anterior segment was examined with a slit lamp and the posterior segment with an indirect ophthalmoscope. All children who may not cooperate should be examined under General Anesthesia.

12.3.7 Visual Outcome

Author reported postoperatively with mean follow-up of 4 months: the visual acuity in the operated eye was >6/60 in 450 (82.7%) and ≥6/12,215 (39.4%) eyes in open globe group and >6/60 in 127 (81.8%) and ≥6/12 36 (28.4%) eyes in closed globe group ($p = 0.143$), and the difference between the groups was not significant in children. Overall, 402 (39.4%) eyes gained ≥6/60 and >6/12 in 238 (35.4%) cases. Surgical treatment caused significant difference in visual outcome ($p = 0.000$) [7–10, 15].

Other results (as well as the experience of several other authors) confirm that good visual outcome is frequently possible following IOL implantation in children. In our patients, 78% achieved a best-corrected visual acuity of 20/40 or better after a mean follow-up of 2.3 years. Koenig et al. reported 20/40 or better visual acuity in 87% (7 out of 8) of eyes undergoing IOL implantation for pediatric traumatic cataracts. The average follow-up in their series was 10 months. Gupta et al. reported that 9 (50%) of 18 children with unilateral traumatic cataract achieved 20/40 (or greater) visual acuity after IOL implantation, with an average follow-up of 12 months [23–39]. These all are very small case series but shah et al. published largest database of 671 cases of traumatic cases in children [10, 13].

According to our study, age of intervention and laterality play important role of visual outcome [4, 10–13].

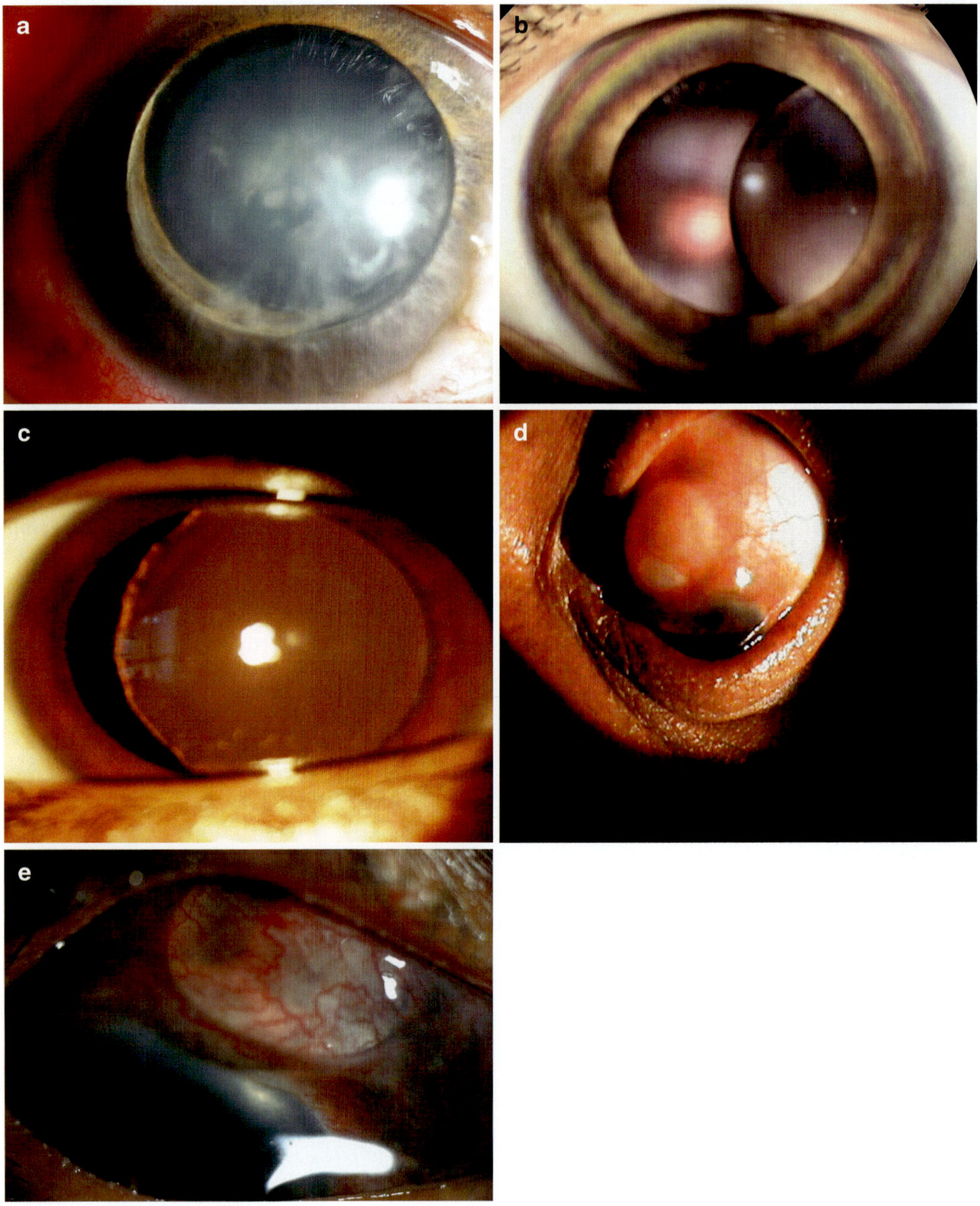

Fig. 12.12 (**a**) Ectopia lentis-1. (**b**) Ectopia lentis-1. (**c**) Temporal subluxation of lens following contusionsl-2. (**d**) Dislocation of crystalline lens in subconjunctival space ac following blunt trauma. (**e**) Dislocation of IOL following blunt trauma and opening of cataract wound

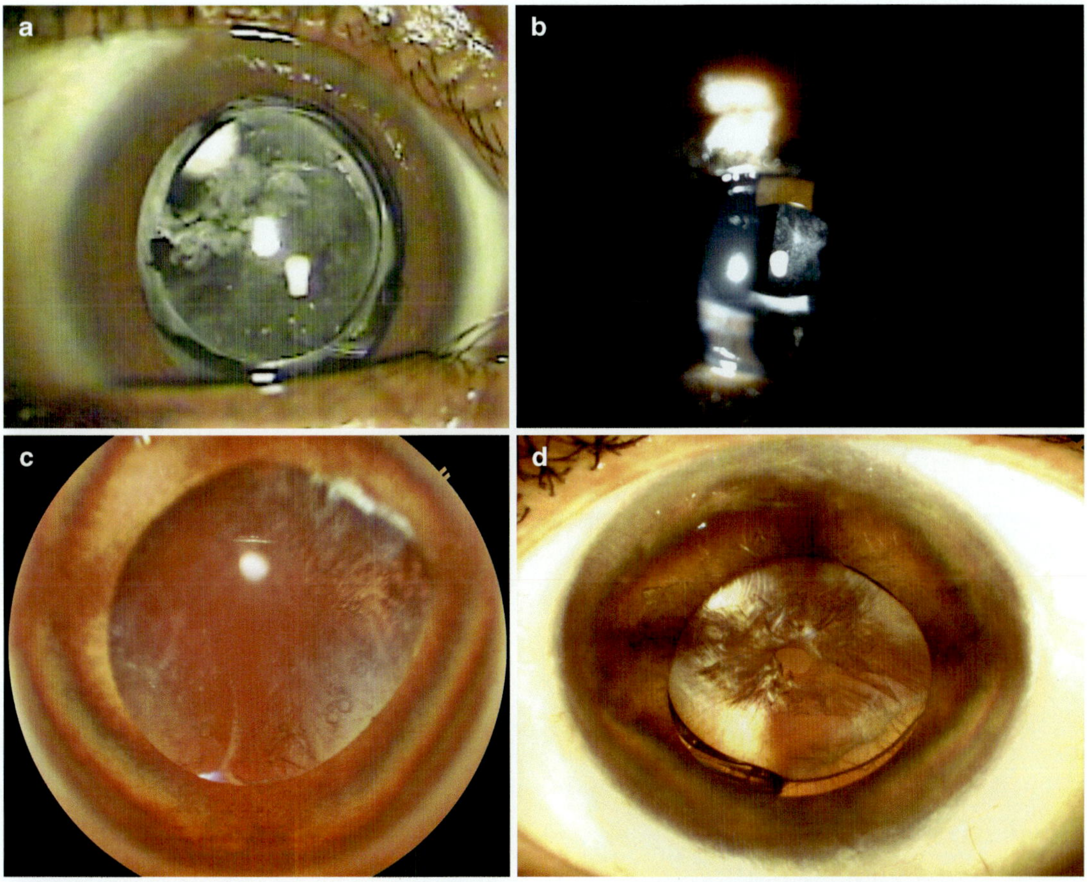

Fig. 12.13 (**a**) After cataract-1. (**b**) After cataract-2. (**c**) After cataract-3. (**d**) Capsular phimosis

12.3.8 Postoperative Complications

Postoperative common complications are [40–42]

1. After cataract (Fig. 12.13a–d)
2. Pupillary capture (Fig. 12.14a–c)
3. Lens precipitates (Fig. 12.15)
4. Recurrent inflammation (Fig. 12.16a, b)
5. Secondary glaucoma
6. Lens mal position (Fig. 12.17a, b)
7. Corneal opacity (Fig. 12.18a, b)

According to our study following are causes of nonimprovement of vision [18] (Table 12.1).

12.4 Summary

Cataract formation is a well-recognized consequence of blunt and penetrating ocular trauma. It results from direct lens injury, contusive ocular damage, or lens; dislocation and is often associated with traumatic injury to the cornea, iris, and vitreous. Traumatic cataract can present many challenges to the ophthalmologist. It adds the challenges presented by childhood cataract Comprehensive examinations, careful planning for surgical management and a close follow-up are necessary for a favorable outcome in these cases. Further prospective studies are probably needed to specifically address the optimum tim-

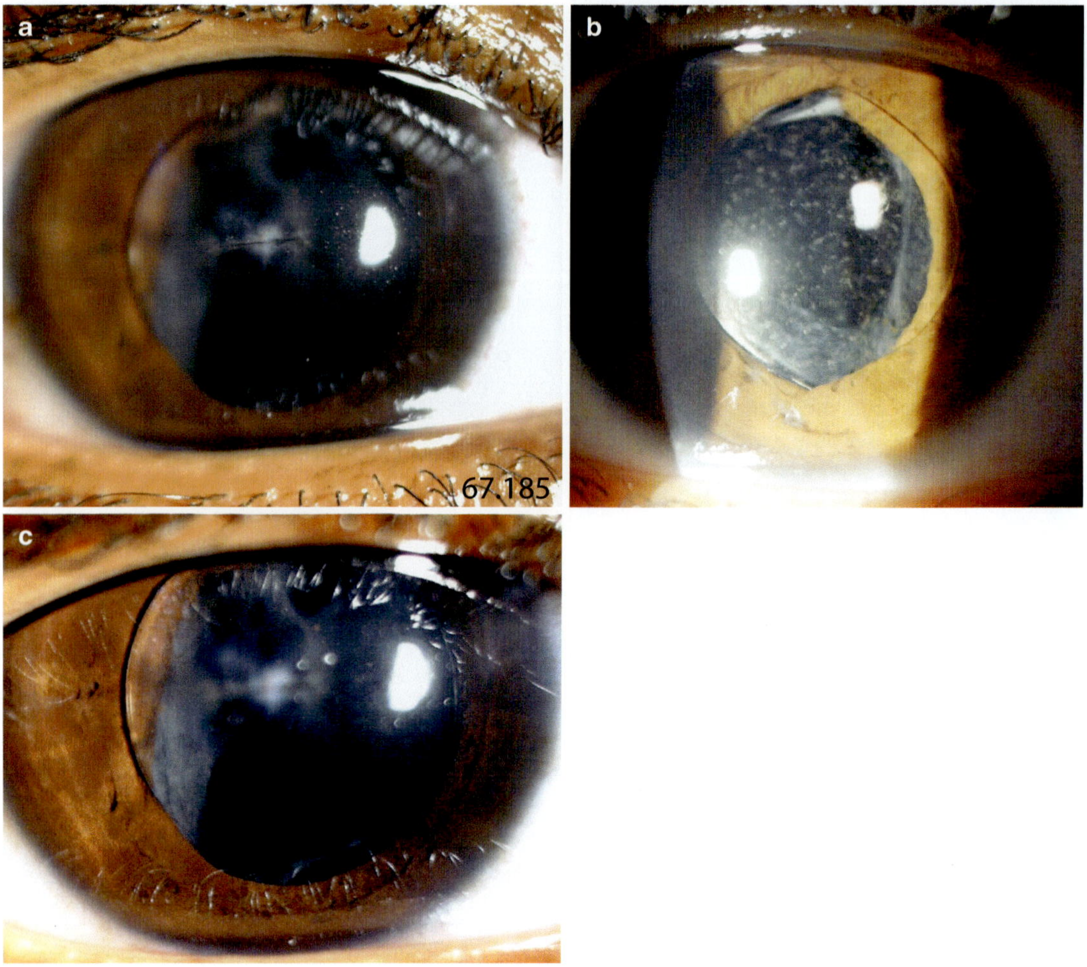

Fig. 12.14 (**a**) IOL capture-1. (**b**) IOL capture-2. (c) IOL capture-3

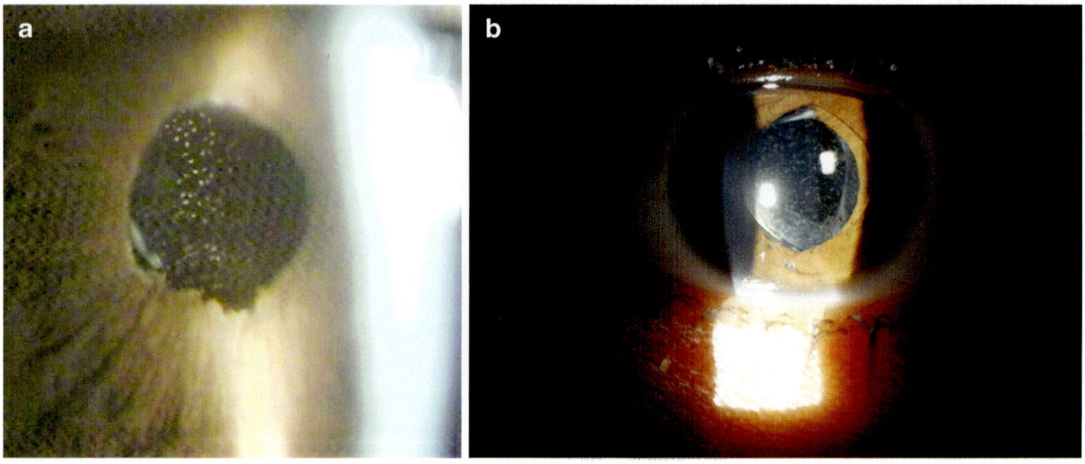

Fig. 12.15 (**a**) Lens precipitates-1. (**b**) Lens precipitates-2

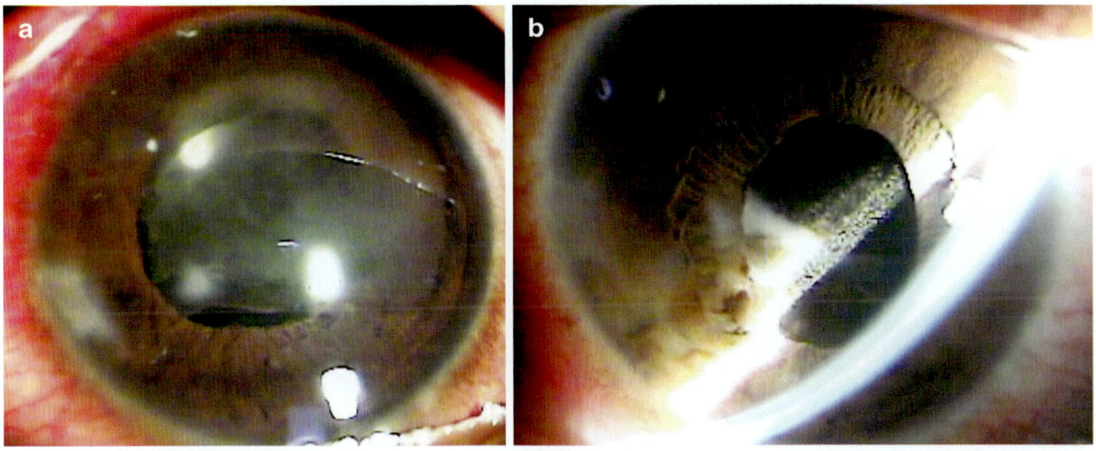

Fig. 12.16 (**a**) Postoperative inflammation-1. (**b**) Postoperative inflammation-2

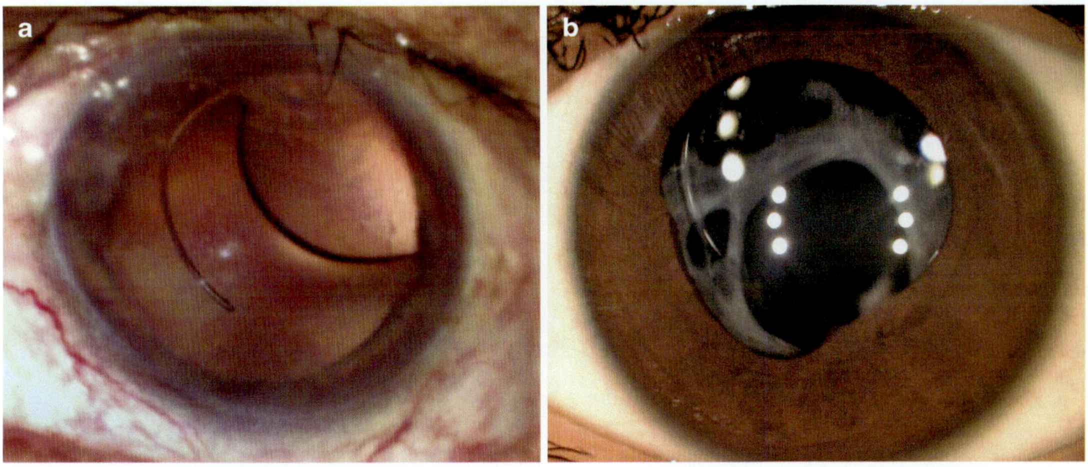

Fig. 12.17 (**a**) Lens malposition-1. (**b**) Lens malposition-2

ing of cataract surgery in cases of pediatric traumatic cataract.

However, based on our experience, we suggest primary repair of the injury first, and cataract surgery after a 2–4 weeks of topical and systemic steroids, primary posterior capsulotomy and anterior vitrectomy and deferring surgery 2–4 weeks of ocular injury. This delay may be helpful in achieving the optimum surgical outcome by reducing the postoperative inflammation in these eyes and allowing healing to occur.

Successful surgery requires a wide variety of techniques to the particular occasion and case. These factors include the history and circumstances of the ocular trauma, hypotony or the elevation of IOP, inflammation, and the extent of associated anterior segment trauma. We support the continued use of IOLs in children in eyes with traumatic cataract.

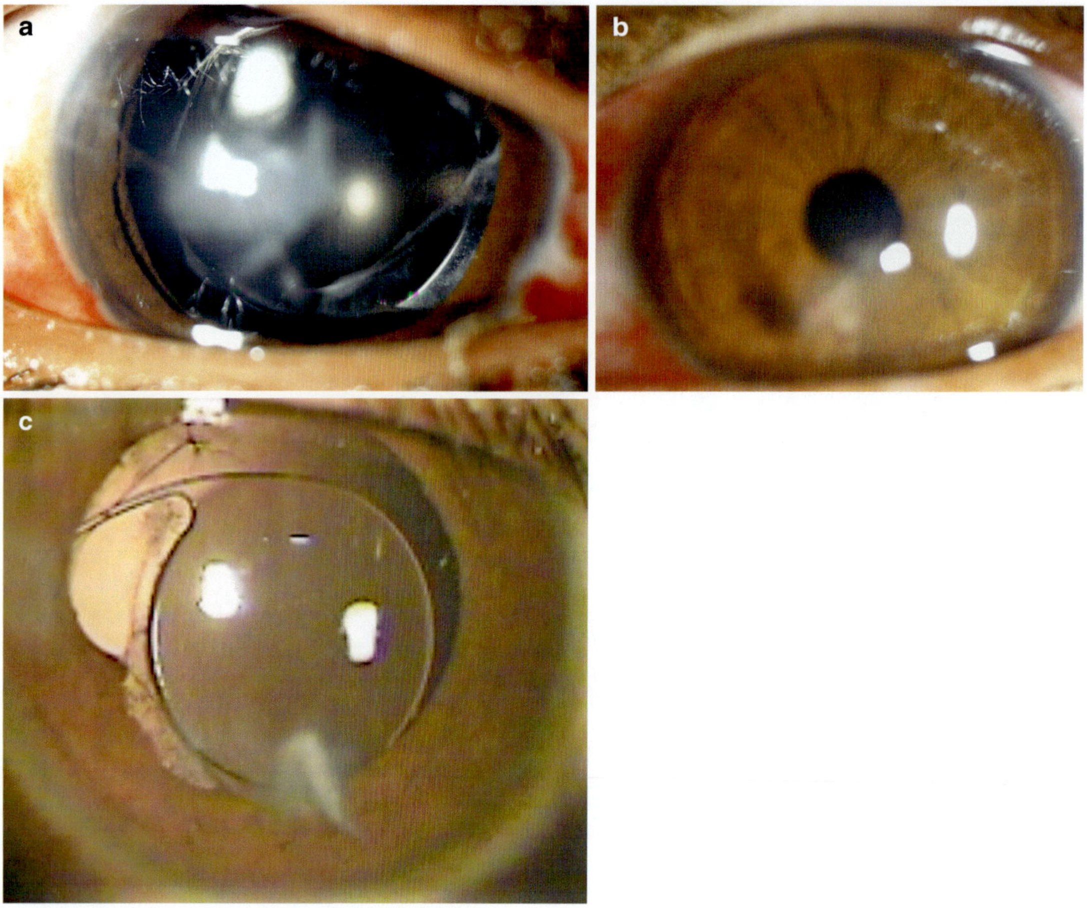

Fig. 12.18 (**a**) Corneal opacity-1. (**b**) Corneal opacity-2. (**c**) Corneal opacity-3

Table 12.1 Complications affected visual outcome

	Number (*n*)	Percent (%)
Corneal opacity	32	3.0
Lens Malposition	13	1.3
Endophthalmitis	5	0.5
Inflammation	18	1.7
Iridodialysis	2	0.2
Secondary glaucoma	6	0.6
Optic capture	6	0.6
Painful blind eye	1	0.1
Phthisis	5	0.5
Retinal detachment	8	0.8

Acknowledgments No financial support received from any company or institution. This study is not presented at any conference or meeting. No conflicting relationship exists for any author.

References

1. Khatry SK, Lewis AE, Schein OD, Thapa MD, Pradhan EK, Katz J. The epidemiology of ocular trauma in rural Nepal. Br J Ophthalmol. 2004;88:456–60.
2. Abraham DI, Vitale SI, West SI, Isseme I. Epidemiology of eye injuries in rural Tanzania. Ophthalmic Epidemiol. 1999;6:85–94.
3. Alfaro DV, Jablon EP, Rodriguez Fontal M, Villalba SJ, Morris RE, Grossman M, Roig-Melo E. Fishing-related ocular trauma. Am J Ophthalmol. 2005;139:488–92.
4. Shah M, Shah S, Khandekar R. Ocular injuries and visual status before and after their management in the tribal areas of Western India—a historical cohort study. Grafes Arch Clin Exp Ophthalmol. 2008;246:191–7.
5. Kuhn F, Morris R, Witherspoon CD, Mester V. The Birmingham Eye Trauma Terminology system (BETT). J Fr Ophtalmol. 2004;27:206–10.

6. Shah M, Shah S, Gupta L, Jain A, Mehta R. Predictors of visual outcome in traumatic cataract. World J Ophthalmol. 2014;4(4):152–9.
7. Shah M, Shah S, Upadhyay P, Agrawal R. Controversies in traumatic cataract classification and management: a review. Can J Ophthalmol. 2013;48:251–8. https://doi.org/10.1016/j.jcjo.2013.03.010.
8. Agrawal R, Shah M, Mireskandari K, Yong GK. Controversies in ocular trauma classification and management: review. Int Ophthalmol. 2013;33(4):435–45. https://doi.org/10.1007/s10792-012-9698-y. Epub 2013 Jan 22.
9. Shah MA, Shah SM, Shah S, et al. Morphology of traumatic cataract: does it play a role in final visual outcome? BMJ Open. 2011;1:e000060.
10. Shah MA, Shah SM, et al. Visual outcome of traumatic cataract in pediatric age group. Eur J Ophthalmol. 2012;22(6):956–63.
11. Shah MA, Shah SM, Shah SB, et al. Effect of interval between time of injury and timing of intervention on final visual outcome in cases of traumatic cataract. Eur J Ophthalmol. 2011;21:760–5.
12. Shah MA, Shah SM, Shah SB, et al. Comparative study of final visual outcome between open- and closed-globe injuries following surgical treatment of traumatic cataract. Graefes Arch Clin Exp Ophthalmol. 2011;249:1775–81.
13. Shah MA, Shah SM, Chaudhry AH, Pannu S. Traumatic cataracts in children: visual outcome. World J Ophthalmol. 2015;5(2):80–5.
14. American Society of Ocular Trauma. Ocular trauma score (OTS). 2000. http://www.asotonline.org/ots.html. Accessed 12 Oct 2019.
15. Shah M, Shah S, Shah SB, et al. Visual recovery and predictors of visual prognosis after managing traumatic cataracts in 555 patients. Indian J Ophthalmol. 2011;59(3):217–22.
16. Kuhn F, Maisiak R. The ocular trauma score (OTS). Ophthalmol Clin N Am. 2002;15:163–5.
17. Sharma HE, Sharma N. Comment on a new ocular trauma score in pediatric penetrating eye injuries. Eye (Lond). 2011;25:1240–1.
18. Shah MA, Shah SM, Applewar A, Chintan P, Krunal P. Ocular trauma score as a predictor of final visual outcomes in traumatic cataract cases in pediatric patients. J Cataract Refract Surg. 2012;38:959–65.
19. Lili Z, Wu Z, Feng D, Jia F, Dinghua L, Chixin D, Peifang R. Two kinds of ocular trauma score for paediatric traumatic cataract in penetrating eye injuries. Injury. 2015;46:1828–33.
20. Shah MA, Agrawal R, Teoh R, Shah SM, Patel K, Gupta S, Gosai S. Pediatric ocular trauma score as a prognostic tool in the management of pediatric traumatic cataracts. Graefes Arch Clin Exp Ophthalmol. 2017;255(5):1027–36.
21. Shah MA, et al. Innovative methods of anesthesia for eye surgery in children. J Anesth Surg. 2015;2:1–3.
22. Vajpayee RB, Sharma N, Dada T, Gupta V, Kumar A, Dada VK. Management of posterior capsule tears. Surv Ophthalmol. 2001;45:473–88.
23. Shah MA, Shah SM, Patel KD, Shah AH, Pandya JS. Maximizing the visual outcome in traumatic cataract cases: the value of a primary posterior capsulotomy and anterior vitrectomy. Indian J Ophthalmol. 2014;62:1077–81.
24. Khokhar S, Gupta S, et al. Epidemiology and intermediate-term outcomes of open- and closed-globe injuries in traumatic childhood cataract. Eur J Ophthalmol. 2014;24(1):124–30.
25. Shah MA, Shah SM, Gosai SR, Gupta SS, Khanna RR, Patel KB, Rathod CD. Comparative study of visual outcome between open- and closed-globe injuries following surgical treatment of traumatic cataract in children. Eur J Ophthalmol. 2018;28(4):406–11.
26. Wos M, Mirkiewicz-Sieradzka B. Traumatic cataract—treatment results. Klin Ocz. 2004;106:31–4.
27. Baklouti K, Mhiri N, Mghaieth F, El Matri L. Traumatic cataract: clinical and therapeutic aspects. Bull Soc Belge Ophtalmol. 2005;298:13–7.
28. Krishnamachary M, Rathi V, Gupta S. Management of traumatic cataract in children. J Cataract Refract Surg. 1997;23:681–7.
29. Gradin D, Yorston D. Intraocular lens implantation for traumatic cataract in children in East Africa. J Cataract Refract Surg. 2001;27:2017–25.
30. Morgan KS. Cataract surgery and intraocular lens implantation in children. Curr Opin Ophthalmol. 1993;4:54–60.
31. Cheema RA, Lukaris AD. Visual recovery in unilateral traumatic pediatric cataracts treated with posterior chamber intraocular lens and anterior vitrectomy in Pakistan. Int Ophthalmol. 1999;23:85–9.
32. Kumar S, Panda A. Safety of primary intraocular lens insertion in unilateral childhood traumatic cataract. JNMA J Nepal Med Assoc. 2008;47:179–85.
33. Bienfait MF, Pameijer JH. Intraocular lens implantation in children with unilateral traumatic cataract. Int Ophthalmol. 1990;14:271–6.
34. Anwar M, Bleik JH. Posterior chamber lens implantation for primary repair of corneal lacerations and traumatic cataracts in children. J Pediatr Ophthalmol Strabismus. 1994;31:157–61.
35. Eckstein M, Vijayalakshmi P. Use of intraocular lenses in children with traumatic cataract in south India. Br J Ophthalmol. 1998;82:911–5.
36. Zou Y, Yang W. Primary posterior chamber intraocular lens implantation in traumatic cataract with posterior capsule breaks. Yan Ke Xue Bao. 1995;11:140–2.
37. Vajpayee RB, Angra SK. Pre-existing posterior capsule breaks from perforating ocular injuries. J Cataract Refract Surg. 1994;20:291–4.
38. Gupta AK, Grover AK. Traumatic cataract surgery with intraocular lens implantation in children. J Pediatr Ophthalmol Strabismus. 1992;29:73–8.

39. Karim A, Laghmari A. Therapeutic and prognostic problems of traumatic cataracts. Apropos of 45 cases. J Fr Ophtalmo. 1998;21:112–7.
40. Brar GS, Ram J. Postoperative complications and visual results in uniocular pediatric traumatic cataract. Ophthalmic Surg Lasers. 2001;32:233–8.
41. Knight-Nanan D, O'Keefe M. Outcome and complications of intraocular lenses in children with cataract. J Cataract Refract Surg. 1996;22:730–6.
42. Lesniak SP, Bauza A. Twelve-year review of pediatric traumatic open globe injuries in an urban U.S. population. J Pediatr Ophthalmol Strabismus. 2012;49:73–9.

Uveitic and Complicated Cataract 13

Parmanand Kumar, Chirakshi Dhull,
and Sudarshan Kumar Khokhar

13.1 Management of Pediatric Uveitic Cataract

Uveitis is a condition wherein inflammation affects different components of the uvea, i.e., the iris, ciliary body, and choroid. Uveitis in pediatric age group is relatively rare compared to adults [1, 2]. The incidence and prevalence rates of uveitis in pediatric age group is 4.3/100,000 and 27.9/100,000, respectively [1, 2]. Pediatric uveitis accounts for merely 5–10% of all uveitis cases [3]. The visual loss is more severe with up to 22% of all affected children developing at least one blind eye and 3% becoming legally bilateral blind [4–10].

Uveitis in children has unfavorable outcome as compared to adults. This may be due to the difficult routine examination, no symptom in many patients, delayed recognition and, persistent chronic inflammation. Adding to this, ophthalmologist and parents are reluctant to treat children with systemic medication as there are multiple side effects associated with them. Management with systemic corticosteroids can have a negative effect on skeletal maturity. So, it is advisable to collaborate with a pediatrician before starting with systemic medications. At the same time, it is important to rule out an infectious origin before prescribing immunosuppressive therapy. Also, all ophthalmic surgery such as cataract and glaucoma are more challenging in children with uveitis [11]. Finally, the cataracts associated with uveitis if not treated in time have the risk of developing amblyopia in children less than 8 years of age. Long standing uveitis disease and added risks of complications can lead to major ophthalmic morbidity, and severe vision loss [2].

13.1.1 Classification

Uveitis can be classified on the basis of anatomical location (Table 13.1), clinical presentation (Table 13.2), etiology (Table 13.3), and histology (*granulomatous or non-granulomatous*).

Non-infectious uveitis is either related to systemic disease or believed to be immune modulated [4–10, 13]. In most of the uveitis cases, the reason remains unspecified and this is stated as idiopathic uveitis [2–10, 13]. In pediatric patients, anterior uveitis is seen in 30–40%, posterior uve-

Supplementary Information The online version of this chapter (https://doi.org/10.1007/978-981-16-0212-2_13) contains supplementary material, which is available to authorized users.

P. Kumar
R P Center, AIIMS, New Delhi, India

C. Dhull
Eye Q Hospital, Rohtak, Haryana, India

S. K. Khokhar (✉)
Professor Ophthalmology, Dr. RP Centre for Ophthalmic Sciences, All India Institute of Medical Sciences, New Delhi, India

S. K. Khokhar, C. Dhull (eds.), *Essentials of Pediatric Cataract Surgery*,
https://doi.org/10.1007/978-981-16-0212-2_13

itis 40–50%, intermediate uveitis 10–20%, and panuveitis 5–10% [3]. In pediatric age group, the most common cause for uveitis is juvenile idiopathic arthritis (JIA) and it causes mostly anterior uveitis [14]. JIA is responsible for chronic type of uveitis and in most of the cases problems are already present at the time of examinations. Other systemic diseases responsible for causing uveitis in children are sarcoidosis and tubulointerstitial nephritis and uveitis (TINU) syndrome[15]. Blau syndrome is a hereditary form of sarcoidosis occur in young, having clinical features similar to uveitis with JIA like rash, arthritis, and uveitis, so one may face difficulty in differentiating from uveitis with JIA [16]. TINU syndrome is a rare condition occurs in younger

Table 13.1 The SUN working group divides anatomical classification into four groups—anterior, intermediate, posterior and pan-uveitis [12]

Type	Primary site of inflammation	Includes
Anterior uveitis	Anterior chamber	Iritis Iridocyclitis Anterior cyclitis
Intermediate uveitis	Vitreous	Pars planitis Posterior cyclitis
Posterior uveitis	Choroid or retina	Focal, multifocal or diffuse choroiditis Chorioretinitis Retinochoroiditis Neuroretinitis
Panuveitis	Anterior chamber, vitreous and retina or choroid	

Table 13.2 Classification based of on clinical presentation [12]

Category	Descriptor	Comment
Onset	Sudden	
	Insidious	
Durations	Limited	<3 months durations
	Persistent	>3 months durations
Course	Acute	Episode characterized by sudden onset and limited duration
	Recurrent	Repeated episode separated by periods of inactivity without treatment ≥3 months duration
	Chronic	Persistent uveitis with re lapse in <3 months after discontinuing treatment

Table 13.3 Classification of uveitis based on etiology [4–10, 13–20]

Idiopathic		
Infectious	Congenital	Toxoplasmosis Syphilis Rubella virus Herpes simplex virus Cytomegalovirus
	Acquired	Tuberculosis Toxoplasmosis Toxocariasis Varicella zoster Leprosy Lyme disease (Borrelia burgdorferi)
Non-infectious	Systemic	Juvenile idiopathic arthritis (JIA) Sarcoidosis Behcets disease Vogt-Koyanagi-Harada syndrome (VKH) Systemic lupus syndrome Multiple sclerosis Wegener granulomatis Psoriasis Inflammatory bowel disease Tubulointerstitial nephritis and uveitic syndrome Kawasaki disease Chronic infantile neurologic cutaneous and articular/neonatal onset Multisystem inflammatory disease syndrome (CINCA/NOMID) Blau syndrome
	Ocular	Fuchs heterochromic uveitis
	Diseases	Sympathetic ophthalmia Retinal vasculitis Acute posterior multifocal placoid pigment epitheliopathy (APMPPE) Diffuse unilateral sclerosing neuroretinitis (DUSN) Traumatic uveitis
	Toxic	Drug induced (Rifabutin)

Table 13.3 (continued)

Idiopathic		
Masquerade	Neoplastic	Retinoblastoma Leukemia Juvenile xanthogranuloma Post transplantation lymphoproliferative disease (PTLD)
	Non-neoplastic	Intraocular foreign body Retinal detachment

population with peak incidence at the age of 14, characterized by tubulointerstitial nephritis and uveitis [15].

13.1.2 Clinical Presentation

Most of the cases are asymptomatic and hence therefore detected late in the progression of disease. JIA patients generally present with systemic involvement first.

- Redness in eye with photophobia is complained of usually, older children may complain of pain in the eyes (Fig. 13.1). In patients of JIA there may be absence of redness.
- Anterior segment examination in acute stage may show cells, flare and keratic precipitates (KPs). Hypopyon might be there in the anterior chamber (Fig. 13.2). So, it is important to rule out a masquerade syndrome or endophthalmitis in this type of presentation.
- As acute phase begins to resolve posterior synechiae may start showing up, which in early stage may be filiform (Fig. 13.3) and may break by intensive cycloplegic treatment (Fig. 13.4). A festooned appearance of pupil may be seen due to multiple posterior synechiae formations (Fig. 13.5).
- Koeppe's nodules may be seen in cases of granulomatous uveitis (Fig. 13.6). Tuberculosis and sarcoidosis are the most common systemic diseases responsible for granulomatous type of uveitis. These systemic diseases usually cause panuveitis (Fig. 13.7).
- Cataract is one of the complications of long-standing uveitis. It may vary from mild poste-

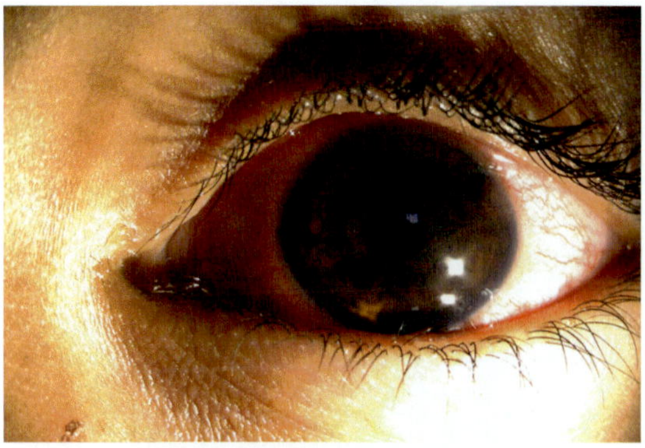

Fig. 13.1 Red eye can be noticed in torch light examination. Flare in the chamber is also noticeable

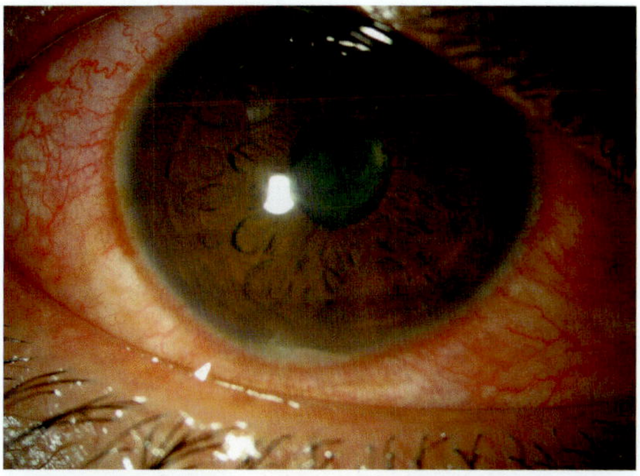

Fig. 13.2 Circumcorneal congestion with fibrinous membrane in anterior chamber with hypopyon

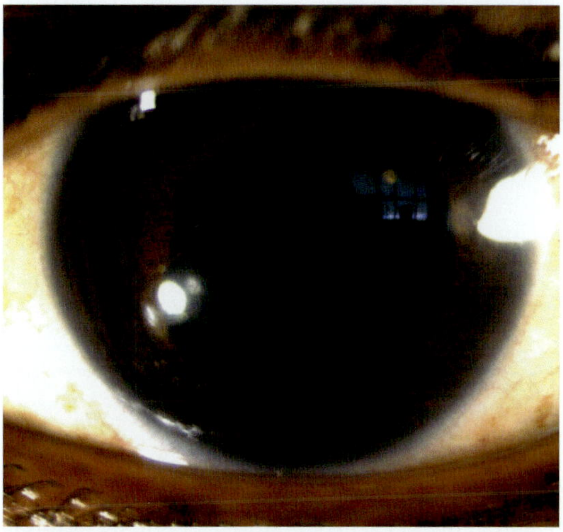

Fig. 13.3 Filiform synechiae seen from 9 to 12 O'clock position

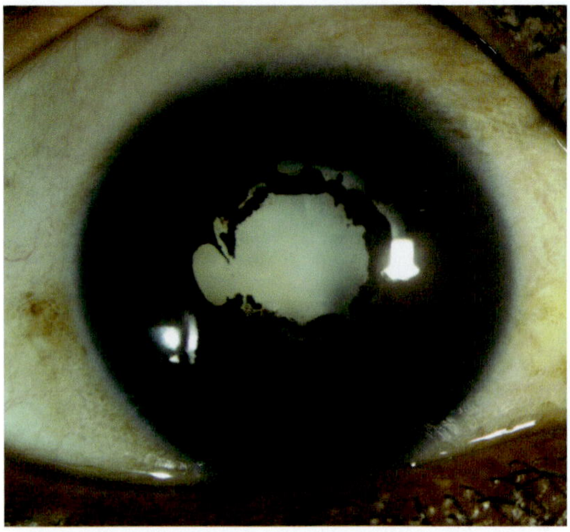

Fig. 13.4 Multiple incompletely broken posterior synechiae with pigment impression on anterior capsule with total cataract

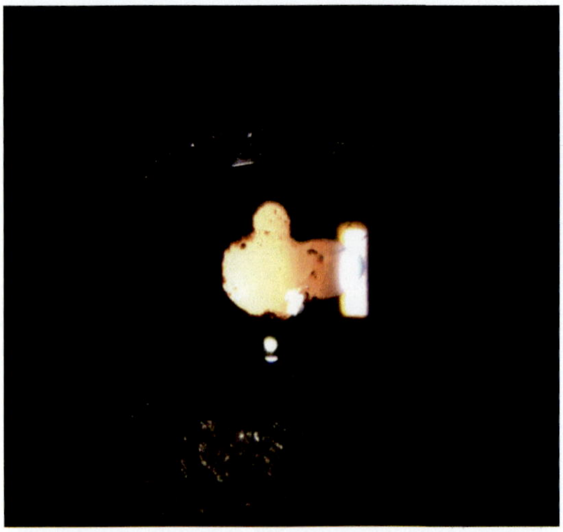

Fig. 13.5 Festooned pupil with clear lens

rior subcapsular cataract with polychromatic luster (Fig. 13.8) to total cataract (Fig.13.9).

13.2 Investigation

Investigations often turn out to be negative in many patients, so instead of performing a battery of screening tests, investigation should be tailored to each patient, directed by clinical features.

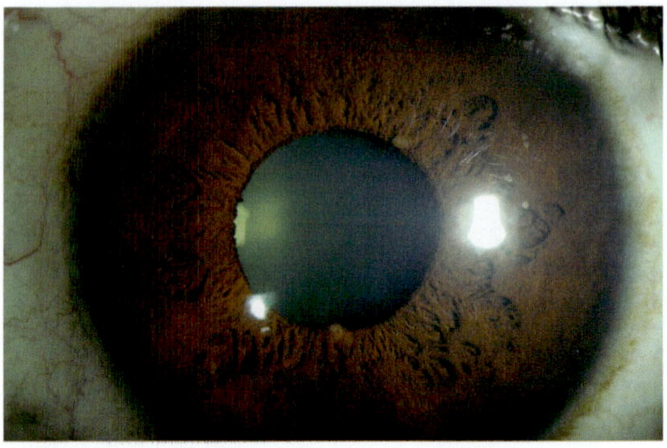

Fig. 13.6 Koeppe's nodules at 2 and 6 O'clock position in granulomatous uveitis

The following investigations may be considered:

Complete blood count: There may be leukocytosis which may point toward an infection and, exceptionally, hematological malignancy. Eosinophilia may be found in parasitic infection [21, 22].

Erythrocyte sedimentation rate (ESR) and C-reactive protein (CRP): These are acute-phase reactants which are probably of limited value as they may be elevated in a range of systemic inflammatory disorders [21, 22].

Chest X-ray: may show features which may be suggestive of sarcoidosis or tuberculosis [21, 22].

Sacroiliac joint X-ray: may show evidence of sacroiliitis in ankylosing spondylitis and other seronegative.

Spondylo-arthropathies [21, 22].

CT of chest: to look for features of sarcoidosis [21, 22].

CT/MRI of brain and orbits: to look for any evidence of sarcoidosis, CNS lymphoma, toxoplasmosis [21, 22].

HLA tissue typing: to look for connective tissue disorder and immunological disorders [21, 22] (Table 13.4).

AAALA type Associated disease.

Antinuclear antibody (ANA) is done for connective tissue disorder like in juvenile idiopathic arthritis [21, 22].

Rheumatoid factor is done to rule out rheumatoid arthritis and juvenile idiopathic arthritis [21, 22].

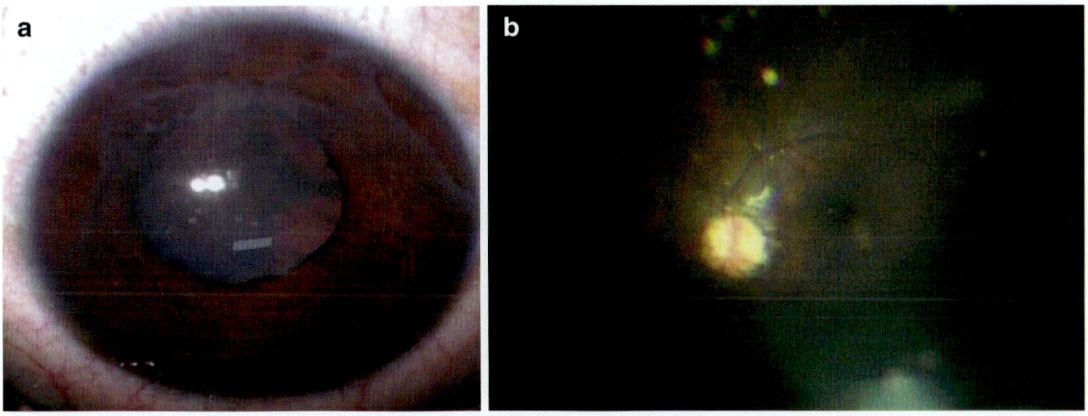

Fig. 13.7 An 8-year-old girl with sarcoidosis. (**a**) Showing band-shaped keratopathy with posterior subcapsular cataract, (**b**) intraoperative fundus image displaying hazy media, disc granuloma, and sclerosed vessels

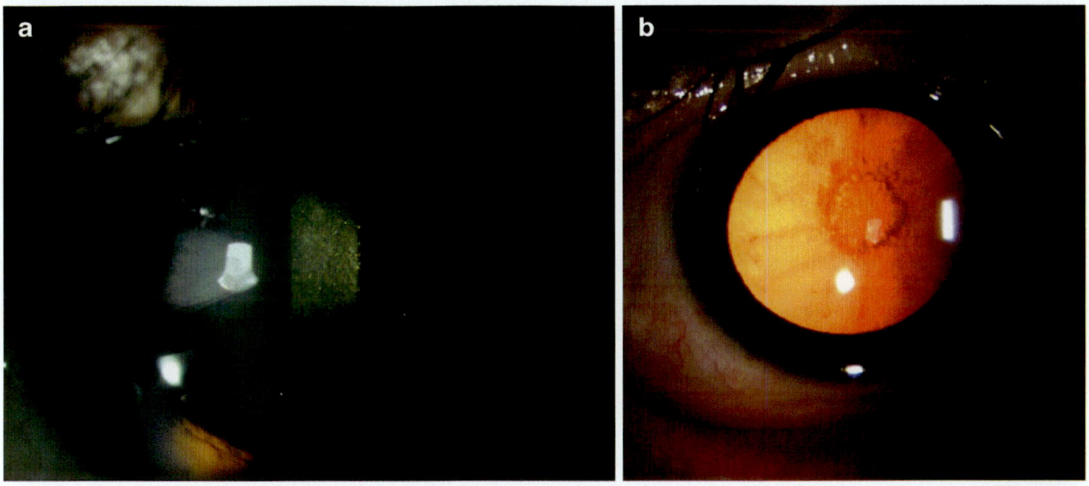

Fig. 13.8 Posterior subcapsular cataract in a patient with intermediate uveitis. (**a**) Slit illumination displaying polychromatic luster, (**b**) retro illumination of the same displaying central involvement

Angiotensin converting enzyme done mainly to rule out sarcoidosis [21, 22].

Serum calcium to corroborate diagnosis of sarcoidosis [21, 22].

VDRL/RPR to find any evidence of syphilis [21, 22].

Lyme disease serology to rule out Lyme disease [21].

Toxoplasma antibody to rule out Toxoplasma [21].

Herpes simplex virus, Rubella virus, Varicella zoster virus and Cytomegalovirus serology to rule any viral cause of viral uveitis.

Rubella serology to confirm the Fuchs heterochromatic iridocyclitis [23].

CSF studies (Proteins, glucose, CSF VDRL cytology, cultures, Gram stain)—are done if following diseases are suspected in patients like VKH syndrome, infection, malignancy, syphilis, lymphoma etc [21].

Intraocular fluid analysis (aqueous humor and vitreous humor tap) [24, 25] for

- Local antibody production—Rubella virus, Herpes simplex virus, Varicella zoster virus, cytomegalovirus, toxoplasma organisms.

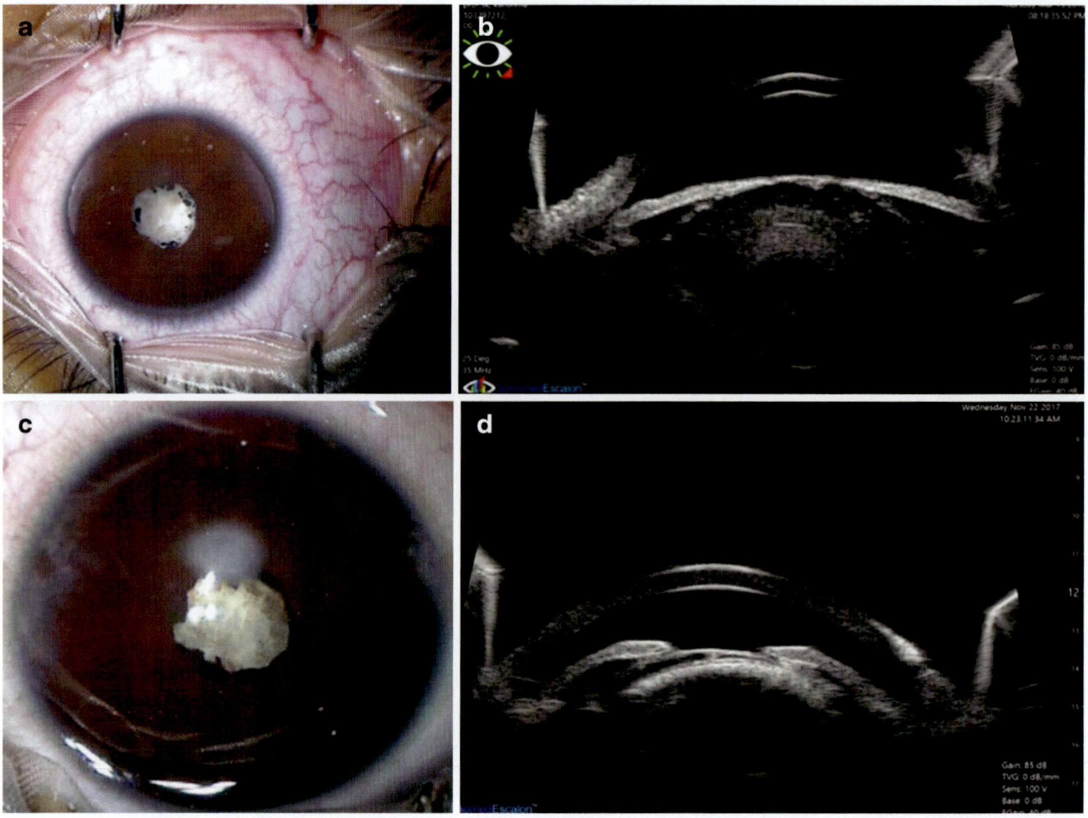

Fig. 13.9 Patient with JIA OD and OS. (**a**, **c**) Figure showing BSK, total cataract, and posterior synechiae, (**b**, **d**) UBM of the same showing OD seclusion-pupillae while OS showing early iris bombe formation

Table 13.4 HLA in different types of diseases

HLA type	Associated disease
HLA- B27	Seronegative spondyloarthropathy
HLA-A29	Birdshot retinochoroidopathy
HLA-B51 and HLA B5	Behcet syndrome
HLA-B7 and HLA-DR2	Ocular histoplasmosis
HLA-DR4	Sympathetic ophthalmitis and VKH

- PCR—for viral—HSV, VZV, CMV.
- Bacteria—Staphylococcus, Bacillus, Streptococcus, Pseudomonas, *Mycobacterium tuberculosis* and non tuberculus mycobacteria, Borrelia burgdorferi.

Ocular imaging [26, 27]-

B-scan ultrasonography—Enables visualization of the posterior segment including the status of retina.

Optical coherence tomography—aids to find out in posterior segment like epiretinal membrane and cystoid macular edema (Fig. 13.10).

Fundus fluorescein angiography—It is an imaging modality to evaluate eyes with chorioretinal disease and structural complications which are caused by posterior uveitis.

Fundus autofluorescence—can demonstrate any suspected posterior segment pathology.

Ultrasound bio microscopy—done in cases of chronic ocular hypotony where ciliary body atrophy can be seen. It may also help to demonstrate

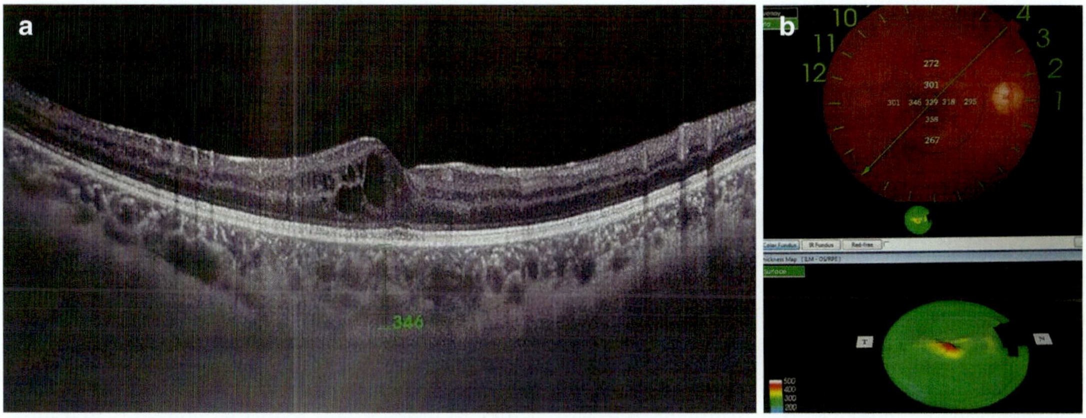

Fig. 13.10 (**a**, **b**) OCT showing macular edema in JIA with panuveitis

conditions such as subtle choroidal effusion, cyclodialysis cleft and cyclitis membrane.

13.2.1 Pathophysiology of Cataract Development in Uveitis

Cataract is a frequently encountered complication of chronic uveitis [28]. It occurs in 52% of children with.

Uveitis [9] and is the most frequent cause of vision loss [9]. In patients with uveitis, cataract surgery is one of the most common procedures done [29].

Uveitis predisposes the Patients to develop cataract particularly due to two reasons—the persistent inflammation which promote development of cataract and also the use of corticosteroids for immunosuppression [30–40] which causes-

1. Inhibition of Na+ k+ ATPase pump of lens
2. Increase cation permeability
3. Hydration of lens fibers
4. Decrease in GSH reductase level
5. Aberrant migration and differentiation of lens epithelial cells
6. Nonenzymatic alterations of lens proteins

Cataract extraction in these patients indeed poses a challenge and requires meticulous care during the perioperative period. Anisometropia either induced by cataract or by lack of optical rehabilitation in postoperative period may lead to development amblyopia. Surgeons must be proficient with the pre, peri, and postoperative management of these patients.

13.2.2 Management of Uveitic Cataract

13.2.2.1 Management of Uveitis

Early diagnosis and prompt initiation of treatment is the primary goal of management so as to attain complete inactivity of disease to avoid sight-threatening complications.

13.2.3 First-Line Treatment

Includes giving a course of topical corticosteroids accompanied by short-acting mydriatics and cycloplegics under surveillance. In severe anterior segment involvement or posterior segment involvement, sub-tenon triamcinolone, intravitreal triamcinolone, or dexamethasone implants can be given. The main concern for giving periocular steroids is the requirement of general anesthesia or sedation in children and hazard of cataract formation. Systemic corticosteroids may also be considered in some cases. Steroids have to be given cautiously because of their possible complications like formation of cataract, ocular-hypertension and multiple generalized side effects [41–43]. Multiple studies have shown less than BID dosing of prednisolone acetate is a reasonable frequency that does not lead to cataract formation [39]. Systemic corticosteroids have added threats in children like it can lead to growth retardation along with the usual side effects observed in adults such as peptic ulcers disease, increases sugar level, increased blood pressure, altered mental status, intracranial hypertension and increased risk of infection.

Systemic immunomodulatory therapy (IMT) should be started in those cases in which steroids cannot be tapered to a secure level or there is systemic cause of the underlying inflammation. IMT can take away the need for steroid therapy in such cases. All immunomodulators are known to have side effects, which has to be monitored for when administered. Supervision with a pediatric rheumatologist is strongly recommended before starting IMT. It is also vital to make sure that the parents and child acknowledge the risks related to inflammation, its treatment and at the same time remain compliant with the prescribed treatment. Extended use of mydriatics and cycloplegics can lead to formation of synechiae in dilated state of the pupils which have to be looked for and managed effectively when found.

Methotrexate is the maximally used and well-known drug to control inflammation in children with uveitis. It has been in used since long time for JIA-associated uveitis and is proven to be well tolerated.

Side effects of methotrexate include gastrointestinal disturbance which is most common and this could frequently be decreased through switching to the subcutaneous form of the medication. Folic acid supplementation reduces some of the side effects. Mycophenolate mofetil, sulfasalazine and azathioprine are other antimetabolites that can be used in place of methotrexate.

Similarly, to antimetabolites, certain biologic agents are getting used now a day to help with immunosuppression. These are antibodies which targets particular to the inflammatory cascade. Most common monoclonal antibodies are infliximab and adalimumab, which acts by inhibiting tumor necrosis factor alpha (TNF-α) [44, 45]. Other medications that can be used are abatacept, which blocks T-cell stimulation by targeting CD80 and CD86 signal molecules, and rituximab, which is an antibody to the CD20 protein found on B cells triggering cell death [46, 47].

13.2.4 Measures to Prevent Cataract Formation

Uveitis screening: It is important to develop strategies to prevent and identify cataract. Cataract is the most frequent ophthalmic complication of uveitis. This includes adherence to early screening and compliance to treatment and regular follow-up for uveitis.

Immunosuppressive therapy: It has been found that early treatment with methotrexate decrease the rate of cataract formation in JIA-uveitis [48].

13.2.5 Cataract Surgery

To begin with it includes a thorough anterior and posterior segment examination of the patient. Underlying deformities like band shape keratopathy, mitotic pupils, narrow anterior chamber, iris abnormality, and posterior synechiae are some of the features to be specifically looked for in these patients. In patients who have a mature cataract making a direct posterior segment examination difficult, imaging modalities like as B-scan ultrasonography should be done to assess for choroidal thickening, vitritis, or retinal detachment. Optical coherence tomography (OCT) can be done (if media enough is enough clear to capture) to look for any macular edema.

Counseling of the patient/parents Parents and patients need to be counseled regarding the visual prognosis, usual risks involved in surgery, like infection and various other intraoperative complications. It is vital to clarify that due to the presence of complications like band keratopathy, synechiae and membranes surgery may be prolonged and may also be difficult and that these factors may contribute to postoperative inflammation, delaying the visual recovery (Figs. 13.11, 13.12, and 13.13).

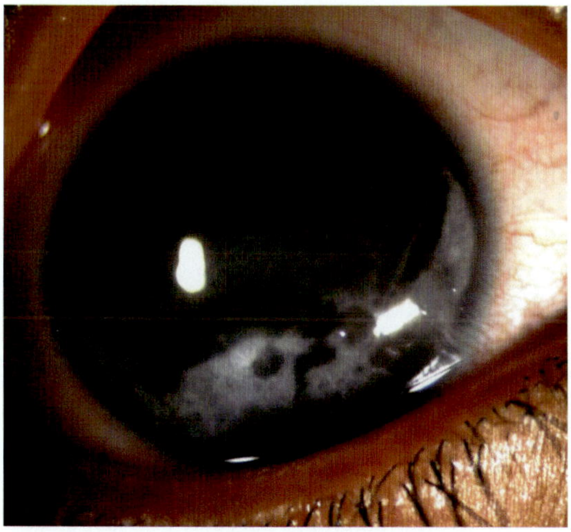

Fig. 13.11 Structural abnormalities in uveitis leading to difficult surgery. Showing band-shaped keratopathy

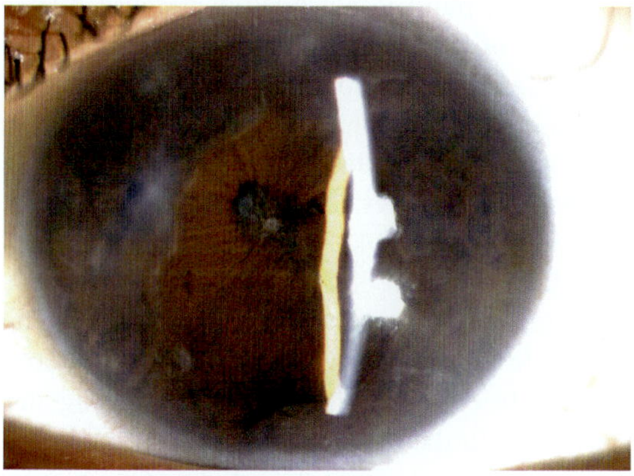

Fig. 13.12 Structural abnormalities in uveitis leading to difficult surgery. Showing extensive peripheral anterior synechiae with complicated cataract

Emphasis ought to additionally give on need for strict compliance of medications (systemic immunosuppression may need to be adjusted) and regular follow-up. Another frequent complication encountered postoperatively is posterior capsule opacification and because of the young age additional surgery may be needed in future.

13.2.6 Control of Inflammation

Preoperative control of inflammation and the underlying systemic disease is of utmost importance for successful outcomes in cataract surgery with uveitis. Patients should have at least 3 months of quiescence before proceeding to surgery [40]. Preoperative intensification of immunosuppressive treatment with systemic or local corticosteroid is recommended to avoid intensive postoperative inflammation. Oral prednisolone is given at a dose of 0.5–1.0 mg/kg 3–7 days before surgery. This can be added with a regime of topical steroids six to eight times per day up to surgery. After surgery, oral and topical corticosteroid should be tapered cautiously based on disease activity [40]. Intravenous or periocular corticosteroids or intensification of corticosteroid-sparing immunosuppression may be needed in patients developing uveitis flare-up after surgery.

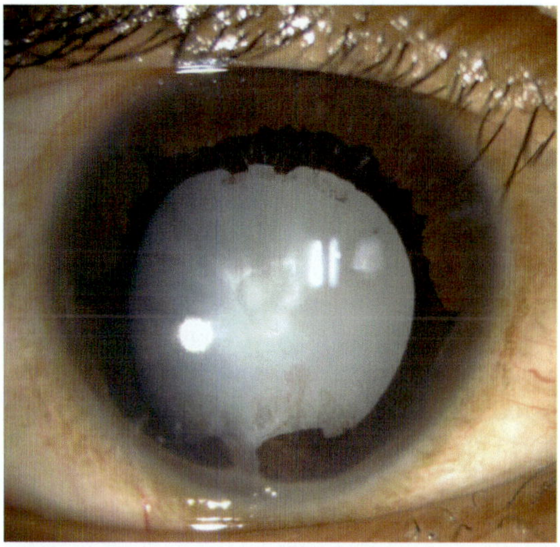

Fig. 13.13 Structural abnormalities in uveitis leading to difficult surgery. Showing ectropion uvea with vascularization of anterior lens capsule

13.2.7 Surgical Techniques

The technique of cataract surgery choice varies according to the individual surgeon's skill and experience. As less minimal inflammation is desired in postoperative period in uveitis cataracts, removal of cataract by phacoemulsification/lens aspiration is a safer method than that by a manual extracapsular cataract extraction.

Attempt should also be made to restore the anterior segment anatomy as close to normal as possible during the surgery.

13.2.8 Intraoperative Management

Postures—Supine position with face parallel to floor is required for cataract surgery. In patients with ankylosing spondylitis especially when the cervical spine is involved with a fixed flexion deformity, have difficulty in lying flat on the operating table. In such cases, Trendelenburg position is used, wherein their lower limbs are raised above the level of their head, so as to keep the plane of the face parallel to the floor. In order to lift the head high up pillow may be stacked up under the head. There are chances that the patient may tend to slide down the bed in which case in order to prevent the slippage a strap is locked around the trunk of the body.

Anesthesia—In adults' local anesthesia may be enough for operating but in children and in patients in whom surgical time is expected to be long surgery is done under general anesthesia.

Incision—To begin with, two paracentesis incisions are made almost 180° apart using MVR in nasal and temporal area. It is so constructed that it gives approach to through of the anterior chamber and lens with comfort. It can be used for both bimanual surgery as well as injection of viscoelastic devices. Then main incision is made superior which can be either clear corneal or scleral tunnel. Both incision techniques have shown to cause similar surgically induced astigmatism (SIA) and are acceptable [49]. In pediatric age group it is preferable to have a superior incision to protect against inadvertent trauma. In adults and older children to reduce the SIA, the incision can be made in the steeper axis but it should not be at the cost of sacrificing the operating comfort of surgeon [50]. Care should be taken to make incision of sufficient length in order to avert iris prolapse in eyes with small or stretched pupils.

13.2.9 Small Pupil Management

Pupil enlargement—Pupils that are not bound by synechiae or membranes an effort to dilate pupil may be made by injection of adrenaline diluted in balance salt solution (1:1000 0.5 mL adrenaline in 500 mL) into the anterior chamber of eyes. Heavy molecular weight viscoelastic like Healon 5 (sodium hyaluronate 2.3%, Abbott Medical Optics) can mechanically open the pupil and maintain it in dilated state as long as the aspiration flow rate is kept at minimum level.

Synechiolysis—Breaking the synechiae and achieving a pupil expansion can be a challenging task in uveitis cataracts surgery. A viscoelastic device, specifically a high molecular weight, can increase mydriasis by means of direct mechanical stress at the pupillary margin during instillation. When pupil is not dilating because of the presence of posterior synechiae and if there is enough zonular support, the surgeon may pass the viscoelastic cannula between the anterior capsule and the pupillary margin and then instill viscoelastic in order to break the iridocapsular adhesions (Fig. 13.14). The cannula of viscoelastic is inserted in an oblique manner to produce a wave of viscoelastic, which will break the synechiae. In this manner, it is done at multiple sites to fully free the pupil. Following breaking the synechiae, further dispersive viscoelastic may be injected in the center of the pupil to obtain even extra dilation of the pupillary margin.

Pupil dilating hooks and expansion rings—If extensive synechiae is present, a bent Kuglen hook can be used to break them off once the pupillary margin has been viscodissected from the anterior capsule. This is "push–pull" instrument which is used for safe release of posterior synechiae, varying from mild to extensive. It permits the surgeon to push or pull the iris, which facilitates to detach the iris from the anterior lens capsule, in spite of an intact pupillary membrane. After making the pupil free, the pupillary membrane can be taken out using a pair Kelman-Mcpherson forceps. Many times it has been seen

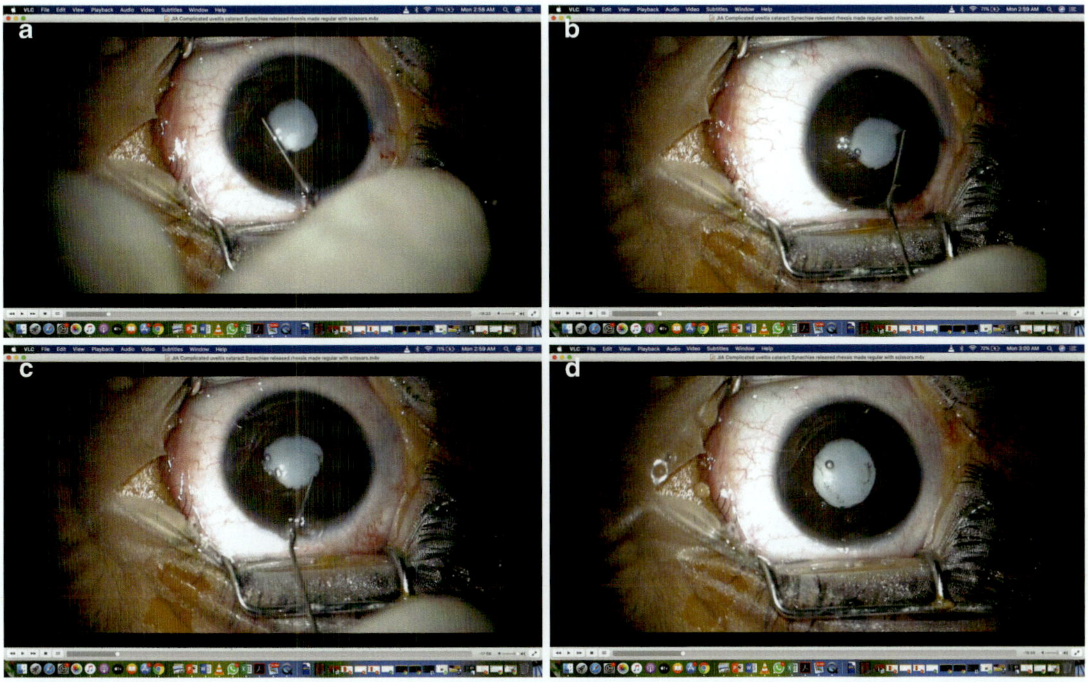

Fig. 13.14 (**a–d**) Use of viscoelastic canula for synechiolysis in pediatric uveitis cataract figure. (**d**) Final pupil size after synechiolysis with viscoelastic

that once the pupillary membrane has been taken out, the pupil begins to expand with viscoelastic (Fig. 13.15). However, if this is not enough, the pupil may be expanded using a pair of angled Kuglen hooks. It is inserted through the main superior incision, and then engaged it to pupillary margin and pulled the iris toward the limbus side till there is suspicion of sphincter tear. This is again repeated in a direction opposite to the first stretch.

Self-retaining Iris hooks (titanium or nylon) is also used for mechanical dilatation of pupil, in fact it is most commonly used as pupil expander. It is placed in anterior chamber through paracentesis and pupillary margin of iris is hooked toward paracentesis side so that the pupil can be kept dilated in a triangular or square shape and thus permitting the surgeon to proficiently complete phacoemulsification irrespective of the initial size of the pupil (Fig. 13.16). However, this method is time taking and also causes significant fluid loss from the anterior chamber during phacoemulsification. However, it is an efficient technique of pupillary expansion and visualization of the structures for phacoemulsification. Iris hooks is removed after placement of intraocular lens before removing viscoelastic substance.

Continuous curvilinear capsulorhexis—Anterior capsule is stained with trypan blue dye under air. The anterior chamber is filled with viscoelastics specially heavy molecular weight to keep the anterior capsule flattened in order to prevent extension of capsulorhexis. The anterior capsule stab incision is given by a 26- or 27-gauge bent cystitome and rhexis is completed by using a modified vitreoretinal forceps which is inserted from the side port. Capsulorhexis should be of adequate size and circular to decrease the incidence of posterior capsule opacification.

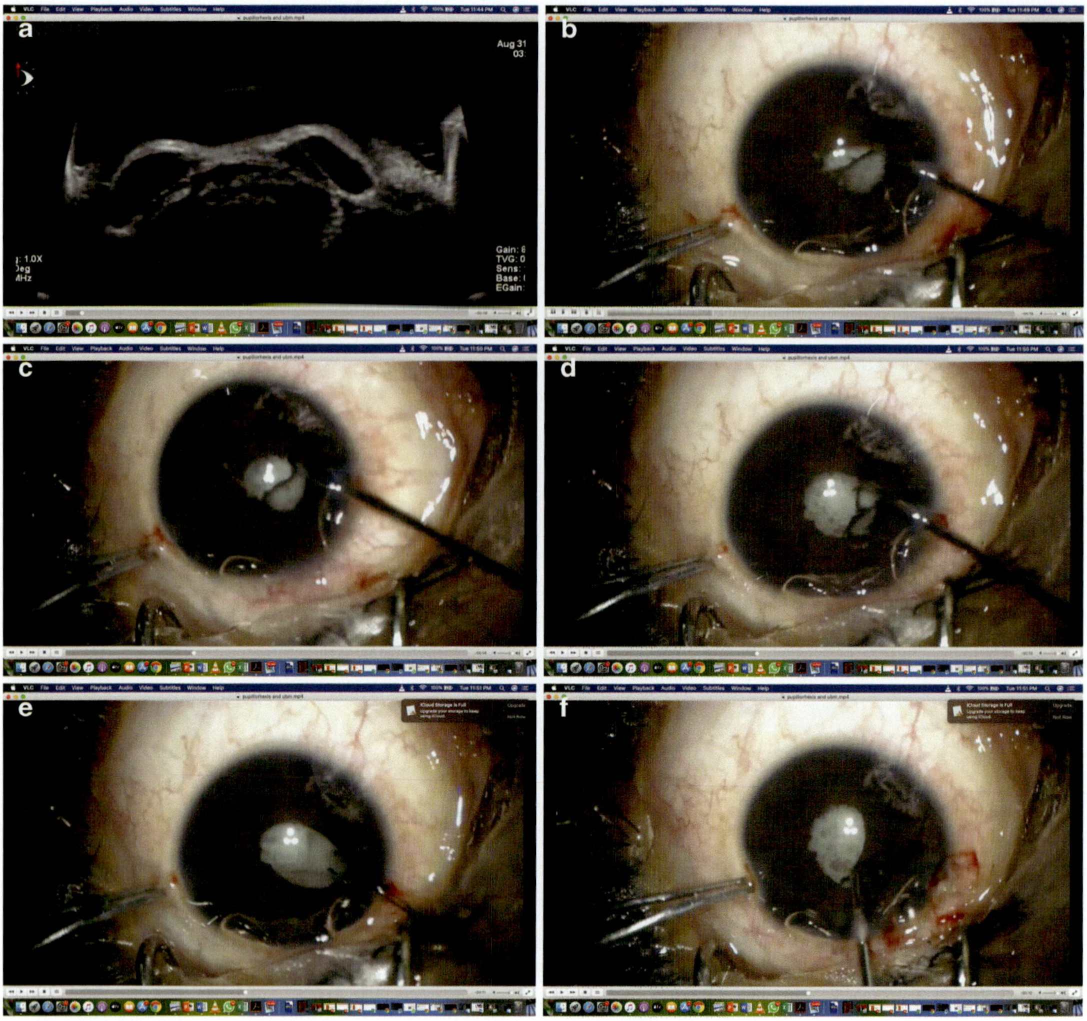

Fig. 13.15 (**a**–**f**) Pediatric uveitic cataract with 360° posterior synechiae with pupillary membrane. (**a**) UBM shows iris bombae. (**b**–**f**) Shows steps of pupillorhexis in same patient with 23 gauge Alcon intravitreal forceps. Membrane at pupillary margin grasped with forceps and pulled centrally

Hydrodissection and lens aspiration—Mild hydrodissection in all quadrants aids in lowering surgical time period and improving the cortical clean up [51]. Lens matter can be removed by either coaxial and bimanual techniques. Bimanual technique of lens matter removal is better as it helps in complete removal of lens matter including sub incisional one and also anterior chamber remains maintained.

IOL implantation—In children above the 2 years of age, intraocular lens (IOL) implantation is a standard way of optics management in non-uveitis cataract surgery but it is controversial to implant IOL in cases of cataracts with uveitis. In patients with uveitis IOL acts as a scaffold for the buildup of inflammatory cells and IOL itself can incite ocular inflammation with the consequent development of a membrane in visual axis [52]. Although, in cases, with satisfactory control of perioperative inflammation and regular follow-up, IOL can be well tolerated even in JIA patients [28, 53–61](Table 13.5). In all uveitis cataracts it is better to implant IOL in the capsular bag to avoid the physical contact of IOL with the iris.

Acrylic IOLs offers a higher visual outcome and lesser complication rate than IOLs of different

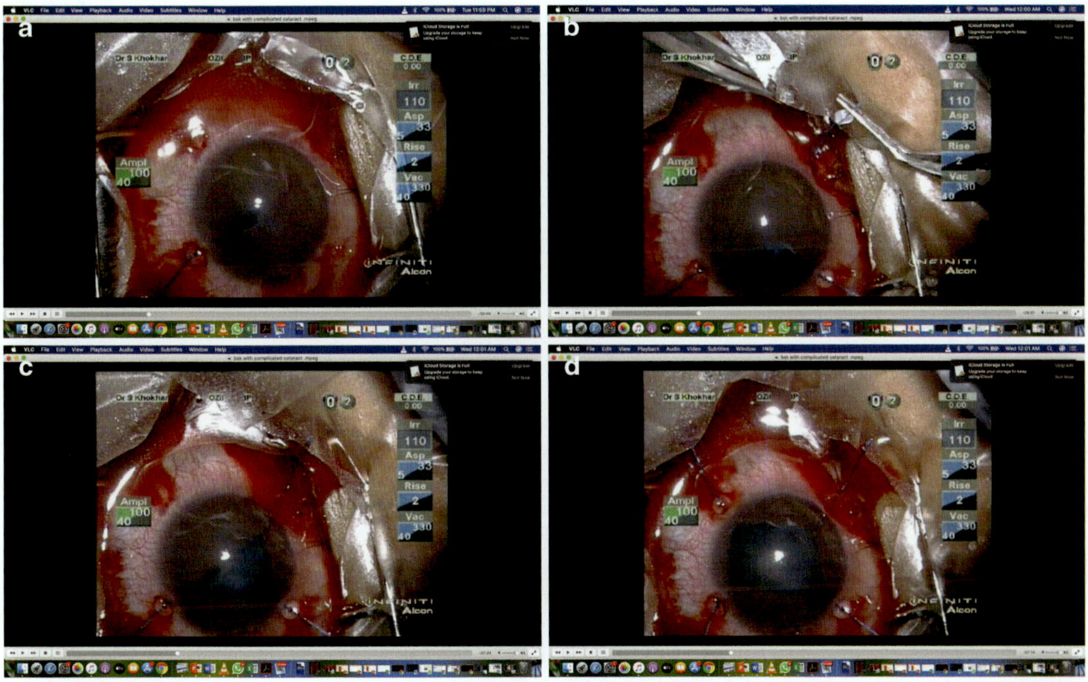

Fig. 13.16 (**a–d**) Pediatric uveitis cataract with non-dilating pin point pupil. Intraoperative still video clip shows placement of self-retaining nylon iris hooks

other materials in uveitis [62, 63]. Silicone lens is less suitable for cataract management in the setting of uveitis in view of increased risk of posterior capsular opacification and its potential of interfering with vitreoretinal instrumentation [62].

Removal of viscoelastic from anterior chamber—Viscoelastic should be removed completely in order to alleviate postoperative inflammation. Subconjunctival injection of antibiotic, steroid and atropine further helps to decrease the amount of inflammation.

13.2.10 Complications of Uveitic Cataract Surgery (Table 13.6)

13.2.10.1 Intraoperative

Zonular dialysis—It is an infrequent intraoperative complication seen in uveitis cases. It is encountered especially in eyes with long standing uveitis. In such cases, intraoperative placement of a capsular tension ring (CTR) is usually required to prevent IOL decentration. Fixation of the ring to the sclera by means of a modified Cionni may be done, if the overall zonular strength is weak. Capsular phimosis may occur if CTR is not implanted in presence of weak zonules because of unopposed capsular bag fibrosis and shrinkage. Failure to apply a CTR in the presence of weak zonules may result in capsular phimosis due to unopposed fibrosis and shrinkage of capsular bag.

Retained Lens Fragments. Small lens material may lodge in the posterior chamber during phacoemulsification specially in small pupil. These lens material may cause persistent inflammation in eye when come out in anterior chamber. For this reason, at the end of phacoemulsification sideways jerky movement to eye should be given or aspiration probe must be gently swept sideways in the bag so that no lens materials are accidently left behind in the bag or posterior chamber. Any amount of lens matter left inside the eye should be removed surgically as soon as possible [64].

Table 13.5 Cataract surgery with IOL implantation in JIA versus non-JIA type of uveitis: comparison of major studies

Study	Number of patients	Etiology	PCIOL in bag (*n* = eyes)	Aphakia (*n* = eyes)	Complication (n = eyes)	Visual outcomes (*n* = eyes)		Conclusion
						Pseudophakia	aphakia	
Probst and Holland [53] (1996)	7 (8 eyes)	JIA	8	0	Glaucoma (4) PCO (5)	All >6/12		JIA-associated uveitis can be treated by the standard surgical procedure with IOL implantation and can have excellent results.
Lundvall and Zetterstorm [54] (2000)	7 (10 eyes)	JIA	10	0	Glaucoma (7) PCO (5) Second surgery for membranes (8)	6/6–6/15 (8) <6/15 (2)		Heparin sulfated PMMA IOL can be used in patients with JIA and can have better results.
BenEzra and Cohen [55] (2000)	17 (20 eyes)	JIA 9 Non-JIA 11	10	7	Glaucoma (4) PS (3) CME (3)	*JIA* 6/9–6/6 (1) 6/60 (1) 6/240(1) LP (1) HM (1) Non-JIA 6/6 (1) 6/9 (1) 6/21(1) 6/60(2)	*JIA* 6/9–6/6 (1) NLP (1) HM (2) Non-JIA 6/6 (1) 6/9 (2) 6/21 (1) 6/60 (1)	IOL implantation is preferable in those needing unilateral cataract surgery. In JIA-associated uveitis, the final visual outcomes remain guarded because of irreversible amblyopia and a more complicated postoperative course.
Lam et al. [56] (2003)	5 (6 eyes)	JIA	7	0	PCO (6) Glaucoma (2) CME (1)	All >6/12		With good perioperative control of inflammation, JIA-associated uveitis can have favorable surgical outcomes with posterior chamber IOL.
Nemet et al. [28] (2007)	18 (19 eyes)	JIA 10 Non-JIA 9	19	0	PCO (10) Glaucoma (4) CME (1) Second surgery (11)	>6/12 (13) <6/12 (6)		IOL implantation is not contraindicated in those with pediatric uveitis, including uveitis associated with JIA.
Quinones et al. [57]	34 (41 eyes)	JIA 27 Non-JIA 14	13	28	Glaucoma (3) RD (3) PCO (4) CME (4) Membranes (2)	>6/12 (8) 6/15–6/24 (4) <6/120 (1)	>6/12 (9) 6/15–6/24 (6) 6/24–6/60 (5) <6/120 (8)	IOL implantation was well tolerated in most cases, which may result in optimal vision.

Sijssens [58] (2010)	29 (48 eyes)	JIA	29	19	Ocular HTN Glaucoma CME	>6/12 (25) 6/12–6/60 (3) <6/60 (1)	>6/12(13) 6/12–6/60 (4) <6/60 (2)	In JIA-associated uveitis IOL implantation in well-selected cases is not associated with increased risk of complications as compared to aphakic patients.
Terrada et al. [59] (2011)	16 (22 eyes)	JIA 9 Non-JIA 7	22	0	PCO (2) CME (3) Glaucoma (4)	>6/12		Uveitis is not a contraindication to primary IOL implantation in cases with full control of intraocular inflammation.
Ganesh et al. [60] (2016)	16 (21 eyes)	JIA 8 Non-JIA 13	21	0	PCO (15) Glaucoma (2) BSK (1)	JIA 6/6 (1), 6/9 (3) 6/12 (1), 6/15 (1) 6/75 (1), 6/24 (1) Non-JIA 6/6 (2), 6/9 (5) 6/12 (1), 6/24 (2) 6/36(1), 3/60 (1) CF (1)		Strict perioperative inflammatory control with immunosuppression can result in good vision after surgery and IOL implantation.
Yangzes s et al. [61] (2019)	37 (58 eyes)	JIA 30 Non-JIA 28	27	31	PCO (23) CME (18) Glaucoma (17) ERM (5) RD (2) Hypotony (2) VH (1) CNVM (2)	>6/12 (19)	>6/16 (13)	Although number of secondary procedures were more in pseudophakic group, Precise surgical technique and satisfactory immunosuppression lead to a gain of visual acuity in children undergoing IOL implantation in uveitis.

JIA juvenile idiopathic arthritis, *PCO* posterior capsular opacification, *CME* cystoid macular edema, *RD* retinal detachment, *BSK* band shape keratopathy, *IOL* intra ocular lens, *ERM* epiretinal membrane, *VH* vitreous hemorrhage, *CNVM* choroidal neovascular membrane, *CF* counting finger, *NLP* no light perception, *HM* hand movement

13.2.10.2 Postoperative

Excessive Postoperative Inflammation. It is the most common complication of uveitis cataract surgery, which can vary in terms of severity or duration. It can be controlled by increasing the frequency of topical steroids and readjust the dose of oral immunosuppressant. One may consider of giving oral pulse of steroids or injection of periocular steroids if no prophylactic oral steroids have been given in the preoperative period. In case of persistent inflammation intravitreal injection of triamcinolone acetonide can be given, thus avoiding the need to adjust the systemic immunosuppression [65]. Posterior synechiae, pupillary membrane may be formed during the postoperative period due to excessive inflammation (Fig. 13.17). Uveitis control and keeping the pupil mobile during this period are important.

Table 13.6 Perioperative complication of uveitis cataract surgery

Intraoperative	Postoperative
Zonular dialysis	Excessive postoperative inflammation
Retained lens fragment	Glaucoma
	Recurrence of uveitis
	CME
	Posterior capsular opacification
	Amblyopia
	Membrane formation

Glaucoma: Glaucoma is an important complication of uveitis. After uveitis cataract surgery transient increase in IOP may be seen most of the patients because of exaggerated postoperative inflammation with already compromised trabecular meshwork and anterior chamber angles. It can be controlled by good postoperative inflammation management aided with topical and systemic glaucoma medications. In intractable cases glaucoma surgery may be required.

Recurrence of uveitis. Recurrence of uveitis after cataract surgery is very common. This is mainly due to the two reasons—poor pre- and postoperative control of inflammation and intraoperative manipulation of intraocular tissue. The relapse rate has been reported to be as high as

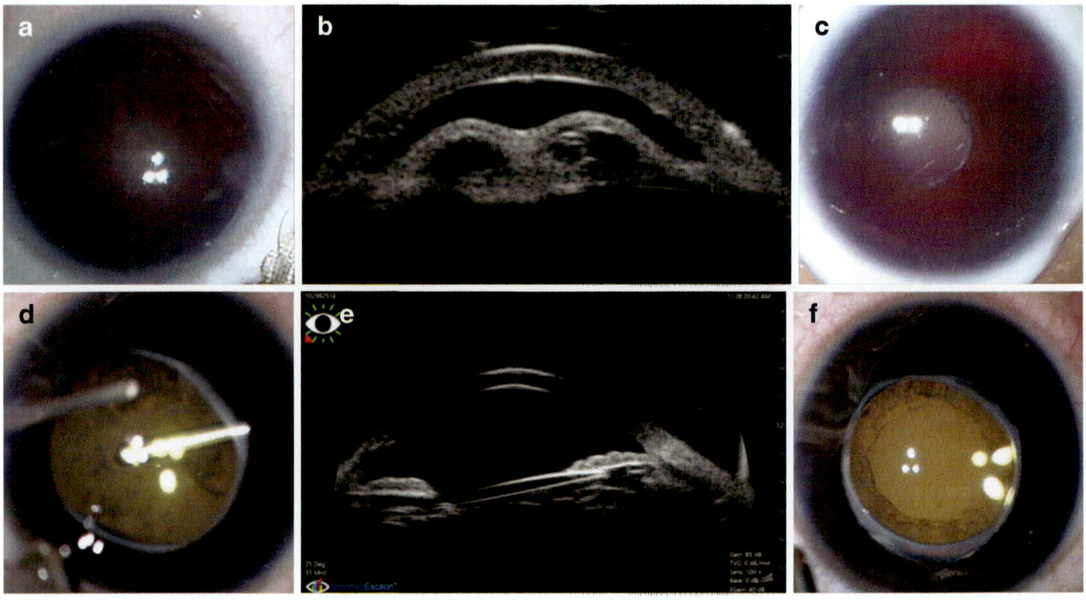

Fig. 13.17 (**a**) Postoperative picture of pediatric uveitis showing visual axis opacification (VAO). (**b**) UBM of the same patient showing iris bombe formation with VAO with aphakia. (**c**). Post-surgery picture of uveitis cataract from anterior route showing clear media. (**d**) Showing intraoperative picture of par plana membranectomy for posterior VAO. (**e**) UBM showing IOL in place with posterior VAO. (**f**) Postoperative picture of uveitis cataract showing clear media and IOL in bag

41% [66]. Hence, in that case, long-term immunosuppression may be required to prevent future relapse.

CME: In any intraocular procedure, CME may occur due to persistent of inflammation. In uveitis, the chances of CME increase because of exaggerated postoperative inflammation. It can be prevented by good pre- and postoperative inflammation control with immunosuppression. In some cases, periocular or intravitreal corticosteroids may be required.

Posterior capsular opacification (PCO): It is one of the most common late complications of any type of cataract surgery. To prevent posterior capsular opacification, it is advised to create a well-centered circular capsulorhexis that is smaller than the optic size of IOL, use an acrylic IOL with a square-edged optic design, complete aspiration of viscoelastic from within the capsular bag and confirmed that optic is stuck on to the posterior capsule at the end of surgery and in last very important in uveitis cataract surgery is control of postoperative inflammation.

Amblyopia management: Following any type of pediatric cataract surgery, visual rehabilitation is the most important. Patients should be prescribed glasses after doing refraction. In unilateral cataract surgery occlusion therapy should be given. Parents must be educated about the importance of compliance and proper follow-up.

13.3 Conclusion

Pediatric cataracts surgery with uveitis is a challenge to ophthalmologist in terms of perioperative management control. But, now a day it is possible to achieve good visual outcomes because of an increased understanding of the uveitis disease and management. Control of inflammation in perioperative period is very important for postoperative outcome. Cataract surgery should only be performed when the inflammation is well controlled. IOL should be implanted in every patients but it depends upon age of the child and ocular conditions. At last, judicious postoperative immunosuppressive therapy is required to reduce postoperative complications. Eyes with uveitis cataracts can achieve good visual outcomes with proper management.

References

1. Paivonsalo-Hietanen T, Tuominen J, Saari KM. Uveitis in children: population-based study in Finland. Acta Ophthalmol Scand. 2000;78(1):84–8.
2. Nagpal A, Leigh JF, Acharya NR. Epidemiology of uveitis in children. Int Ophthalmol Clin. 2008;48(3):1–7.
3. Edelsten C, Reddy MA, Stanford MR, Graham EM. Visual loss associated with pediatric uveitis in English primary and referral centres. Am J Ophthalmol. 2003;135:676–80.
4. Cunningham ET Jr. Uveitis in children. Ocul Immunol Inflamm. 2000;8(4):251–61.
5. Azar D, Martin F. Paediatric uveitis: a Sydney clinic experience. Clin Exp Ophthalmol. 2004;32(5):468–71.
6. Tugal-Tutkun I, Havrlikova K, Power WJ, Foster CS. Changing patterns in uveitis of childhood. Ophthalmology. 1996;103(3):375–83.
7. Smith JA, Mackensen F, Sen HN, Leigh JF, Watkins AS, Pyatetsky D, et al. Epidemiology and course of disease in childhood uveitis. Ophthalmology. 2009;116(8):1544–51.
8. De Boer J, Wulffraat N, Rothova A. Visual loss in uveitis of childhood. Br J Ophthalmol. 2003;87(7):879–84.
9. Rosenberg KD, Feuer WJ, Davis JL. Ocular complications of pediatric uveitis. Ophthalmology. 2004;111(12):2299–306.
10. Paroli MP, Spinucci G, Liverani M, Monte R, Pezzi PP. Uveitis in childhood: an Italian clinical and epidemiological study. Ocul Immunol Inflamm. 2009;17(4):238–42.
11. Foster CS. Diagnosis and treatment of juvenile idiopathic arthritis associated uveitis. Curr Opin Ophthalmol. 2003;14(6):395–8.
12. The Standardization of Uveitis Nomenclature (SUN) Working Group. Standardization of uveitis nomenclature for reporting clinical data. Results of the First International Workshop. Am J Ophthalmol. 2005;140(3):509–16.
13. Clarke LA, Guex-Crosier Y, Hofer M. Epidemiology of uveitis in children over a 10-year period. Clin Exp Rheumatol. 2013;31(4):633–7.
14. O'Brien JM, Albert DM, Foster CS. Juvenile rheumatoid arthritis. In: Albert DM, Jakobiec FA, editors. Principles and practice of ophthalmology: clinical practice, vol. 5. Philadelphia: WB Saunders; 1994. p. 2873–86.
15. Mandeville JT, Levinson RD, Holland GN. The tubulointerstitial nephritis and uveitis syndrome. Surv Ophthalmol. 2001;46(3):195–208.

16. Sfriso P, Caso F, Tognon S, Galozzi P, Gava A, Punzi L. Blau syndrome, clinical and genetic aspects. Autoimmun Rev. 2012;12(1):44–51.
17. Perkins ES. Pattern of uveitis in children. Br J Ophthalmol. 1966;50(4):169–85. https://doi.org/10.1136/bjo.50.4.169.
18. Smith C, Ashton N. Studies on the aetiological problem of uveitis. Br J Ophthalmol. 1955;39(9):545–56. https://doi.org/10.1136/bjo.39.9.545.
19. BenEzra D, Cohen E, Maftzir G. Uveitis in children and adolescents. Br J Ophthalmol. 2005;89(4):444–8. https://doi.org/10.1136/bjo.2004.050609.
20. Rothova A, Suttorp-van Schulten MS, Frits Treffers W, Kijlstra A. Causes and frequency of blindness in patients with intraocular inflammatory disease. Br J Ophthalmol. 1996;80(4):332–6. https://doi.org/10.1136/bjo.80.4.332.
21. Bansal R, Gupta V, Gupta A. Current approach in the diagnosis and management of panuveitis. Indian J Ophthalmol. 2010;58(1):45–54. https://doi.org/10.4103/0301-4738.58471.
22. Sinha R, Naithani P, Garg S. Newer investigations and management guidelines in uveitis. Indian J Ophthalmol. 2010;58(1):88–91.
23. Quentin CD, Reiber H. Fuchs heterochromic cyclitis: rubella virus antibodies and genome in aqueous humor. Am J Ophthalmol. 2004;138(1):46–54.
24. Matos K, Muccioli C, Belfort R Jr, Rizzo L. Correlation between clinical diagnosis and PCR analysis of serum, aqueous, and vitreous samples in patients with inflammatory eye disease. Arq Bras Oftalmol. 2007;70(1):109–14.
25. Harper TW, Miller D, Schiffman JC, Davis JL. Polymerase chain reaction analysis of aqueous and vitreous specimens in the diagnosis of posterior segment infectious uveitis. Am J Ophthalmol. 2009;147(1):140–7.
26. Ciardella AP, Prall FR, Borodoker N, Cunningham ET Jr. Imaging techniques for posterior uveitis. Curr Opin Ophthalmol. 2004;15(6):519–30.
27. Gupta V, Gupta A. Ancillary investigations in uveitis. Indian J Ophthalmol. 2013;61(6):263–8. https://doi.org/10.4103/0301-4738.114093.
28. Nemet AY, Raz J, Sachs D, et al. Primary intraocular lens implantation in pediatric uveitis: a comparison of 2 populations. Arch Ophthalmol. 2007;125(3):354–60.
29. Llop SM, Papaliodis GN. Cataract surgery complications in uveitis patients: a review article. Semin Ophthalmol. 2018;33(1):64–9. https://doi.org/10.1080/08820538.2017.1353815.
30. Mayman CI, Miller D, Tijerina ML. In vitro production of steroid cataract in bovine lens: part II, measurement of sodium potassium adenosine triphosphatase activity. Acta Ophthalmol. 1979;57:1107–1116.
31. Harris JE, Gruber L. The electrolyte and water balance of the lens. Exp Eye Res. 1962;l:372–84.
32. Beswick HT, Harding JJ. Conformational changes induced in bovine lens alpha-crystallins by protein carbamylation. Biochem J. 1984;223:221–7.
33. Harding JJ, Rixon KC. Carbamylation of lens proteins: a possible factor in cataractogenesis in some tropical countries. Exp Eye Res. 1980;31:567–71.
34. Monnier VM, Stevens VJ, Cerami A. Nonenzymatic glycosylation, sulphydral oxidation, and aggregation of lens proteins in experimental sugar cataracts. J Exp Med. 1979;150:10981107.
35. Greiner JV, Chylack LT Jr. Posterior subcapsular cataracts: histopathologic study of steroid-associated cataracts. Arch Ophthalmol. 1979;97:135–44.
36. Eshaghian J. Human posterior subcapsular cataracts. Trans Ophthalmol Soc UK. 1982;102:364–8.
37. Eshaghian J, Streeten BW. Human posterior subcapsular cataract: an ultrastructural study of the posteriorly migrating cells. Arch Ophthalmol. 1980;98:134–43.
38. Dickerson JE Jr, Dotzel E, Clark AF. Steroid-induced cataract: new perspective from in vitro and lens culture studies. Exp Eye Res. 1997;65:507–16.
39. Thorne JE, Woreta FA, Dunn JP, Jabs DA. Risk of cataract development among children with juvenile idiopathic arthritis related uveitis treated with topical corticosteroids. Ophthalmology. 2010;117:1436–41.
40. Blum-Hareuveni T, Seguin-Greenstein S, Kramer M, Hareuveni G, Sharon Y, Friling R, Sharief L, Lightman S, Tomkins-Netzer O. Risk factors for the development of cataract in children with uveitis. Am J Ophthalmol. 2017;177:139–43.
41. Slabaugh MA, Herlihy E, Ongchin S, van Gelder RN. Efficacy and potential complications of difluprednate use for pediatric uveitis. Am J Ophthalmol. 2012;153(5):932–8.
42. Kothari S, Foster CS, Pistilli M, Liesegang TL, Daniel E, Sen HN, Suhler EB, Thorne JE, Jabs DA, Levy-Clarke GA, Nussenblatt RB, Rosenbaum JT, Lawrence SD, Kempen JH. The risk of intraocular pressure elevation in pediatric noninfectious uveitis. Ophthalmology. 2015;122(10):1987–2001.
43. Biester S, Deuter C, Michels H, et al. Adalimumab in the therapy of uveitis in childhood. Br J Ophthalmol. 2007;91(3):319–24.
44. Feldmann M, Maini RN. Lasker clinical medical research award. TNF defined as a therapeutic target for rheumatoid arthritis and other autoimmune diseases. Nat Med. 2003;9(10):1245–50.
45. Lerman MA, Burnham JM, Chang PY, Daniel E, Foster CS, Hennessy S, Jabs DA, Joffe MM, Kacmaz RO, Levy-Clarke GA, Mills MD, Nussenblatt RB, Rosenbaum JT, Suhler EB, Thorne JE, Kempen JH. Response of pediatric uveitis to TNFa inhibitors. J Rheumatol. 2013;40(8):1394–403.
46. Korhonen R, Moilanen E. Abatacept, a novel CD80/86-CD28 T cell co-stimulation modulator, in the treatment of rheumatoid arthritis. Basic Clin Pharmacol Toxicol. 2009;104(4):276–84.
47. Rudnicka D, Oszmiana A, Finch DK, Strickland I, Schofield DJ, Lowe DC, Sleeman MA, Davis DM. Rituximab causes a polarization of B cells that augments its therapeutic function in NK-cell-mediated antibody-dependent cellular cytotoxicity. Blood. 2013;121(23):4694–702.

48. Sarsens KM, Rothova A, Van De Viewer DA, Stigma JS, De Boer JH. Risk factors for the development of cataract requiring surgery in uveitis associated with juvenile idiopathic arthritis. Am J Ophthalmol. 2007;144(4):574–9.
49. Bar-Sela SM, Spierer A. Astigmatism outcomes of scleral tunnel and clear corneal incisions for congenital cataract surgery. Eye (Lond). 2006;20:1044–8.
50. Matsumoto Y, Hara T, Chiba K, et al. Optimal incision sites to obtain an astigmatism-free cornea after cataract surgery with a 3.2 mm sutureless incision. J Cataract Refract Surg. 2001;27:1615–9.
51. Vasavada AR, Trivedi RH, Apple DJ, et al. Randomized, clinical trial of multiquadrant hydrodissection in pediatric cataract surgery. Am J Ophthalmol. 2003;135:84–8.
52. Foster CS, Barrett F. Cataract development and cataract surgery in patients with juvenile rheumatoid arthritis associated iridocyclitis. Ophthalmology. 1993;100:809–17.
53. Probst LE, Holland EJ. Intraocular lens implantation in patients with juvenile rheumatoid arthritis. Am J Ophthalmol. 1996;122(2):161–70. https://doi.org/10.1016/s0002-9394(14)72007-0.
54. Lundvall A, Zetterström C. Cataract extraction and intraocular lens implantation in children with uveitis. Br J Ophthalmol. 2000;84(7):791–3. https://doi.org/10.1136/bjo.84.7.791. PMID: 10873997; PMCID: PMC1723524.
55. BenEzra D, Raz J, Cohen E. IOL implantation following cataract extraction in children with uveitis; surgery and immediate followup. Ocular Immunol Inflamm. 1993;1:167–70.
56. Lam LA, Lowder CY, Baerveldt G, Smith SD, Traboulsi EI. Surgical management of cataracts in children with juvenile rheumatoid arthritis-associated uveitis. Am J Ophthalmol. 2003;135(6):772–8. https://doi.org/10.1016/s0002-9394(03)00123-5.
57. Quiñones K, Cervantes-Castañeda RA, Hynes AY, Daoud YJ, Foster CS. Outcomes of cataract surgery in children with chronic uveitis. J Cataract Refract Surg. 2009;35(4):725–31. https://doi.org/10.1016/j.jcrs.2008.12.014.
58. Sijssens KM, Los LI, Rothova A, Schellekens P, Does P, Stilma JS, et al. Long term ocular complications in aphakic versus pseudophakic eyes of children with juvenile idiopathic arthritis-associated uveitis. Br J Ophthalmol. 2010;94:1145–9.
59. Terrada C, Julian K, Casoux N, Prieur AM, Debre M, Quartier P, et al. Cataract surgery with primary intraocular lens implantation in children with uveitis: long term outcomes. J Cataract Refract Surg. 2011;37:1977–83.
60. Ganesh SK, Mistry S. Phacoemulsification with intraocular lens implantation in pediatric uveitis: a retrospective study. Ocular Immonol Inflamm. 2016;26:305–12.
61. Yangzes S, Seth NG, Singh R, et al. Long-term outcomes of cataract surgery in children with uveitis. Indian J Ophthalmol. 2019;67(4):490–5. https://doi.org/10.4103/ijo.IJO_846_18.
62. Alio JL, Chipont E, BenEzra D, Fakhry MA. Comparative performance of intraocular lenses in eyes with cataract and uveitis. J Cataract Refract Surg. 2002;28:2096–108.
63. Papaliodis GN, Nguyen QD, Samson CM, Foster CS. Intraocular lens tolerance in surgery for cataracta complicata: assessment of four implant materials. Semin Ophthalmol. 2002;17:120–3.
64. Teo L, Chee SP. Retained lens fragment in the anterior segment as a cause of recurrent anterioruveitis. Int Ophthalmol. 2010;30(1):89–91.
65. Degenring RF, Jonas JB. Intravitreal injection of triamcinolone acetonide as treatment for chronic uveitis. Br J Ophthalmol. 2003;87(3):361.
66. Foster RE, Lowder CY, Meisler DM, Chauhan R. Extracapsular cataract extraction and posterior chamber intraocular lens implantation in uveitis patients. Ophthalmology. 1992;99(8):1234–41.

14 Infective Cataract (TORCH)

Parmanand Kumar, Chirakshi Dhull, and Sudarshan Kumar Khokhar

Certain viral and parasitic infections occurring during embryogenesis may predispose to the development of congenital cataract [1, 2]. TORCH group of infections like Toxoplasma, Rubella, Cytomegalovirus (CMV), Herpes Simplex virus (HSV), and Others including syphilis have been associated with congenital cataract formation especially in developing countries [3–5]. The pathogen enters the fetus through the placenta of the infected mother during pregnancy [6]. Following infection, the immune systems produces a series of antibodies in the fetus. Antibodies are transferred to the developing fetus through the placenta from the infected mother and remains for a specific period of time following birth [3]. TORCH infections can be detected by immunoglobulin (Ig) M and Ig G titers in serum [3–5, 7–9]. Mahalakshmi and coworkers have described the presence of IgM antibodies in congenital cataract with infective etiology [3]. They have reported CMV Ig M in 17.8% and rubella virus Ig M in 8.4% among 593 infants with congenital cataract. Various studies have reported Ig M for HSV and Toxoplasma with congenital cataract [4, 5, 7–9]. There can be an overlap in manifestation of these infections. TORCH group of pathogens may additionally affect the ectodermal tissues [10], from which the lens is also derived. Other ocular manifestations of TORCH infections in addition to childhood cataract include microphthalmos, keratitis, glaucoma, iris atrophy, iridocyclitis, optic neuritis, retinitis, and chorioretinitis [11].

P. Kumar
R P Center, AIIMS, New Delhi, India

C. Dhull
Eye Q Hospital, Rohtak, Haryana, India

S. K. Khokhar (✉)
Professor Ophthalmology, Dr. RP Centre for Ophthalmic Sciences, All India Institute of Medical Sciences, New Delhi, India

14.1 Congenital Toxoplasmosis

Congenital Toxoplasmosis has wide-ranging clinical manifestations from being completely asymptomatic at birth to severe neurological and ocular disease. The majority of the infants have no apparent clinical manifestations at birth. These may be identified during routine new born examination and maternal screening [12]

Systemic features includes [12]

- Neurological features such as micro or macrocephaly, seizures, nystagmus, hydrocephalus, cerebral calcifications, meningoencephalitis
- Small for gestational age
- Hepatosplenomegaly
- Generalized lymphadenopathy
- Jaundice
- Thrombocytopenia, anemia, petechiae
- Maculopapular rash

S. K. Khokhar, C. Dhull (eds.), *Essentials of Pediatric Cataract Surgery*,
https://doi.org/10.1007/978-981-16-0212-2_14

Ophthalmic features includes

- Chorioretinitis
- Microphthalmos
- Retinochoroiditis
- Strabismus
- Iridocyclitis
- Cataract
- Glaucoma

Congenital toxoplasmosis is a reason for substantial visual loss and neurologic morbidity in children. Even if treatment is initiated at birth, it may not successfully prevent ocular damage [13–16]. The most common ocular manifestation of congenital toxoplasmosis is chorioretinitis (upto 92%), which is then followed by microphthalmos, squint, iridocyclitis, cataract and glaucoma [17–20]. Congential cataract is featured more commonly in congenital rubella, chorioretinitis is more commonly associated with congenital toxoplasmosis (Fig. 14.1). The pathogenesis of cataract in congenital toxoplasmosis remains unknown. Generally, the retina and choroid are affected first. It is then followed by involvement of iris leading to iridocyclitis and cataract, which can develop as secondary complication of retinochoroiditis. The incidence of cataract was 11.6% in the National Collaborative Chicago-based Congenital Toxoplasmosis Study (NCCCTS), typically occurring in those with the more extreme disease [15]. These infections can affect any part of the lens and cataract can vary in severity from partial to total. Most frequently noted cataract variety is posterior subcapsular; but, nuclear, anterior subcapsular, and anterior polar cataracts have also been reported [16].

Test for diagnosis of toxoplasmosis [12]

- Serological test
- Presence of Toxoplasma specific Ig M and/or Ig A antibodies 10 days after birth.
- Persistent or increasing IgG titer without treatment in infants at or beyond 1 year of age
- Positive PCR for T. gondii DNA or positive Toxoplasma IgM or Ig A antibodies in the CSF
- Positive IgG is indicative of prior or current maternal infection. Repeat IgG testing is done at every 4–6 weeks until complete disappearance in case of clinical suspicion of toxoplasmosis with negative IgM and IgA antibodies.

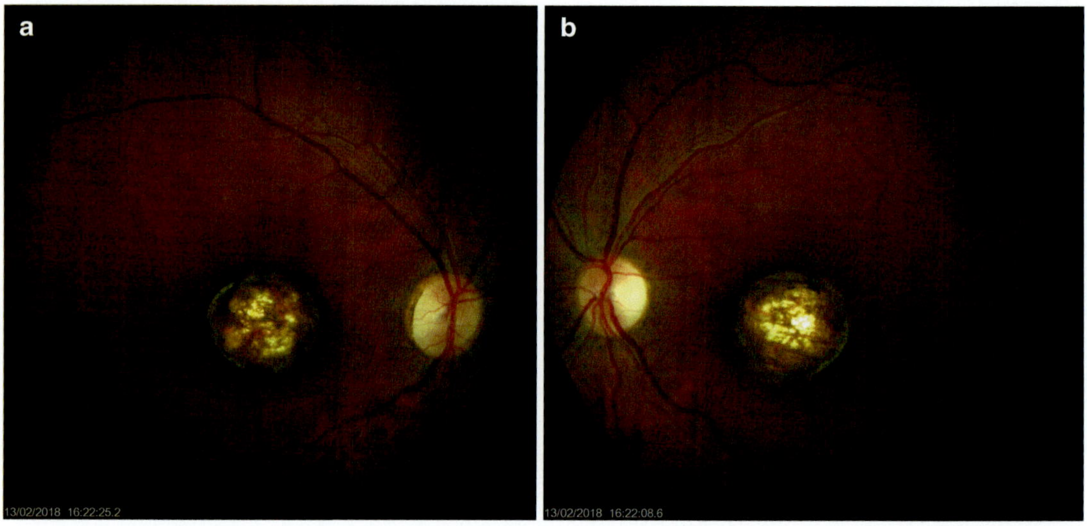

Fig. 14.1 (**a**, **b**) Clinical picture of right and left eye fundus showing typical punched out macular scar suggestive of healed congenital toxoplasma infection

- Negative IgM and IgA antibodies do not exclude the infection. There's a delay within the production of antibodies in the newborn, if the mother is affected later in her pregnancy. When an infection is suspected, the antibodies should be repeated every 2–4 weeks till at least 3 months of age.
- Imaging
- The main findings on computed tomography (CT) of the head include diffuse intracranial periventricular calcifications, brain atrophy or hydrocephalus
- CSF examination—CSF composition is usually abnormal with high protein levels (over 1 g/dl) and mild elevation of WBC with monocyte predominance.
- Hemogram—A complete blood count may demonstrate anemia or thrombocytopenia.

14.2 Congenital Cytomegalovirus (CMV) Infection

CMV is the reason for most common intrauterine infection, varying from 0.5 to 2.4% of live births [21]. However, it is usually subclinical.

14.2.1 Clinical Manifestation [22]

Systemic features

- Neurological features includes intracranial calcification, brain atrophy, ventriculomegaly, microcephaly, seizures, and hypotonia
- Hearing loss
- Hepatosplenomegaly
- Jaundice
- Petechiae
- Ocular features includes chorioretinitis, microphthalmos, microcornea, cataract, optic nerve hypoplasia, disc anomaly, keratitis, and glaucoma

Like congenital toxoplasmosis, chorioretinitis is the most common ophthalmic manifestation seen [11, 23–25].

Test for diagnosis of congenital cytomegalovirus infection includes:

1. Isolation of virus from urine
2. Identification of CMV-DNA by polymerase chain reaction (PCR) in urine, blood (including dried blood spots (DBS)), saliva, and cerebrospinal fluid sampled before 3 weeks of age
3. Detection of antigen or CMV-IgM in blood

Detection of IgM antibodies before 2–3 weeks of age in a new born is indicative of a congenital infection.

14.3 Herpes Simplex Virus (HSV) Infection

HSV strains are of two types—HSV-1 and HSV-2. HSV-1 is the oral strain and HSV-2 is genital strain. HSV-1 causes mouth lesions, eye infections, and encephalitis, while HSV-2 causes genital infection. The HSV-2 IS transmitted venereally [26, 27]. Multiple studies have reported the association of congenital cataracts with HSV infection [4, 28, 29]. Both HSV 1 and 2 were implicated in neonatal infections and more often causes Conjunctivitis, keratitis, iridocyclitis, iris atrophy, cataract, posterior synechiae, Retinitis, chorioretinitis, chorioretinal scarring, optic atrophy, optic neuritis and microphthalmos [11]. Common morphology reported in literature in Herpes congenital cataract is anterior linear cortical cataract and fluid clefts.

Diagnosis of congenital Herpes.

Serological diagnoses can be made with detection of Ig M antibody in infant blood.

14.4 Congenital Rubella Syndrome

Gregg in 1941, during epidemic of rubella in Australia, put forward that Rubella infection can be a cause of congenital cataract [30]. He had given idea of maternally transmitted infections causing ocular and systemic disease in children and it remains a milestone in ophthalmology and epidemiology. Rubella is still an important cause of congenital cataract in developing countries, despite being eradicated from developed countries [3, 31, 32].

14.4.1 Clinical Presentation

Congenital rubella syndrome (CRS) involves multiple systems of patients. Congenital heart disease, deafness, and cataract is the classical triad seen in patients with congenital rubella syndrome [23]. World health organization (WHO) has given the clinical criteria for diagnosing CRS [33] (Table 14.1). Cardiovascular abnormalities seen in this syndrome include patent ductus arteriosus (PDA) (most common), atrial septal defect, pulmonary stenosis, and ventricular septal defect [34].

Neurological abnormalities consist of microcephaly, hearing disorder, developmental delay, mental retardation, seizure disorder, and speech abnormality [34, 35] (Fig. 14.2).

Ocular features are the following, and the presence of these features would raise a suspicion of CRS [35–37]:

- Microphthalmos (Fig. 14.3).
- Opacification or cloudiness of cornea may be present (Fig. 14.4).
- Abnormal iris pattern like atrophy of iris, iritis, iridocyclitis, or iris hypoplasia may be seen. In most of the patients, pupils are non-dilating (Fig. 14.5).
- Lens may be cataractous which include total, nuclear, or membranous type. Sometimes, peripheral clear area around central cataract may be seen (Fig. 14.6).
- Anterior chamber angle abnormalities and glaucoma may be present.

Table 14.1 WHO criteria for diagnosis of CRS

Infection only	Suspected	Probable	Confirmed
Only laboratory evidence of infection demonstrated by- Isolation of rubella virus OR Detection of rubella-specific IgM antibody OR Persistence of rubella antibody at a higher level and for a longer period of time than expected from passive transfer of maternal antibody OR A specimen that is PCR positive for rubella virus	Patient does not meet the criteria for a probable or confirmed case but who has one or more of the following finding: Cataracts Congenital glaucoma Congenital heart disease (PDA or PS) Hearing impairment Pigmentary retinopathy Purpura Hepatosplenomagaly Jaundice Microcephaly Developmental delay Meningoencephalitis Radiolucent bone disease	Patient does not have the laboratory confirmation but has at least two of the following finding: Cataracts Congenital glaucoma Congenital heart disease (PDA or PS) Hearing impairment Pigmentary retinopathy OR Patient does not have the laboratory confirmation but has at least one or more of the following finding: Cataracts Congenital glaucoma Congenital heart disease (PDA or PS) Hearing impairment Pigmentary retinopathy AND one or more of the following: Purpura Hepatosplenomagaly Jaundice Microcephaly Developmental delay Meningoencephalitis Radiolucent bone disease	Patient with at least one of the symptoms clinically consistent with congenital rubella syndrome, and laboratory evidence of congenital rubella infection demonstrated by: Isolation of virus OR Detection of rubella specific IgM OR Persistence of rubella antibody at a higher level and for a longer period of time than expected from passive transfer of maternal antibody OR A specimen that is PCR positive for rubella virus

- Retina may show features of pigmentary retinopathy typically salt and pepper type (Fig. 14.7). Maculopathy may be associated with it. In vitro studies have observed that rubella virus infection of RPE can hamper the phagocytosis function by RPE cells [38]. Subretinal neovascularization may be seen in rare cases [20].
- There might be presence of squint or nystagmus.
- Optic atrophy, optic neuritis, lens absorption, keratoconus, corneal hydrops, or even phthisis bulbi may often be associated [20]

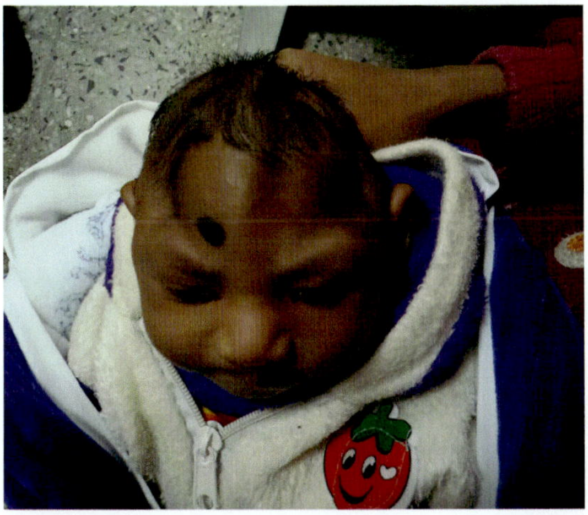

Fig 14.2 Showing 6-month-old child with microcephaly with CRS

14.5 Management

General principles of management remain similar to normal pediatric cataract surgery. Here we discuss about the management specifically related to cataract with infective etiology.

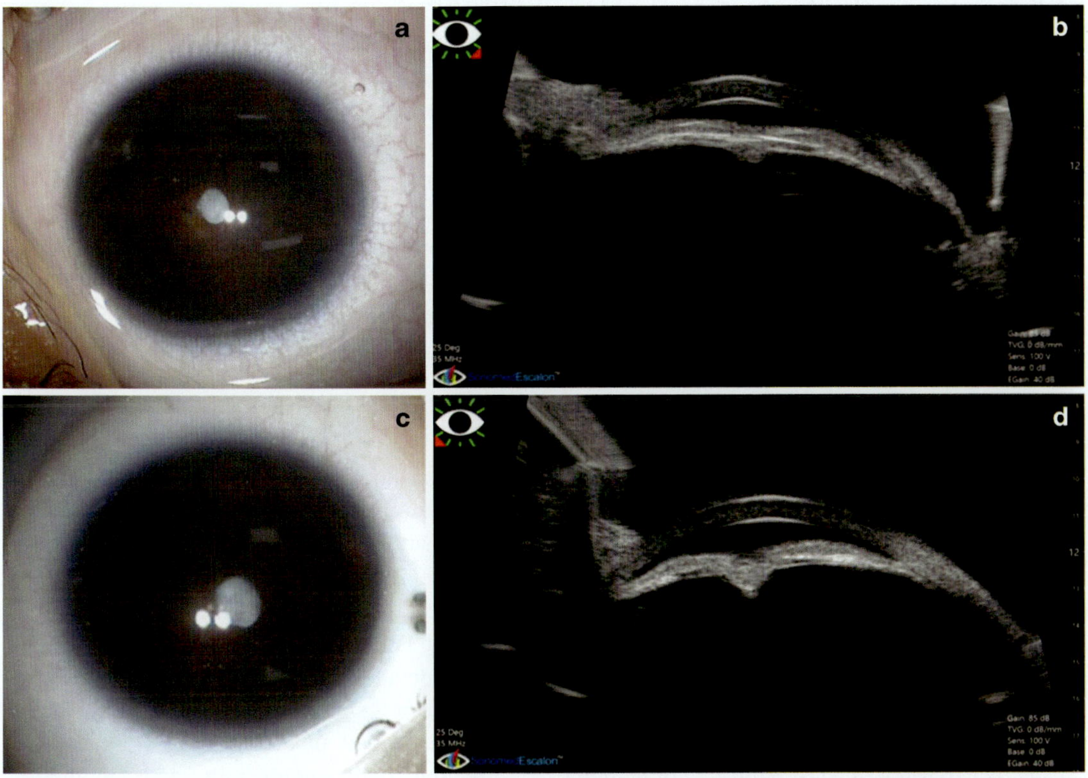

Fig. 14.3 (**a**, **c**) Two-month-old infant with clinical picture showing microphthalmos, small pupil, atrophic iris and cataract of right and left eye, respectively, (**b**, **d**) showing microphthalmos, microcornea, shallow anterior chamber, and membranous cataract on ultrasound biomicroscopy of the same patient

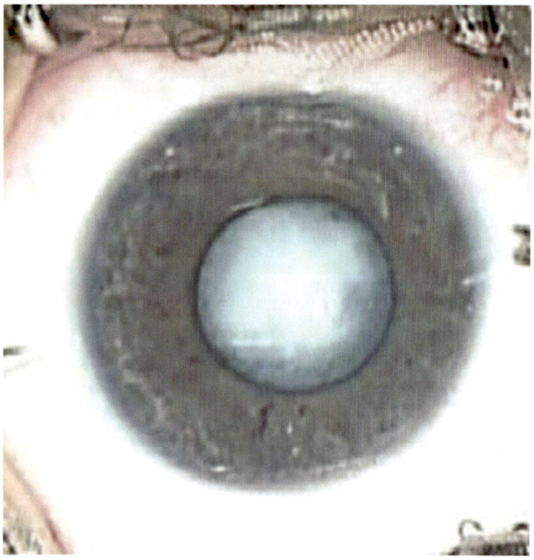

Fig. 14.4 Hazy cornea, atrophic iris, and cataract in infant with CRS

14.5.1 Preoperative Evaluation

It starts with a good history taking, also including various investigations to confirm the diagnosis and prognosticating the disease. It is equally important to emphasize the need for counseling the parents to relieve their anxiety and fear related to the condition in their child.

1. History—a thorough history to rule out the presence of fever with rash in antenatal period should be taken.
2. Investigation—TORCH profile done in cases with bilateral congenital cataract where there is high clinical suspicion based on ocular or systemic findings.

   In children infected with rubella, the specific IgM is present up to 3 months of age in all confirmed cases. It is present in 86% at the age of 3–6 months, 62% at 6 months to 1 year, and 42% at 12–18 months, rarely above 18 months. Maternally transferred rubella specific IgG disappears by around 6 months of age. A persistent level of High IgG or Rubella specific IgG during the age of 1–2 years is an indication to congenital infection by this organism. Antibody levels are higher after congenital infection than after vaccination [37]. In addition, due to multisystem involvement seen in these conditions an appropriate systemic evaluation has to be undertaken in these patients.

   Cardiology evaluation may reveal the presence of patent ductus arteriosus, pulmonary stenosis, ventricular septal defect, and atrial septal defect and any of these if seen have to be tackled accordingly. Neurology evaluation is done in cases with seizure and gross developmental delay. ENT evaluation should be done to rule out sensorineural hearing loss.
3. Parent counseling—It is particularly important in these cases as there is a higher rate of both intraoperative and postoperative surgical complications as compared to normal pediatric cataract surgery with normal axial length. Parents should be explained that in eyes with microphthalmos and or microcornea due to TORCH infection there is a chance of increased tissue manipulation during surgery. This in turn leads to increase in the postoperative complications including anterior chamber inflammation, posterior synechiae, glaucoma, and posterior capsular opacification (PCO). Regarding IOL, parents need to be counseled in cases where no IOL has been inserted regarding visual rehabilitation with aphakic glasses or contact lenses.

14.5.2 Intraoperative

1. Starts with an examination under anesthesia to measure and note the various parameters like corneal diameter, keratometry and axial length. IOL may not be implanted if horizontal corneal diameter is less than 10 mm and axial length is less than 17 mm or at least two standard deviations below the mean for age [39].
2. Anterior segment examination: Gonioscopy is performed in each patient suspected of having shallow angle with Swan Jacob goiniolens to observe for crowding of angle and also to compare the anterior chamber angles between the two eyes. Ultrasound biomi-

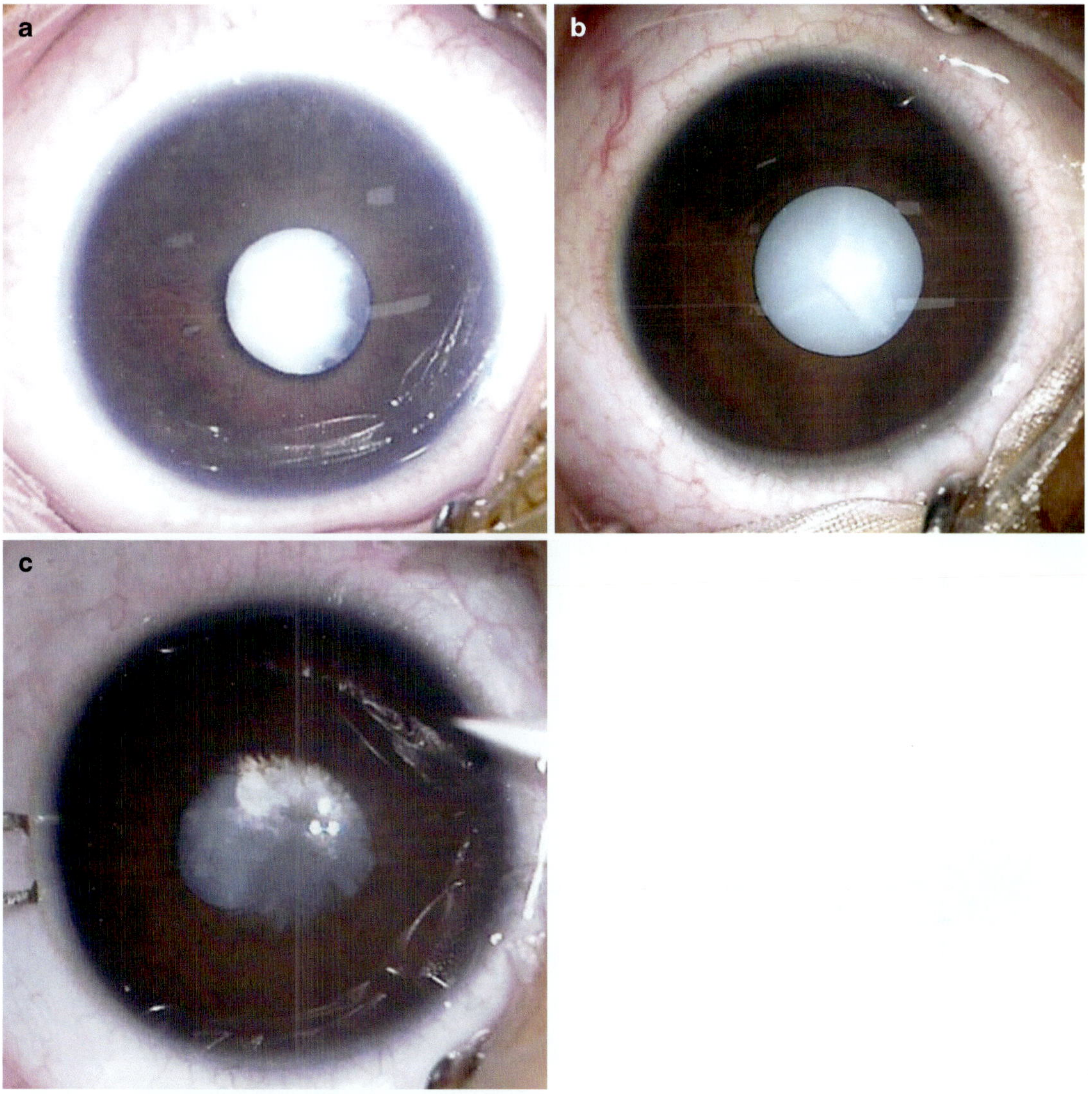

Fig. 14.5 CRS with iris abnormality. (**a**) Patchy iris atrophy with non-dilating pupil with membraneous cataract. (**b**) Loss of normal iris pattern with diffuse iris atrophy along with total congenital cataract with plaque over anterior capsule (**c**) Iris atrophy with posterior synechiae with membranous calcified cataract

croscopy (UBM) may also be done to evaluate the angle, anterior chamber depth, lens thickness, bag to bag diameter, measurement of natural lens and also to know status of posterior capsule of lens.

3. Incision: In eyes with microcornea and microphthalmos—length of clear corneal incision made is kept smaller or scleral entry to anterior chamber can be done to minimize corneal trauma and postoperative decompensation. Two such incisions should be made, 180° apart in nasal and temporal quadrants. The corneal incision must be meticulously built in order to prevent iris prolapse and maintain a stable anterior chamber intra- and postoperatively. In microcornea, IOL is not implanted so it averts the need for a 2.2/2.8 mm superior incision.
4. Anterior chamber depth: In microphthalmos, anterior chamber is on shallower side, so the

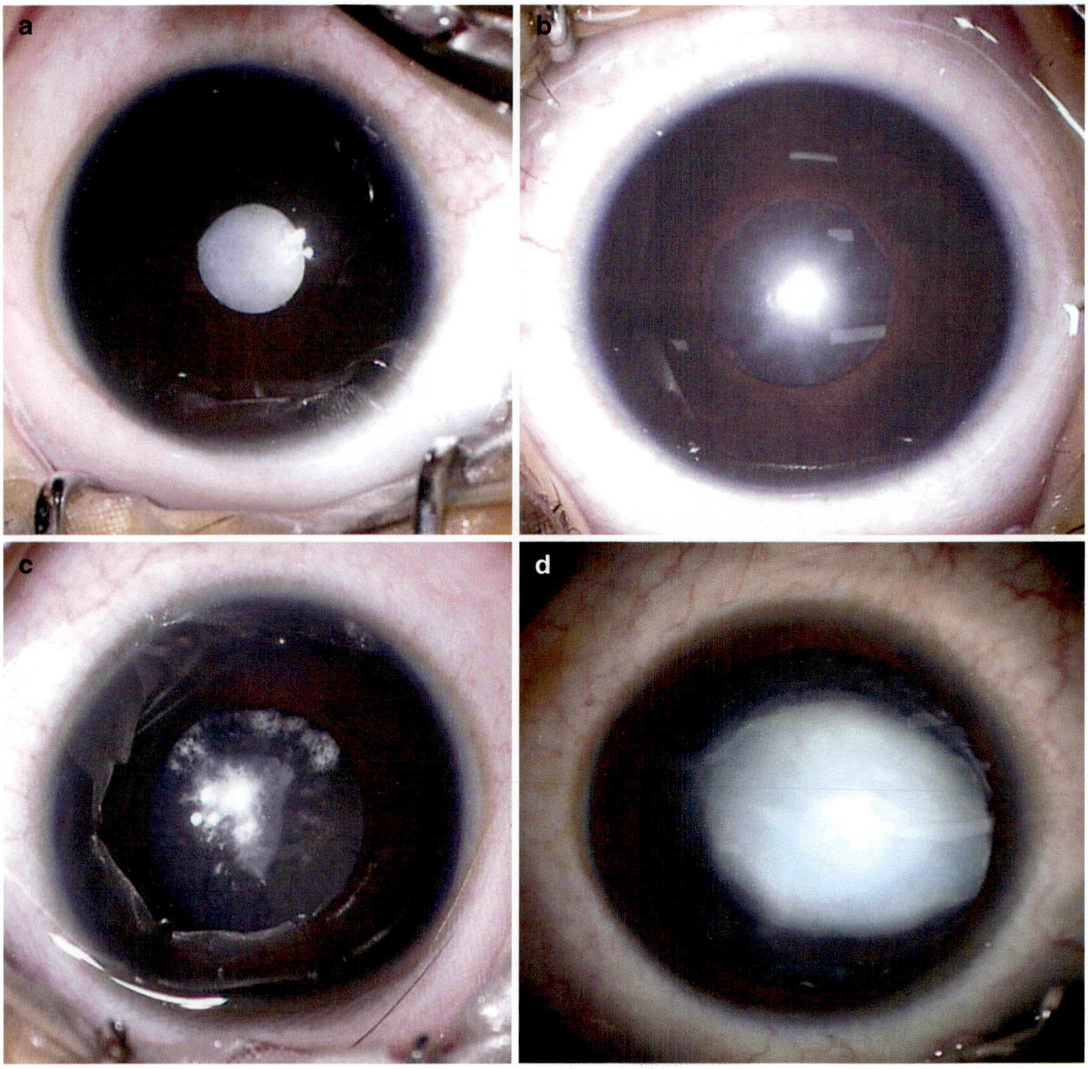

Fig. 14.6 Different type of cataract in CRS. (**a**) Total cataract, (**b**) nuclear cataract, (**c**) absorbed cataract, (**d**) membranous cataract

distance between the lens and corneal endothelium is reduced hence restricting the space for maneuvering during surgery. Arshinoff's soft-shell method may be useful in such cases. First cohesive ophthalmic viscosurgical device (OVD) is injected into the center of the anterior chamber in order to inflate the anterior chamber and then a dispersive OVD is injected on top to protect the corneal endothelium [40].

5. Management of a small pupil: In Cataract due to TORCH infection particularly rubella, children may have poorly or non-dilating pupils and/or posterior synechiae. If adequate pupil dilation is not achieved after intracameral injection of mydriatics and release of posterior synechiae, cohesive OVDs may be used to facilitate mydriasis [41]. If pupil is still not dilating with cohesive OVDs, adequate size pupilloplasty

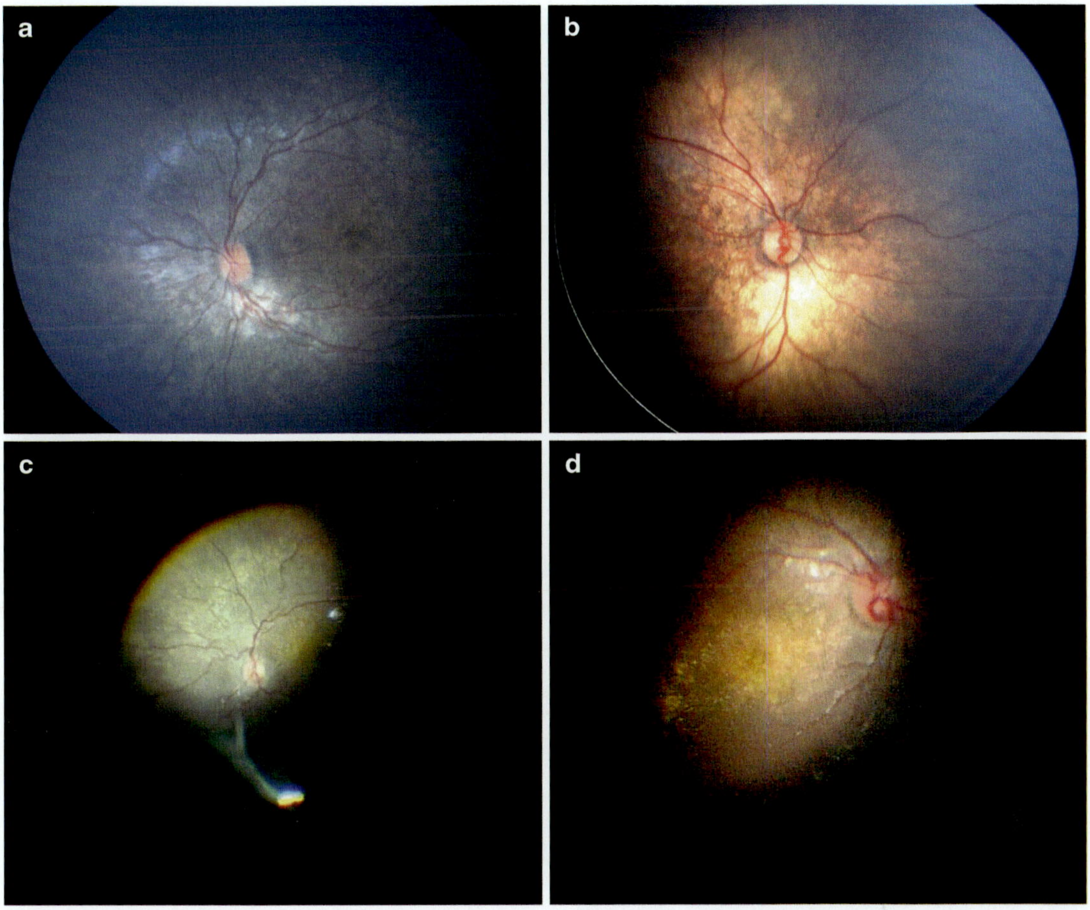

Fig. 14.7 Retinal changes in CRS. (**a**) Retcam picture showing mild salt and pepper retinopathy at macula. (**b**) Chorioretinal atrophy with Salt and pepper retinopathy. (**c**, **d**) Intraoperative fundus view with wide angle viewing system with anterior route showing rubella pigmentary retinopathy (**c**) and maculopathy (**d**)

should be done with vitrectomy cutter. This will also reduce future incidence of VAO.

6. Continuous curvilinear capsulorrhexis (CCC): Anterior continuous curvilinear capsulorhexis in microphthalmic eyes is little challenging and complicated because of shallow anterior chamber, elevated intraocular pressure and extreme elasticity of the anterior capsule in all pediatric cataract [42]. Staining of anterior capsule of lens with trypan blue dye is done under air this is preferred method. This is followed by expanding the anterior chamber by cohesive OVD till the anterior capsule becomes flat and this enables a sufficient operating space and also counteracts the elevated posterior pressure. In some cases, cataract is membranous with fibrosed and fused anterior capsule. In such cases, incision is made on the fibrosed capsule with MVR blade and rhexis is completed 360° with the help of microvitreoretinal scissor (Fig. 14.8).
7. Hydrodissection and lens aspiration: Mild hydrodissection in all quadrants aids in lowering surgical time period and improving the cortical clean up [43]. Lens matter can be aspirated by either Coaxial or bimanual methods. Bimanual method of lens matter

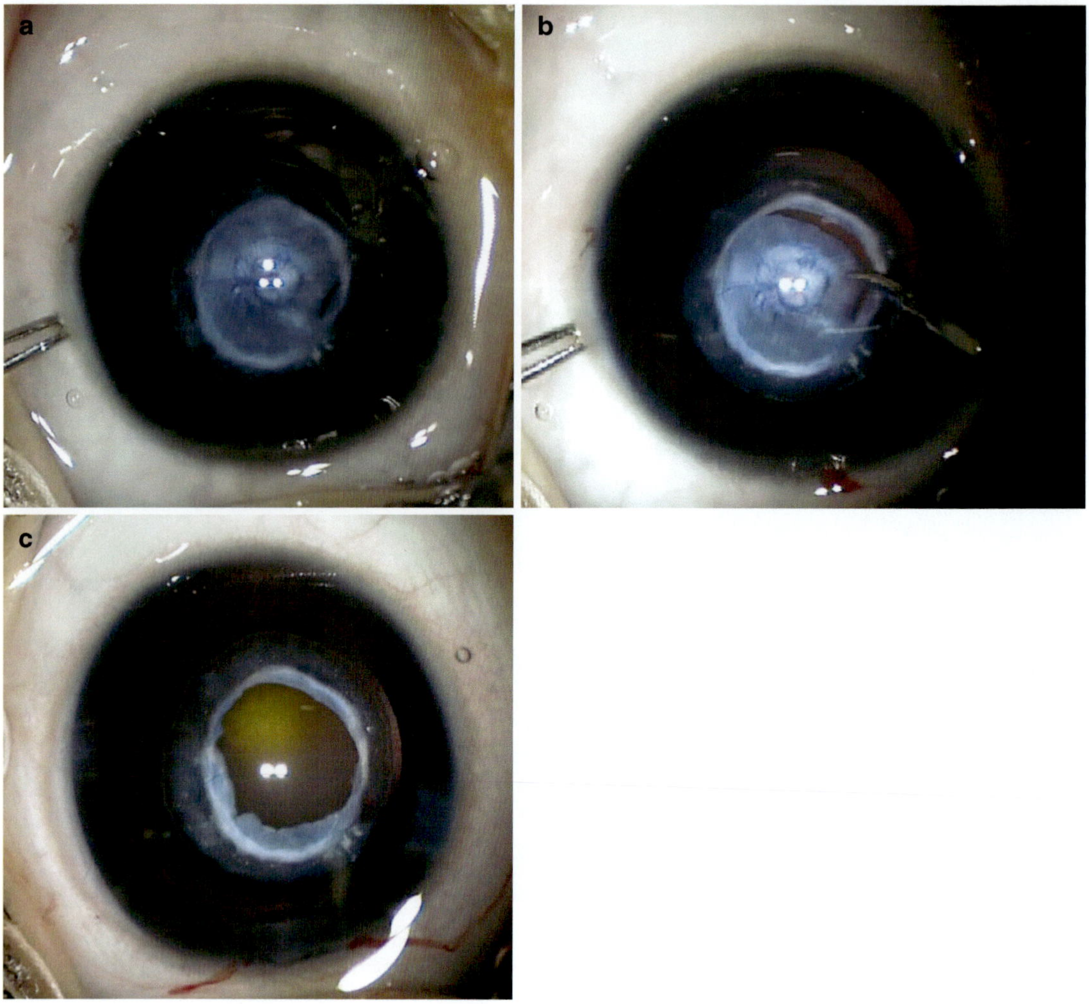

Fig. 14.8 Intraoperative picture of a patient with CRS with absorbed cataract with fibrosis of capsule (**a**) Incision with MVR is made in the fused anterior and posterior capsule. (**b**) Central 4 mm opening is made with microincision. (**c**) Anterior vitrectomy is done after making opening, 360 support is present for IOL insertion in sulcus

aspiration is preferred as it helps in complete removal of lens matter including subincisional one. It additionally provides improve chamber stability and more meticulous lens aspiration.

8. Posterior capsulorhexis and anterior vitrectomy: Pediatric cataract with TORCH infection has high incidence of VAO formation compared to normal [44]. Posterior capsulorhexis with or without anterior vitrectomy has been used to lessen VAO formation since 1980s [45]. This is standard method of prevention of VAO formation in pediatric cataract surgery and it is advocated by many previous studies [46–49]. So, we suggest posterior capsulorhexis in pediatric patients up to 8 years of age and anterior vitrectomy up to 6 years of age specially in cataract with TORCH infection [39, 50]. Procedure has been discussed in detail in Chap. 3.
9. IOL implantation: IOL should not be implanted in eyes with severe microcornea

or microphthalmos. If the Axial Length is >17 mm and white to white distance is >10 mm then IOL can be implanted to reduce the postoperative refractive error and amblyopia [39]. Peripheral iridectomy should be done if IOL is not implanted.

10. Viscoelastic removal and wound suturing: All Viscoelastic substance should be removed from the chamber at the end of surgery. In most of the cases high molecular weight OVD is used, so aspiration is generally easy and fast. In the end main incision which is used for IOL implantation must be sutured with 10-0 nylon suture to prevent wound leakage and thus minimize the risk of hypotony. Side incision is closed with wound hydration and if in cases side wound is leaking then wound must be secured with 10-0 nylon suture.

14.6 Complication

1. Corneal injury: Risk of corneal injury is more in patients with microphthalmic eye because of the shallow anterior chamber which reduces the distance between the instruments and the cornea, making the eye more susceptible to corneal endothelial injury.
2. Posterior synechiae: Posterior synechiae is one of the important postoperative complications of pediatric cataract extraction with infective etiology. In microphthalmos with cataract the incidence of posterior synechiae formation after surgery reported is as much as 35.7–59.5% [51, 52]. The cause of posterior synechiae formation is intense postoperative anterior chamber inflammation. This may be due to release of rubella virus from intralenticular space and thus causes severe inflammation either by direct viral insults or by delayed hypersensitivity reaction. Live rubella virus has been isolated from the lens till 3 years of age [44]. Good postoperative inflammatory control with mydriatics like atropine 1% and intensive topical steroids minimize the formation posterior synechiae.
3. Glaucoma: Pediatric cataract with infective etiology with microphthalmos has a crowding of anterior chamber angle and thus is susceptible to postoperative glaucoma. Incidence of secondary glaucoma in cataract surgery with micropthalmos is 30.9–43.2% of patients [51, 52]. Management includes inclusion of a peripheral iridectomy during cataract surgery and adequate anterior vitrectomy and meticulous control of inflammation in postoperative period.
4. Visual axis opacification: Children have high incidence of visual axis opacification because of younger age and of course in this case incidence increases due to infective etiology of cataract. VAO after cataract surgery in microphthalmos range from 16.6 to 24.3% [51, 52].

14.7 Visual Rehabilitation

It is suggested that in eyes with microphthalmia, IOL implantation should be deferred to lessen the risks of complications such as posterior synechiae and glaucoma [51, 53]. The general management for aphakia after cataract extraction is wearing spectacles or contact lenses and follow up at regular interval. Most important is counseling of parents to encourage the use of glasses. Refraction should be done at regular interval. Parents must ensure that child is wearing glass with latest refractive power. In unilateral aphakia amblyopia therapy should be given. Alternate to spectacles is use of contact lens. In future, Secondary IOL implantation may be planned on the basis of growth of the aphakic eye.

Spectacles: It is the most important form of refractive correction in patients with binocular aphakia specially in developing countries. Advantages of glasses include affordability, safe, easy to wear compared to contact lens, can be replaced readily and monofocal and bifocal design are available.

Disadvantages are:

Cosmetic blemish and cumbersome to wear—Aphakic glasses are thick and heavy, which causes cosmetic blemish. In infant and younger kids, the nose bridge and ears are not fully developed, which makes it tough to achieve a solid suit for the spectacles.

Others problems are image magnification, restricted field of vision, colored vision, spherical aberration, prismatic aberration

Contacts lens—Contact lens is one of the best devices to visually rehabilitate the children with aphakia specially in unilateral cases.

Advantages are less magnification of image, elimination of aberration, wider and better field of view and cosmetically more acceptable.

Disadvantages are compliance in young children is poor, costly, allergic hypersensitivity to lens some may develop corneal infection.

14.8 Conclusion

Cataract with infective etiology is usually bilateral and the children often have systemic association. Most of the patients have other ocular morbidity besides having cataract. So, doing surgery in these cases is challenging. IOL implantation should be delayed in microphthalmos in view of many postoperative complications. Postoperative complications like VAO, posterior synechiae, secondary glaucoma is more in this type of cataract. These complications can be minimized with proper preoperative planning, meticulous surgery and judicious control of inflammation in postoperative period. Most of the patients can achieve good vision with proper management.

References

1. Matoba A. Ocular viral infections. Pediatr Infect Dis. 1984;3:358–68.
2. Cotlier E. Congenital varicella cataract. Am J Ophthalmol. 1978;86:627–9.
3. Mahalakshmi B, Therese KL, Devipriya U, Pushpalatha V, Margarita S, Madhavan HN. Infectious aetiology of congenital cataract based on TORCHES screening in a tertiary eye hospital in Chennai, Tamil Nadu, India. Indian J Med Res. 2010;131:559–64.
4. Raghu H, Subhan S, Jose RJ, Gangopadhyay N, Bhende J, Sharma S. Herpes simplex virus-1-associated congenital cataract. Am J Ophthalmol. 2004;138:313–4.
5. Madhavan HN. Laboratory investigations on viral and chlamydia trachomatis infections of the eye: Sankara Nethralaya experiences. Indian J Ophthalmol. 1999;47:241–6.
6. Li Z, Yan C, Liu P, Yan R, Feng Z. Prevalence of serum antibodies to TORCH among women before pregnancy or in the early period of pregnancy in Beijing. Clin Chim Acta. 2009;403:212–5.
7. Mahalakshmi B, Therese KL, Shyamala G, Devipriya U, Madhavan HN. Toxoplasma gondii detection by nested polymerase chain reaction in lens aspirate and peripheral blood leukocyte in congenital cataract patients - the first report from a tertiary eye hospital in India. Curr Eye Res. 2007;32:653–7.
8. Shyamala G, Sowmya P, Madhavan HN, Malathi J. Relative efficiency of polymerase chain reaction and enzyme-linked immunosorbent assay in determination of viral etiology in congenital cataract in infants. J Postgrad Med. 2008;54:17–20.
9. Lu B, Yang Y. Detection of TORCH pathogens in children with congenital cataracts. Exp Ther Med. 2016;12(2):1159–64.
10. Krummenacher C, Baribaud F, Ponce de Leon M, Baribaud I, Whitbeck JC, Xu R, Cohen GH, Eisenberg RJ. Comparative usage of herpesvirus entry mediator A and nectin-1 by laboratory strains and clinical isolates of herpes simplex virus. Virology. 2004;322:286–99.
11. Mets MB. Eye manifestations of intrauterine infections. Ophthalmol Clin North Am. 2001;14:521–31.
12. Kota AS, Shabbir N. Congenital toxoplasmosis. [Updated 2019 Sep 22]. In: StatPearls [Internet]. Treasure Island: StatPearls Publishing; 2020. https://www.ncbi.nlm.nih.gov/books/NBK545228/
13. McLeod R, Boyer K, Karrison T, Kasza K, Swisher C, Roizen N, et al. Outcome of treatment for congenital toxoplasmosis, 1981-2004: The National Collaborative Chicago-Based, Congenital Toxoplasmosis Study. Clin Infect Dis. 2006;42:1383–94.
14. McAuley J, Boyer K, Patel D, Mets M, Swisher C, Roizen N, et al. Early and longitudinal evaluations of treated infants and children and untreated historical patients with congenital toxoplasmosis. The Chicago Collaborative Treatment Trial. Clin Infect Dis. 1994;18:38–72.
15. Mets M, Holfels E, Boyer KM, Swisher C, Roizen N, Stein L, et al. Eye manifestations of congenital toxoplasmosis. Am J Ophthalmol. 1996;122:309–24.
16. Vutova K, Peicheva Z, Popova A, Markova V, Mincheva N, Todorov T. Congenital toxoplasmosis: eye manifestations in infants and children. Ann Trop Paediatr. 2002;22:213–8.
17. Vutova K, Peicheva Z, Popova A, Markova V, Mincheva N, Todorov T. Congenital toxoplasmosis:

eye manifestations in infants and children. Ann Trop Paediatr. 2002;22:213–8.
18. Datta S, Banerjee DP. Chorioretinitis in congenital toxoplasmosis. Indian Pediatr. 2003;40:790–1.
19. Mittal V, Bhatia R, Singh VK, Sengal S. Low incidence of congenital toxoplasmosis in Indian children. J Trop Pediatr. 1995;41:62–3.
20. O'Neill JF. The ocular manifestations of congenital infection: a study of the early effect and long-term outcome of maternally transmitted rubella and toxoplasmosis. Trans Am Ophthalmol Soc. 1998;96:813–79.
21. Dobbins J, Stewart J, Demmler G. Surveillance of congenital cytomegalovirus disease, 1990-1991: Collaborating Registry Group. MMWR Morb Mortal Wkly Rep. 1992;41:35–9.
22. Malm G, Engman M-L. Congenital cytomegalovirus infections. Semin Fetal Neonatal Med. 2007;12(3):154–9. https://doi.org/10.1016/j.siny.2007.01.012.
23. Boniuk I. The cytomegalovirus and the eye. Int Ophthalmol Clin. 1972;12:169–90.
24. Tarkkanen A, Merenmies L, Holmstrom T. Ocular involvement in congenital cytomegalic inclusion disease. J Pediatr Ophthalmol. 1972;9:82–6.
25. Hittner HM, Desmond MM, Montgomery JR. Optic nerve manifestations of human congenital cytomegalovirus infection. Am J Ophthalmol. 1976;81:661–5.
26. Feigin R, Cherry J. Textbook of pediatric infectious disease, vol. 1. 4th ed. Philadelphia: WB Saunders; 1998.
27. Whitley RJ, Kimberlin DW, Roizman B. Herpes simplex viruses. Clin Infect Dis. 1998;26:541–55.
28. Madhavan HN. Laboratory investigations on viral and chlamydia trachomatis infections of the eye: Sankara Nethralaya experiences. Indian J Ophthalmol. 1999;47:241–6.
29. Shyamala G, Sowmya P, Madhavan HN, Malathi J. Relative efficiency of polymerase chain reaction and enzyme-linked immunosorbant assay in determination of viral etiology in congenital cataract in infants. J Postgrad Med. 2008;54:17–20.
30. Gregg NM. Congenital cataract following German measles in the mother. Trans Ophthalmol Soc Aust. 1941;3:35–46.
31. Papania MJ, Wallace GS, Rota PA, Icenogle JP, Fiebelkorn AP, Armstrong GL, Reef SE, Redd SB, Abernathy ES, Barskey AE, Hao L, McLean HQ, Rota JS, Bellini WJ, Seward JF. Elimination of endemic measles, rubella, and congenital rubella syndrome from the Western hemisphere; the US experience. JAMA Pediatr. 2014;168:148–55.
32. Sheridan E, Aitken C, Jeffries D, Hird M, Thayalasekaran P. Congenital rubella syndrome: a risk in immigrant populations. Lancet. 2002;359:674–5.
33. World Health Organization. Surveillance guidelines for measles, rubella and congenital rubella syndrome in the WHO European Region. http://www.euro.who.int/__data/assets/pdf_file/0018/79020/e93035-2013.pdf?ua=1.
34. Cooper LZ, Ziring PR, Ockerse AB, Fedun BA, Kiely B, Krugman S. Rubella clinical manifestations and management. Am J Dis Child. 1969;118:18–9.
35. Vijayalakshmi P, Kakkar G, Samprathi A, et al. Ocular manifestations of congenital rubella syndrome in a developing country. Indian J Ophthalmol. 2002;50:307–11.
36. Vijayalakshmi P, Rajasundari TA, Prasad NM, et al. Prevalence of eye signs in congenital rubella syndrome in South India: a role for population screening. Br J Ophthalmol. 2007;91:1467–70.
37. Boger WP III, Petersen RA, Robb RM. Spontaneous absorption of the lens in the congenital rubella syndrome. Arch Ophthalmol. 1981;99:433–4.
38. Williams LL, Lew HM, Davidorf FH, et al. Altered membrane fatty acids of cultured human retinal pigment epithelium persistently infected with rubella virus may affect secondary cellular function. Arch Virol. 1994;134:379–92.
39. Khokhar SK, Pillay G, Dhull C, Agarwal E, Mahabir M, Aggarwal P. Pediatric cataract. Indian J Ophthalmol. 2017;65(12):1340–9.
40. Arshinoff SA. Dispersive-cohesive viscoelastic soft shell technique. J Cataract Refract Surg. 1999;25(2):167–73.
41. Jhanji V, Sharma N, Vajpayee RB. Management of intraoperative miosis during pediatric cataract surgery using healon 5. Middle East Afr J Ophthalmol. 2011;18(1):55–7.
42. Yu SY, Lee JH, Chang BL. Surgical management of congenital cataract associated with severe microphthalmos. J Cataract Refract Surg. 2000;26(8):1219–24.
43. Vasavada AR, Trivedi RH, Apple DJ, et al. Randomized, clinical trial of multiquadrant hydrodissection in pediatric cataract surgery. Am J Ophthalmol. 2003;135:84–8.
44. Cordes FC. Surgery of congenital cataracts. Am J Ophthal. 1948;31:1073.
45. Parks MM. Management of the posterior capsule in congenital cataracts. J Pediatr Ophthalmol Strabismus. 1984;21:114–7.
46. BenEzra D, Cohen E. Posterior capsulectomy in pediatric cataract surgery the necessity of a choice. Ophthalmology. 1997;104:2168–74.
47. Vasavada A, Desai J. Primary posterior capsulorhexis with and without anterior vitrectomy in congenital cataracts. J Cataract Refract Surg. 1997;23(Suppl 1):645–51.
48. Alexandrakis G, Peterseim MM, Wilson ME. Clinical outcomes of pars plana capsulotomy with anterior vitrectomy in pediatric cataract surgery. J AAPOS. 2002;6:163–7.
49. Guo S, Wagner RS, Caputo A. Management of the anterior and posterior lens capsules and vitreous in pediatric cataract surgery. J Pediatr Ophthalmol Strabismus. 2004;41:330–7.
50. Lin AA, Buckley EG. Update on pediatric cataract surgery and intraocular lens implantation. Curr Opin Ophthalmol. 2010;21:55–9.

51. Vasavada VA, Dixit NV, Ravat FA, Praveen MR, Shah SK, Vasavada V, Vasavada AR, Trivedi RH. Intraoperative performance and postoperative outcomes of cataract surgery in infant eyes with microphthalmos. J Cataract Refract Surg. 2009;35:519–28.
52. Shah SK, Praveen MR, Vasavada AR, Vasavada VA, Carelli R, Trivedi RH, Rasoebala V. Long-term longitudinal assessment of postoperative outcomes after congenital cataract surgery in children with congenital rubella syndrome. J Cataract Refract Surg. 2014;40(12):2091–8. https://doi.org/10.1016/j.jcrs.2014.04.028.
53. Yu YS, Kim SJ, Choung HK. Posterior chamber intraocular lens implantation in pediatric cataract with microcornea and/or microphthalmos. Korean J Ophthalmol. 2006;20(3):151–5.

Congenital Glaucoma and Anterior Segment Dysgenesis

15

Chirakshi Dhull and Sudarshan Kumar Khokhar

Childhood cataract may occur in association with ocular comorbidities involving cornea, angle structures, and/or iris. These abnormalities may include congenital glaucoma and anterior segment dysgenesis. These associated abnormalities may alter presentation and management of these conditions. In this chapter, we will discuss these two entities in separate section. They have been clubbed together since anterior segment dysgenesis is associated with glaucoma in significant number of cases and few cases of presumed primary congenital glaucoma may actually be secondary to anterior segment dysgenesis.

15.1 Childhood Glaucoma

- Introduction
- Clinical presentation
- Investigations
- Surgical outcomes

Supplementary Information The online version of this chapter (https://doi.org/10.1007/978-981-16-0212-2_15) contains supplementary material, which is available to authorized users.

C. Dhull (✉)
Eye Q Hospital, Rohtak, Haryana, India

S. K. Khokhar
Professor Ophthalmology, Dr. RP Centre for Ophthalmic Sciences, All India Institute of Medical Sciences, New Delhi, India

15.1.1 Introduction

Primary congenital glaucoma (PCG) is an anomaly affecting anterior chamber angle which leads to obstruction of aqueous outflow, increased intraocular pressure (IOP) and optic nerve damage [1]. Buphthalmos is an alternate term used to describe congenital glaucoma. Buphthalmos means "bull's eye." It is used to describe visible enlargement of the eyeball and clouding of cornea at birth or early childhood due to uncontrolled glaucoma [2]. High intraocular pressure (IOP) causes increase in axial length and corneal dimensions of the eye, leading to axial myopia, stretched limbus, corneal thinning and visibly enlarged eyeballs. The common causes of buphthalmos include primary congenital glaucoma (PCG), Sturge-Weber syndrome, neurofibromatosis, and aniridia [2].

Incidence of PCG is one in every 10,000–15,000 live births which accounts for 0.01–0.04% of total blindness [3]. It is bilateral in up to 80% of cases and two-third of cases are males. Most cases are sporadic (90%) [4]. However, in the remaining 10%, there appears to be a strong familial component.

15.1.2 Clinical Presentation

PCG patients may present with corneal haze, enlarged eye size, or abnormal eye move-

S. K. Khokhar, C. Dhull (eds.), *Essentials of Pediatric Cataract Surgery*, https://doi.org/10.1007/978-981-16-0212-2_15

ments. Vision loss in these eyes may occur secondary to uncorrected refractive error, corneal opacity, optic nerve damage, amblyopia, and cataracts. Cataract may be congenital/developmental or as a sequalae to glaucoma filtration surgery. Examination findings may be variable.

- Progressive myopia and high astigmatism may be seen.
- Cornea may be hazy and presence of Haab striae is a common finding (Fig. 15.1).
- Cataract may be anterior or posterior subcapsular cataract, total or less commonly cortical or zonular cataract (Fig. 15.2). Cataract may be primary or more commonly secondary to trabeculectomy in 6–58% cases [5–7]. Zonular weakness may be present.
- Bleb in post trabeculectomy eyes with buphthalmos may be thin cystic and rarely associated with other complications (Fig. 15.3).
- Fundus examination may reveal advanced cupping. The cupping may be reversible in small children. Features associated with pathological myopia may be seen.

15.1.3 Investigations

In addition to usual investigations, Ultrasound biomicroscopy (UBM) can be used for measurement of angle to angle and bag diameter and aid in planning of surgery (Fig. 15.4). UBM also helps to assess anterior segment structures, anterior chamber depth (ACD), angle anomalies, abnormal iris insertion, helps assess sulcus-to-sulcus measurement and identifies lax zonules and posterior capsular defect preoperatively [8].

15.1.3.1 Management of Cataract in Buphthalmic Eyes

Apart from the routine challenges encountered, there are additional surgical difficulties faced by surgeon while operating cataract in buphthalmic eyes. These include the following:

- **Corneal haze** may cause difficulty in visualization during surgery (Fig. 15.5). IOP should be controlled before surgery. We recommend use of dye for staining of anterior capsule in such cases. Posterior capsule may also require staining if visibility is low.

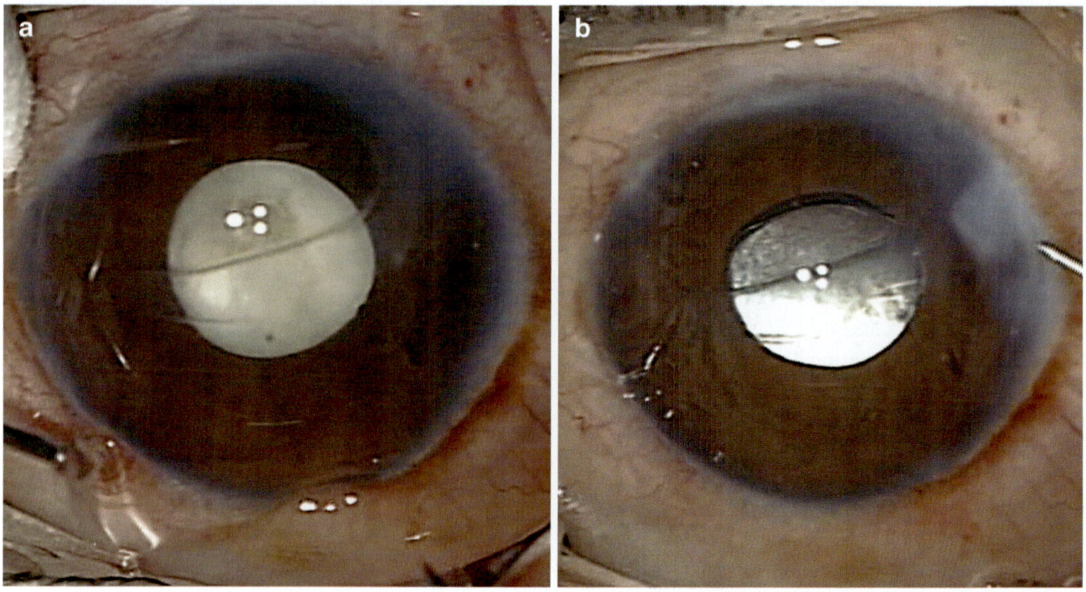

Fig. 15.1 Congenital glaucoma with Haab striae and total cataract. (**a**) Preoperative picture where large superior and multiple peripheral Haab striae. (**b**) Postoperative picture with IOL in situ and more pronounced Haab striae

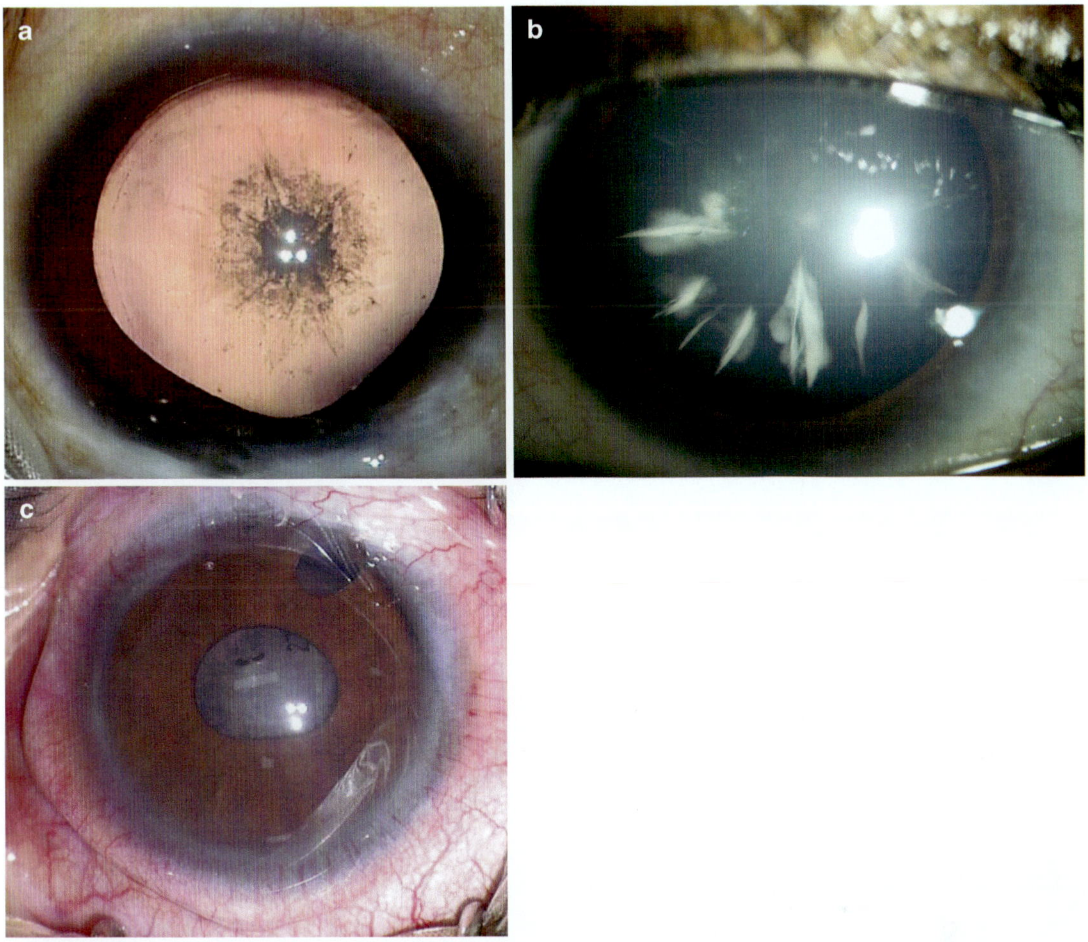

Fig. 15.2 Morphology in cataract with childhood glaucoma post trabeculectomy. (**a**) Posterior subcapsular cataract. (**b**) Cortical cataract. (**c**) Diffuse cataract with large superonasal peripheral iridotomy

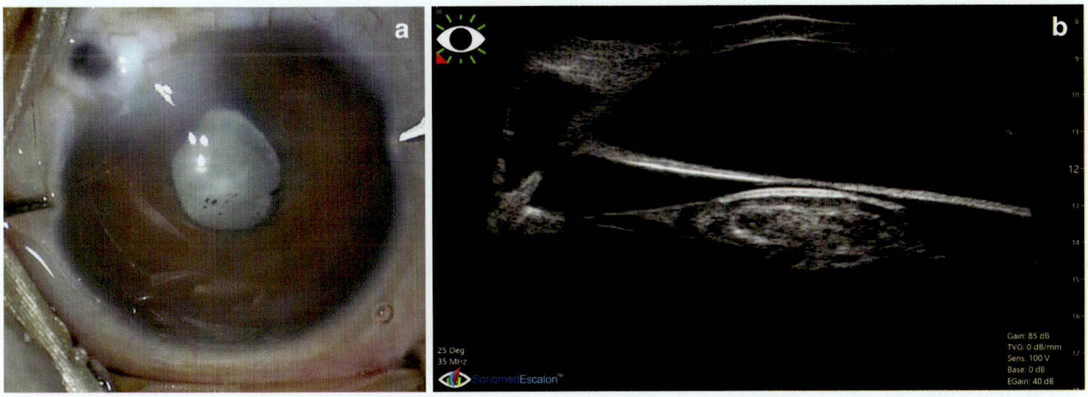

Fig. 15.3 Post trabeculectomy thin cystic bleb with iris prolapse from the ostium and total cataract. (**a**) Clinical picture. (**b**) Ultrasound biomicroscopy of the same showing patent ostium and elevated bleb

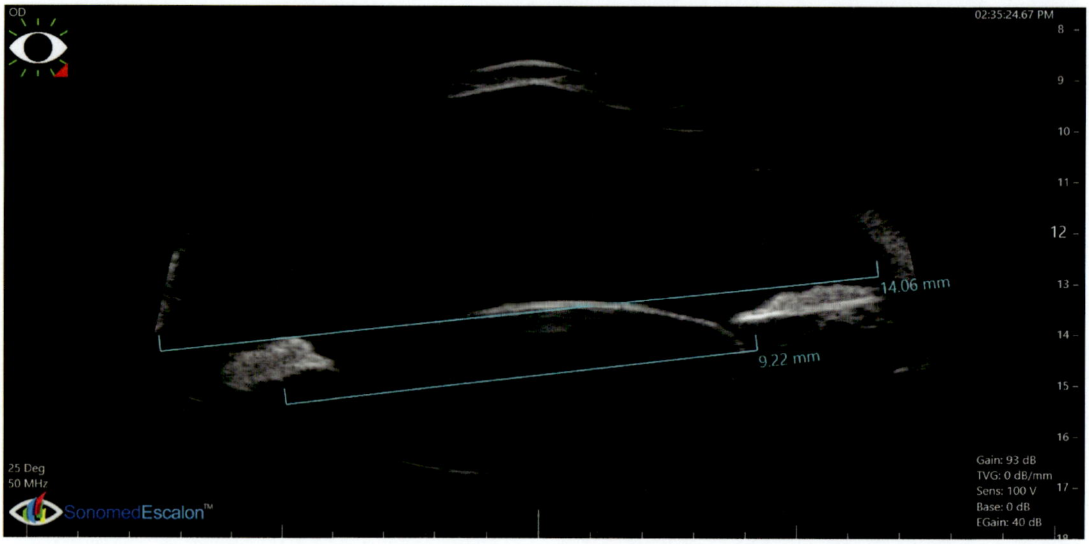

Fig. 15.4 Ultrasound biomicroscopy showing dimensions of buphthalmic eye. Complete white to white examination is not possible in single view. (**a**) Angle to angle distance, (**b**) bag diameter

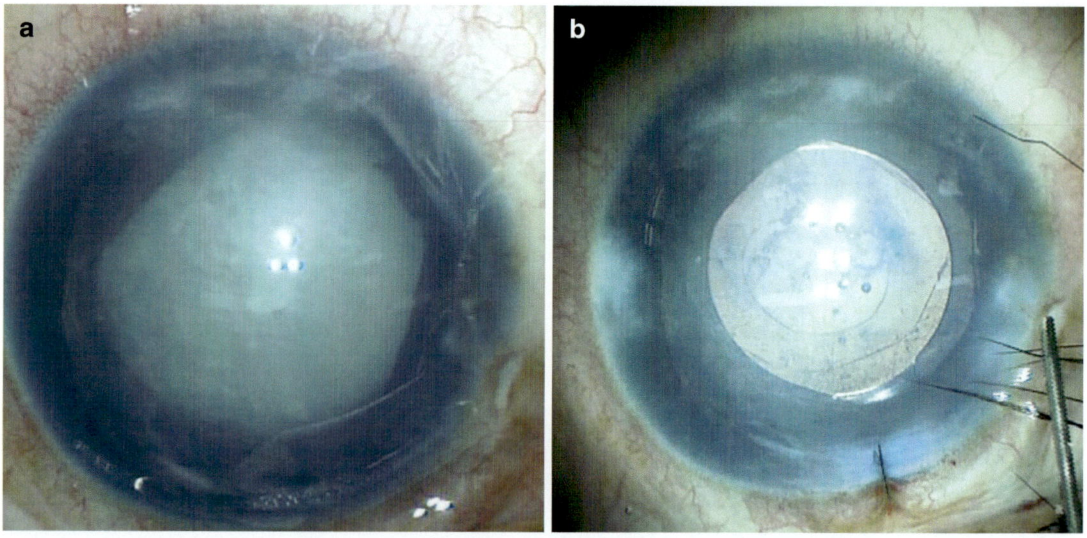

Fig. 15.5 Six-year-old child with congenital glaucoma with corneal haze with atrophic iris. (**a**) Preoperative picture with total cataract. (**b**) Postoperative picture with circular anterior and posterior capsulorhexis and IOL in bag

- **Very deep anterior chamber (AC)** may result in difficult instrumentation. Intraoperatively, anterior chamber depth may show frequent fluctuations due to low scleral rigidity. We use microincision forceps with longer arm compared to utrata's forceps for capsulorhexis. Use of bimanual irrigation and aspiration provides better control to the situation.
- **Zonular weakness:** Phacodonesis, lax lens zonules, liquefied vitreous and, thus, a weak posterior capsular support can lead to inadvertent complications. There is increased risk of vitreous loss in these patients.

- **Wound apposition**: Bupthihalmic eyes have thin sclera and cornea. Hydration alone does not provide sufficient wound closure in most cases. We recommend suturing of main wound as well as side port to prevent postoperative shallow AC.
- **IOL power calculation** remains difficult. Post-trabeculectomy buphthalmic eyes have a shift towards with-the rule astigmatism [9, 10]. As most of these eyes are high myopic, IOL power calculation should be done using appropriate IOL formulae e.g., SRK-T for axial lengths >24.5 mm. Many a times, no single IOL power formulae might be able to predict the correct emmetropic power of implant for buphthalmic eyes. Parents should be counseled preoperatively, regarding use of spectacles for distance and near vision.
- Large eye size and bag dimensions that may lead to postoperative intraocular lens (IOL) decentration [11, 12]. In the bag IOL placement with posterior capsulorhexis has been reported to be associated with decentration. The technique of IOL implantation in the sulcus with optic capture with anterior or both anterior and posterior capsule (i.e., optic in bag and haptic in sulcus) may provide satisfactory anatomical outcome (Fig. 15.6) [12].

15.1.4 Surgical Outcomes

Temporary cessation of ocular growth is reported after adequate IOP control in eyes with AL > 22 mm and in children aged 3 months or older [13].

Our experience with 31 eyes of primary congenital glaucoma (post trabeculectomy) with visually significant cataract undergoing lens aspiration surgery showed a mean best corrected visual acuity of 6/60 (Snellen's) at 1 year postoperatively. Reasonably predictable refractive results were obtained in these eyes, provided glaucoma was well controlled [14].

Thus, besides control of IOP, visual rehabilitation of buphthalmic eyes may involve appropriate management for amblyopia, keratoplasty for corneal opacity in addition to timely cataract surgery for visually significant cataract. Buphthalmic eyes undergoing cataract surgery can achieve successful refractive and visual outcomes if careful preoperative planning is carried out regarding the choice of IOL type and IOL power, taking into consideration the adequacy of intraocular pressure control, accurate biometry, assessment of bag size and use of appropriate IOL power formulae.

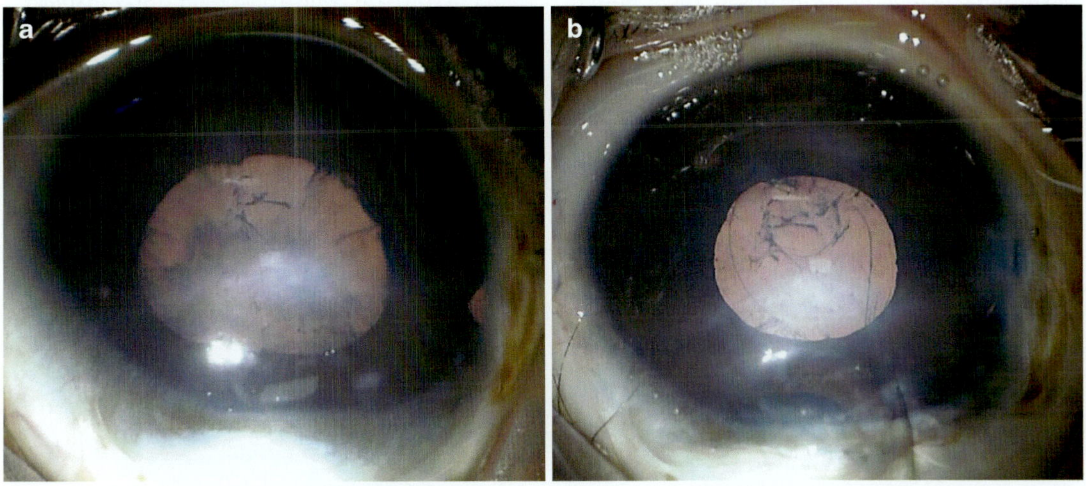

Fig. 15.6 Fifteen-month-old child with congenital glaucoma with corneal haze with Haab striae and large cornea (buphthalmos). (**a**) Preoperative picture with Anterior and posterior subcapsular cataract. (**b**) Postoperative picture with IOL in sulcus with optic capture with anterior and posterior capsulorhexis (bag complex) for better centration

15.2 Anterior Segment Dysgenesis

Anterior segment dysgenesis (ASD) is a group of disorders arising from abnormal development in cornea, iris, lens and angle structures. This includes Axenfeld's anomaly, Rieger's anomaly, Axenfeld-Rieger syndrome (ARS), Peters anomaly, sclerocornea, aniridia, posterior keratoconus, and iridogoniodysgenesis. It occurs due to abnormalities in neural crest differentiation and migration. Various classifications are used for describing ASD depending either on their clinical features or area of involvement [15–17]. Lens abnormalities are not uncommon in cases with ASD. Townsend, Font, and Zimmerman have classified ASD based on involvement as Descemet layer defect alone or associated with lens abnormalities or with iris stromal abnormalities. This involvement of lens suggested the effects of primary mesenchymal defect on the development of lens [17].

15.2.1 Embryology

The surface ectoderm invaginates and forms lens vesicle in the embryonic cup at sixth week of gestation. Then, neural-crest-derived tissue migrates in three waves beneath this surface ectoderm. The surface ectoderm forms the corneal epithelium. The three waves forms endothelium, corneal stroma, and iris stroma. Any arrest in the development of these layers may affect further development of anterior chamber leading to different presentations of ASD [18].

15.2.2 Genetics

Many genes are involved in the ASD with variable degree of penetrance. Forty percent cases occur due to involvement of PITX2 (4q25) and FOXC1 (6p25). Typically, PITX2 disruption is associated with ARS with ocular and dental abnormalities, and FOXC1 is associated with ARS with hearing or cardiac abnormalities. Others associated with ARS include PAX6 (11p13) and FOXO1A (13q14) [19, 20]. ARS has autosomal dominant inheritance pattern in 70% cases. In Peter's anomaly, rare cases have been attributed to PITX2, FOXC1, and PAX6 mutations, but the majority of cases are sporadic [21–23].

15.2.3 Clinical Features

- Axenfeld-Rieger syndrome
- Axenfeld anomaly presents as posterior embryotoxon (Fig. 15.7) (anteriorly displaced

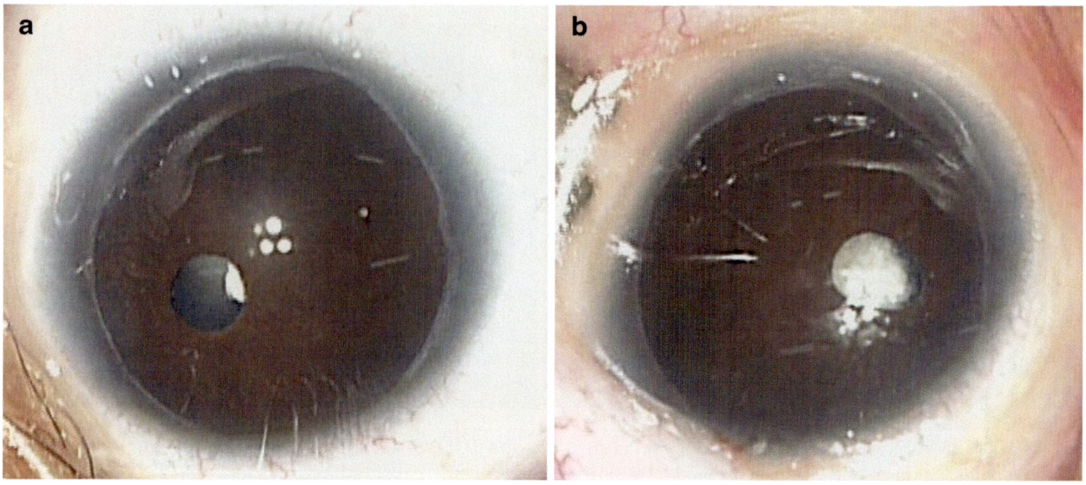

Fig. 15.7 Mild variant of Axenfield-Rieger syndrome (**a**, **b**) Posterior embryotoxon in 9-month-old child with cataract in right and left eye, respectively. Also notice presence of corectopia in both eyes

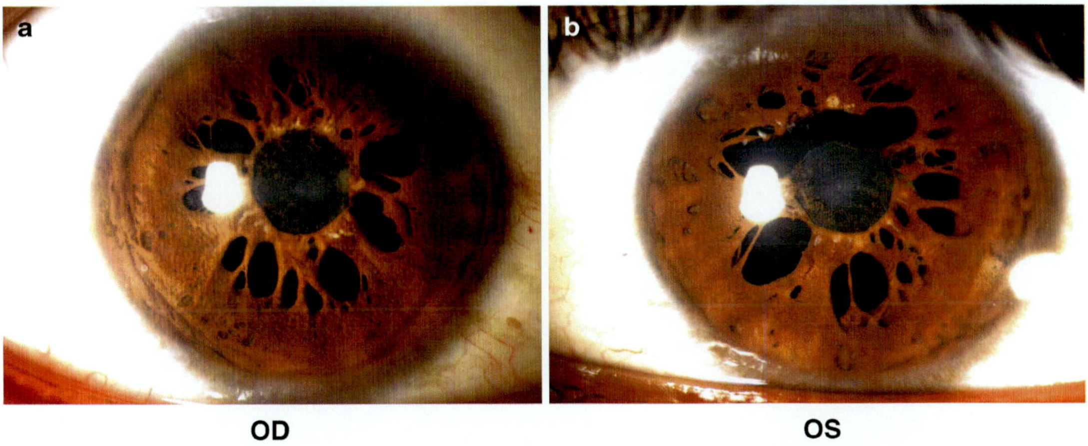

Fig. 15.8 (**a**, **b**) Rieger Anomaly-polycoria and iris atrophy in 7-year-old girl in right and left eye respectively

Schwalbe line) and iris strands adhered to the anteriorly displaced Schwalbe line. Rieger anomaly includes posterior embryotoxon, pseudopolycoria, and iris atrophy (Fig. 15.8) while Rieger syndrome is Rieger anomaly along with systemic findings including facial bone defects, hypertelorism, telecanthus, maxillary hypoplasia, dental abnormalities (microdontia and hypodontia), umbilical abnormalities or pituitary involvement. Thus, they are now considered as a spectrum of disorder termed as Axenfeld-Rieger syndrome (Fig. 15.9). It may vary from subtle changes in the angle to severe ocular changes. Systemic involvement may also include cardiac and endocrine system. Fifty percent cases with ARS are associated with glaucoma [24, 25].

- Peters anomaly
- Peter syndrome is characterized by a shallow anterior chamber, synechiae between iris and cornea and central corneal opacity. It occurs due to defect in endothelium, Descemet membrane and posterior stroma due to the defect in the migration of the neural crest cells. This syndrome can vary in severity with ocular findings ranging from unilateral mild central corneal opacity to severe bilateral microphthalmia, corneal opacification, cataract, and glaucoma. Eighty percent of cases have bilateral presentation. The Peters anomaly has been further divided into type I and type II. Type I Peters anomaly is categorized by central corneal opacity and iridocorneal adhesions (Fig. 15.10). Type II Peters anomaly has a more severe phenotype with corneal opacity and lens involvement with iridocorneal touch with or without cataract (Fig. 15.11). The Peters plus syndrome includes the anterior segment findings with systemic developmental anomalies. These include craniofacial dysmorphism, cleft lip/palate,

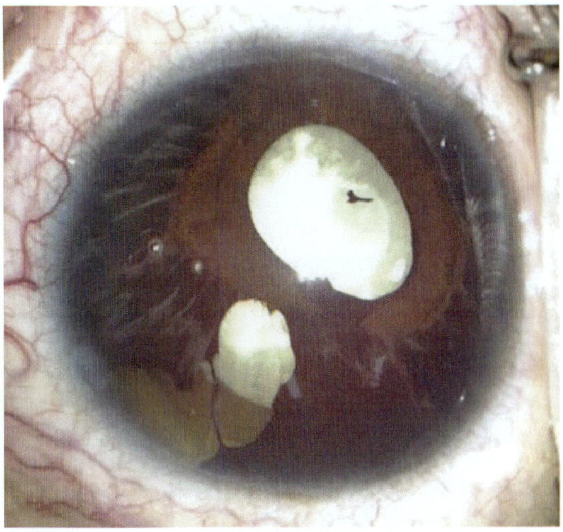

Fig. 15.9 Severe variant of Axenfield-Rieger syndrome—posterior embryotoxon with corectopia, iris atrophy and polycoria along with total cataract

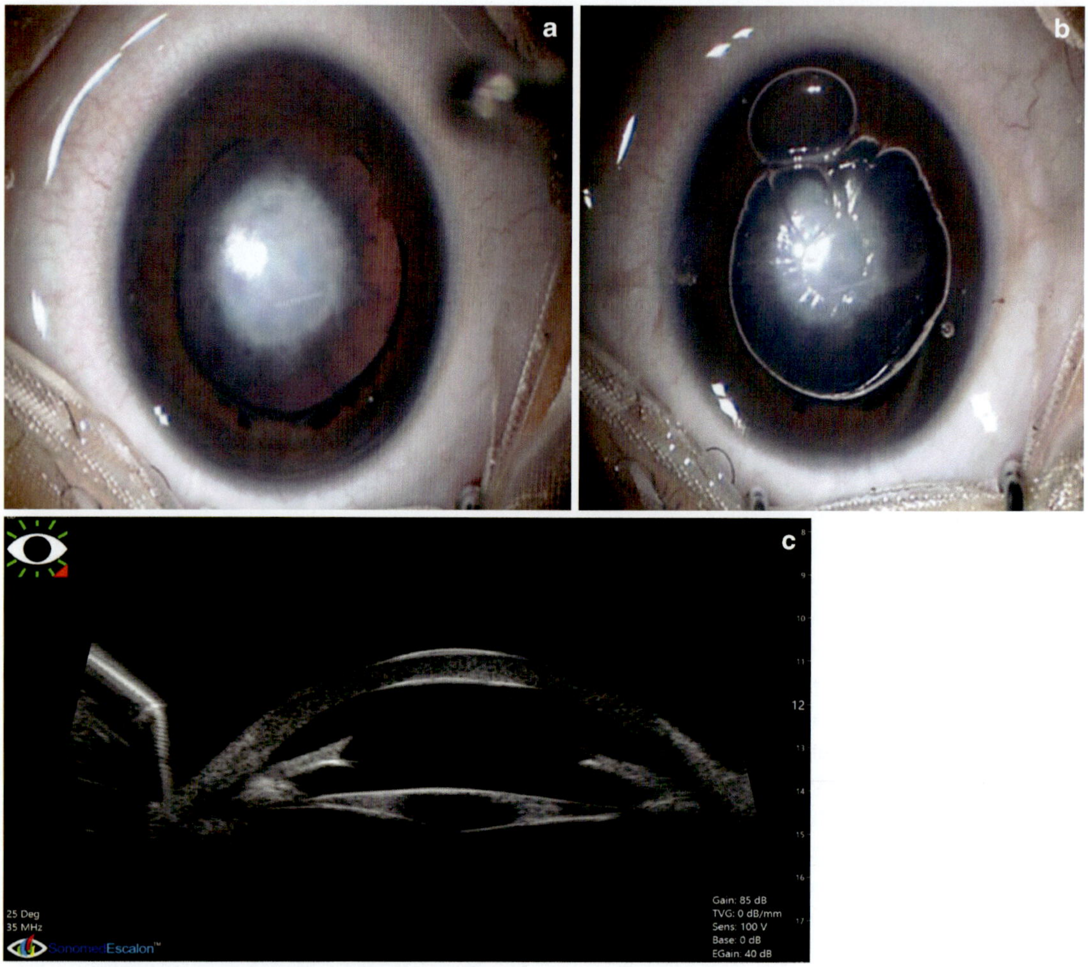

Fig. 15.10 Peter's anomaly type 1 in 2-month-old child. (**a**) Small corneal opacity with iridocorneal adhesions with cataract. (**b**) Intraoperative picture after ingestion of air in anterior chamber, irregular air bubble is seen due to iridocorneal adhesions. (**c**) Ultrasound biomicroscopy of the same showing fine central iridocorneal adhesions

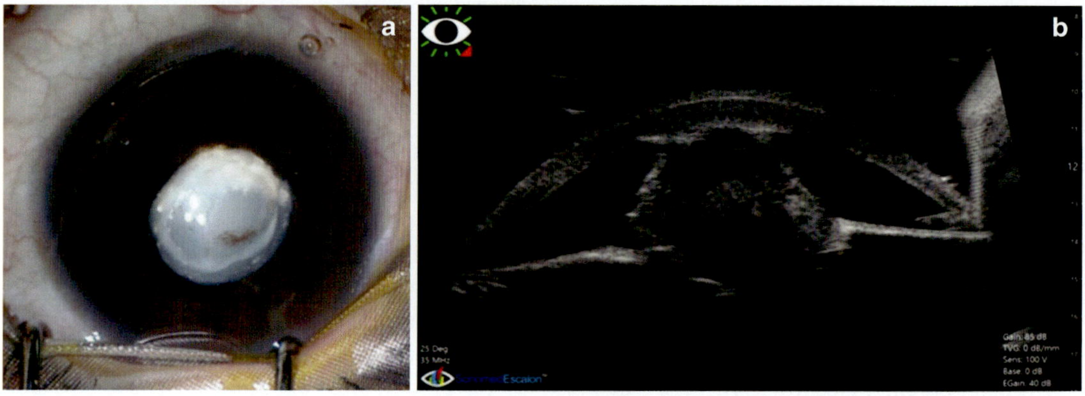

Fig. 15.11 Peter's anomaly type 2 in 4-month-old child. (**a**) Central corneal opacity with total cataract. (**b**) Ultrasound biomicroscopy of the same showing iridolenticular adhesions with anterior displacement of lens

short stature, brachydactylyl, ear abnormalities, and mental retardation [26, 27].

- Aniridia

  Aniridia is a rare congenital disorder characterized by iris hypoplasia along with other abnormalities of the eye [28]. Ocular abnormalities include dry eye, aniridia associated keratopathy (AAK) (Fig. 15.12), angle abnormalities, glaucoma, cataract, foveal hypoplasia, optic nerve hypoplasia, nystagmus, or strabismus [29–31]. Cataract morphology may be anterior or posterior subcapsular, lamellar, cortical, total or a combination of the above [28] (Fig. 15.13). Zonular weakness may be seen and ectopia lentis may be associated in some patients [28]. This can be managed with placement of capsular tension ring in mild cases (Fig. 15.14). Anterior polar or pyramidal cataract may be associated with aniridia along with remnants of persistent fetal vasculature [32] (Fig. 15.15).

15.2.4 Differential Diagnosis

The differential diagnosis of ASD includes obstetric trauma, congenital glaucoma, intrauterine infections like rubella, herpes simplex virus and bacterial infections, iridocorneo-endothelial syndrome (Fig. 15.16), metabolic diseases like mucopolysaccharidosis, mucolipidoses and tyrosinosis, congenital hereditary endothelial dystrophy, congenital hereditary stromal dystrophy and dermoids.

15.2.5 Investigations

Apart from usual investigations ultrasound biomicroscopy may allow us to preoperatively assess the area beneath the corneal opacity. It helps us to determine the area of corneal opacity, depth of opacity, presence of iris adhesion, anterior chamber depth and angle details in the involved area. The lens can be visualized and observed for kerato-lenticular adhesion or presence of any tilting of the lens (Figs. 15.10b, 15.11b, and 15.13d, e). This can help us in the planning of the cataract surgery and a better outcome.

15.2.6 Surgical Pearls

Patients with ASD should be screened for glaucoma and managed appropriately. They require optimization of visual function which includes refractive error prescription and tinted contact lenses for photophobia. This is important for prevention and treatment of amblyopia. Few patients may also require surgery for corneal opacity, lens abnormality or glaucoma management. Various challenges may be involved in the cataract surgery in cases with ASD.

- Corneal abnormalities: Corneal opacity or AAK may cause difficulty in visualization. Staining of the anterior capsule enhances its visualization during capsulorhexis. Other methods like use of illumination techniques

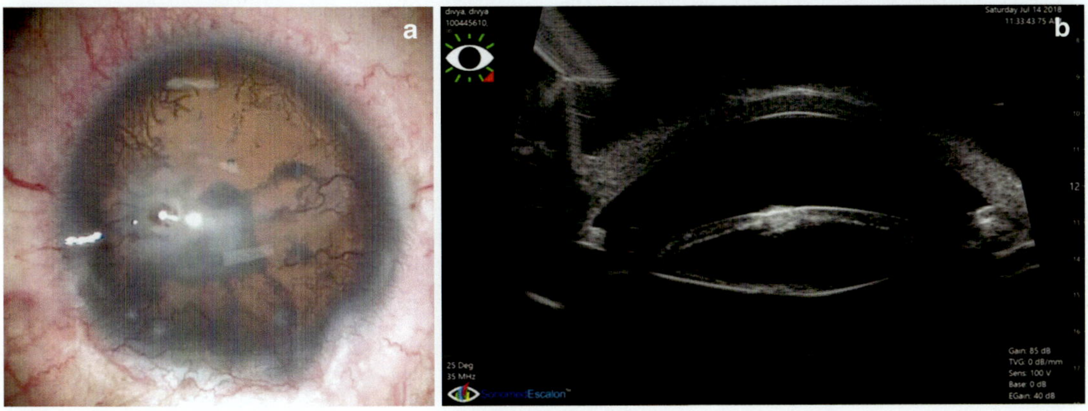

Fig. 15.12 Aniridia associated keratopathy with corneal opacity with 360° pannus. (**a**) Clinical picture. (**b**) Ultrasound biomicroscopy of the same showing anterior subcapsular cataract, not clearly seen clinically

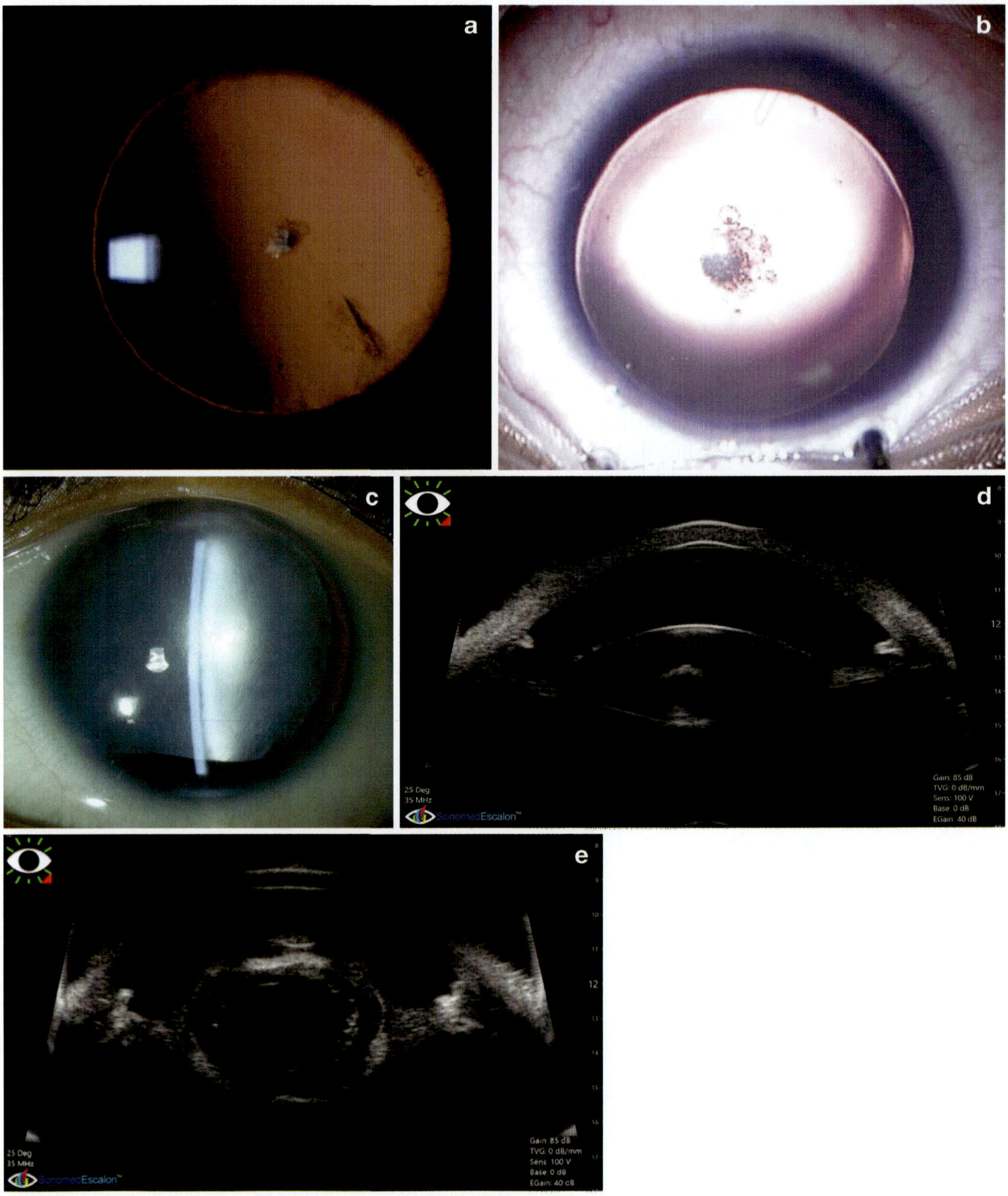

Fig. 15.13 Aniridia with cataract. (**a**) Clinical picture of insignificant anterior polar with cortical cataract. (**b**) Clinical picture of posterior subcapsular cataract. (**c**) Clinical picture of total cataract with inferior notching due to zonular laxity (Pseudo-coloboma). (**d**) UBM of aniridia patient showing minimal cataract and remnant of iris stump clearly with no subluxation. (**e**) UBM of aniridia patient with anterior polar and zonular cataract with zonular laxity causing increase in lens globularity

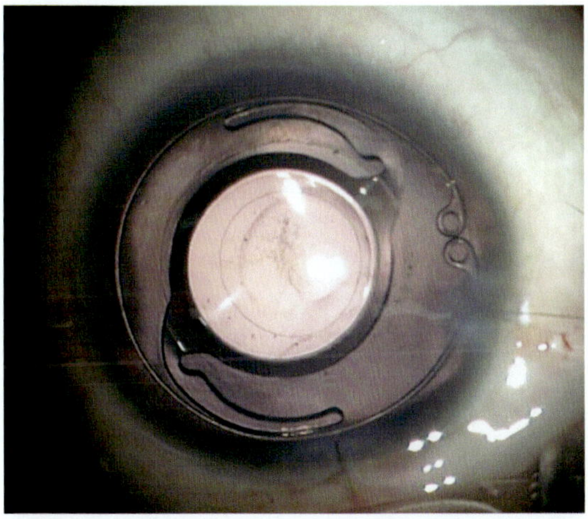

Fig. 15.14 Postoperative picture of aniridia with mild subluxation. Notice anterior and posterior capsulorhexis with well-centered IOL in bag with capsular tension ring

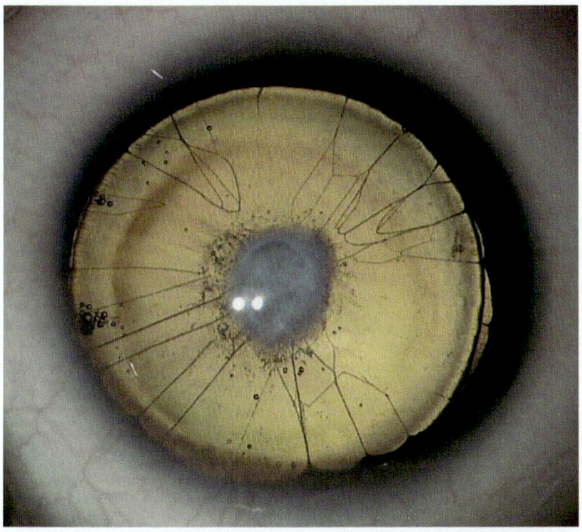

Fig. 15.15 Aniridia with anterior polar cataract with remnant of persistent fetal vasculature

like transcorneal oblique illumination or endoscope assisted surgery can help in better visualization but are time-consuming methods with a greater learning curve [33–35]. Image-guided surgery using femtosecond laser for cataract surgery in peter syndrome has also been recently used [36]. However, the depth and height of the femtosecond laser should be

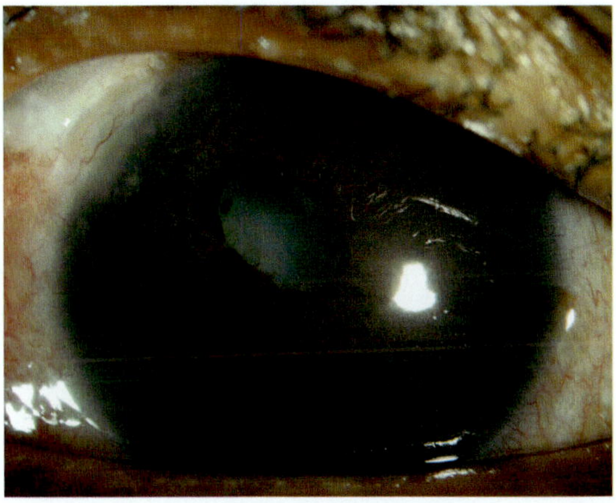

Fig. 15.16 Sixteen-year-old girl with Cogan Reese syndrome. Notice atophic iris and corectopia with iris nodules

cautiously adjusted to avoid damage to the endothelium.

- Presence of kerato-lenticular adhesion increases difficulty in surgical maneuvering. There may be risk of Descemet and endothelial damage during release of the keratolenticluar adhesions and difficulty to achieve appropriate size regular capsulorhexis. We have also noticed "irregular air bubble" in anterior chamber as a sign of presence of adhesions when they are not clearly visible (Fig. 15.17a, b).
- Iris abnormalities like corectopia, polycoria, iridocorneal adhesion, posterior synechiae between iris and lens may require anterior segment reconstruction may be required with synechiae release, anterior chamber formation or pupilloplasty along with the cataract surgery. Aniridia patients require use of tinted glasses or contact lens. Iris prosthetic devices may be used [37]. There is risk of secondary glaucoma, corneal decompenstion, band shaped keratopathy and device displacement [38] (Fig. 15.18).
- Zonular weakness: Aniridia cases have been reported with zonular laxity and lens subluxation. Use of capsular tension ring in cases with mild zonular laxity may give more desirable anatomical outcomes.

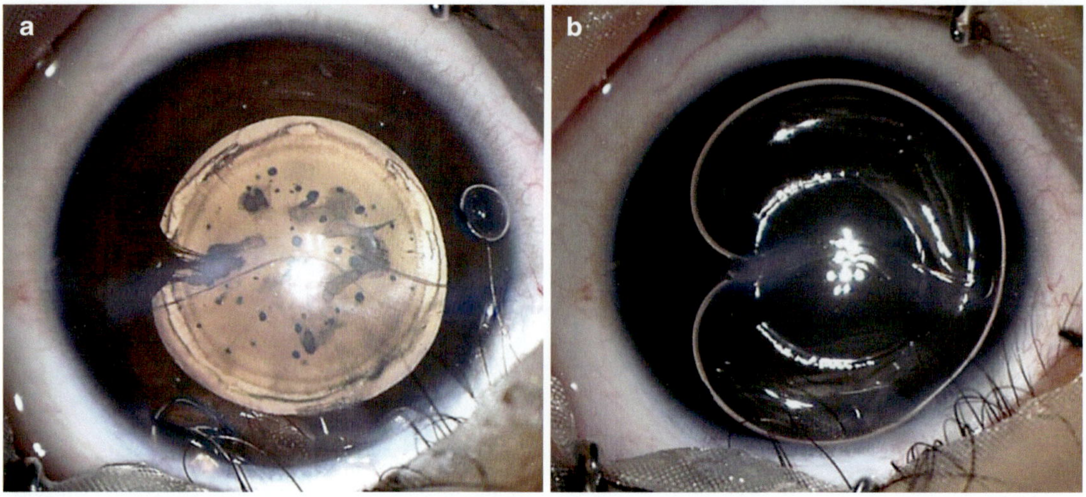

Fig. 15.17 Irregular air bubble sign in Anterior segment dysgenesis with glaucoma. (**a**) Corneal opacity with iridocorneal adhesions with Haab striae with anterior capsular pigments and zonular cataract. (**b**) Intraoperative picture after ingestion of air in anterior chamber, irregular air bubble is seen. Iridocorneal adhesions which were not clearly seen preoperatively are enhanced

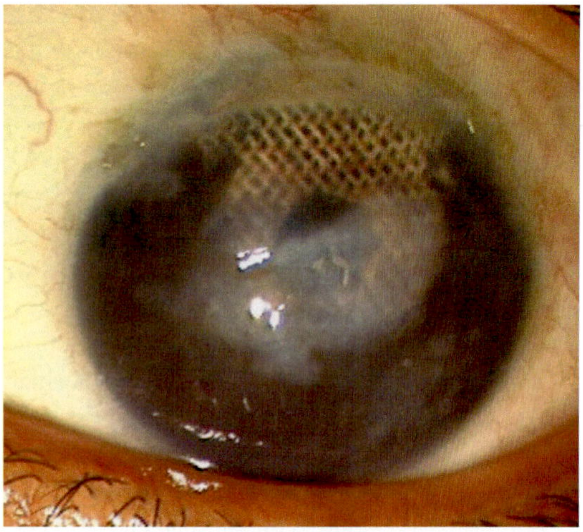

Fig. 15.18 One year postoperative picture of patient operated with Iris implant (outside center) with acquired aniridia (traumatic) with band shaped keratopathy and corneal decompensation

- Glaucoma management in cases with ASD is of importance and may include medical management, surgical management or both. Thus a regular follow-up with monitoring of visual acuity and the intraocular pressure is crucial.

Challenges in surgery in patients with ASD have to be carefully dealt with, in order to achieve satisfactory visual outcome. In addition to cataract surgery, glaucoma management is of utmost importance in these cases.

References

1. Wiggs JL, Damji KF, Haines JL, Pericak-Vance MA, Allingham RR. The distinction between juvenile and adult-onset primary open-angle glaucoma. Am J Hum Genet. 1996;58(1):243–4.
2. Feroze KB, Patel BC. Buphthalmos. In: StatPearls [Internet]. Treasure Island: StatPearls Publishing; 2018. http://www.ncbi.nlm.nih.gov/books/NBK430887/.
3. Yanoff M, Duker JS. Ophthalmology. 3rd ed. Philadelphia: Mosby Elsevier; 2009.
4. Basic and clinical science course (2011–2012). Glaucoma. American Academy of Ophthalmology.
5. Edmunds B, Thompson JR, Salmon J, Wornald RP. The national survey of trabeculectomy III. Early and late complications. Eye. 2002;16:297–303.
6. Adelman RA, Brauner SC, Afshari NA, Grosskreutz CL. Cataract formation after initial trabeculectomy in young patients. Ophthalmology. 2003;110:625–9.
7. Daugeliene L, Yamamoto T, Kitazawa Y. Cataract development after trabeculectomy with mitomycin C: a 1-year study. Jpn J Ophthalmol. 2000;44:52–7.
8. Khokhar SK, Pillay G, Agarwal E, Mahabir M. Innovations in pediatric cataract surgery. Indian J Ophthalmol. 2017;65(3):210–6.
9. Hugkulstone CE. Changes in keratometry following trabeculectomy. Br J Ophthalmol. 1991;75(4):217–8.

10. Chan HHL, Kong YXG. Glaucoma surgery and induced astigmatism: a systematic review. Eye Vis [Internet]. 2017;4. https://www.ncbi.nlm.nih.gov/pmc/articles/PMC5691392/.
11. Vaz FM, Osher RH. Cataract surgery and anterior megalophthalmos: custom intraocular lens and special considerations. J Cataract Refract Surg. 2007;33(12):2147–50.
12. Sukhija J, Kaur S, Pandav SS, Kaushik S, Raj S, Ram J. Cataract surgery in children with buphthalmos. Clin Experiment Ophthalmol. 2016;44(8):739–40.
13. Dietlein TS, Jacobi PC, Krieglstein GK. [Eyeball growth after successful glaucoma surgery in the 1st year of life--follow-up values for primary congenital glaucoma]. Klin Monbl Augenheilkd. 1998;213(2):67–70.
14. Khokhar S, Yadav D, Gupta S, Chaurasia AK, Gupta A, Gupta V. Refractive outcomes of cataract surgery in primary congenital glaucoma. Eye (Lond). 2018; https://doi.org/10.1038/s41433-018-0253-6.
15. Waring GO, Rodrigues MM, Laibson PR. Anterior chamber cleavage syndrome. A stepladder classification. Surv Ophthalmol. 1975;20:3–27.
16. Shields MB, Buckley E, Klintworth GK, Thresher R. Axenfeld-Rieger syndrome. A spectrum of developmental disorders. Surv Ophthalmol. 1985;29:387–409.
17. Townsend WM, Font RL, Zimmerman LE. Congenital corneal leukomas. 2. Histopathologic findings in 19 eyes with central defect in Descemet's membrane. Am J Ophthalmol. 1974;77:192–206.
18. Beauchamp G, Knepper P. Role of the neural crest in anterior segment development and disease. J Pediatr Ophthalmol Strabismus. 1984;21:209–14.
19. Glaser T, Walton DS, Maas RL. Genomic structure, evolutionary conservation and aniridia mutations in the human PAX6 gene. Nat Genet. 1992;2:232–9.
20. Phillips JC, et al. A second locus for Rieger syndrome maps to chromosome 13q14. Am J Hum Genet. 1996;59:613–9.
21. Dahl E, Koseki H, Balling R. Pax genes and organogenesis. Bioessays. 1997;19:755–65.
22. Doward W, Perveen R, Lloyd IC, Ridgway AE, Wilson L, Black GC. A mutation in the RIEG1 gene associated with Peters' anomaly. J Med Genet. 1999;36(2):152–5. PMID: 10051017; PMCID: PMC1734311.
23. Iseri SU, et al. Seeing clearly: the dominant and recessive nature of FOXE3 in eye developmental anomalies. Hum Mutat. 2009;30:1378–86.
24. Fitch N, Kaback M. The Axenfeld syndrome and the Rieger syndrome. J Med Genet. 1978;15:30–4.
25. Chang TC, Summers CG, Schimmenti LA, Grajewski AL. Axenfeld-Rieger syndrome: new perspectives. Br J Ophthalmol. 2012;96:318–22.
26. Bhandari R, Ferri S, Whittaker B, Liu M, Lazzaro DR. Peters anomaly: review of the literature. Cornea. 2011;30:939–44.
27. Harissi-Dagher M, Colby K. Anterior segment dysgenesis: Peters anomaly and sclerocornea. Int Ophthalmol Clin. 2008;48:35–42.
28. Nelson LB, Spaeth GL, Nowinski TS, Margo CE, Jackson L. Aniridia. A review. Surv Ophthalmol. 1984;28:621–42.
29. Eden U, Riise R, Tornqvist K. Corneal involvement in congenital aniridia. Cornea. 2010;29:1096–102.
30. Chang JW, Kim JH, Kim SJ, Yu YS. Congenital aniridia: long-term clinical course, visual outcome, and prognostic factors. Korean J Ophthalmol. 2010;28:479–85.
31. Singh B, Mohamed A, Chaurasia S, Ramappa M, Mandal AK, Jalali S, Sangwan VS. Clinical manifestations of congenital aniridia. J Pediatr Ophthalmol Strabismus. 2014;51:59–62.
32. Khokhar S, Sinha G, Sharma R, Patil B, Mahabir M, Nayak B. Anterior pyramidal cataract: a rare association. JAMA Ophthalmol. 2015;133(4):e144626. https://doi.org/10.1001/jamaophthalmol.2014.4626.
33. Farjo AA, Meyer RF, Farjo QA. Phacoemulsification in eyes with corneal opacification. J Cataract Refract Surg. 2003;29:242–5.
34. Moore JE, Herath GD, Sharma A. Continuous curvilinear capsulorhexis with use of an endoscope. J Cataract Refract Surg. 2004;30:960–3.
35. Al Sabti K, Raizada S, Al Abduljalil T. Cataract surgery assisted by anterior endoscopy. Br J Ophthalmol. 2009;93:531–4.
36. Hou JH, Crispim J, Cortina MS, Cruz Jde L. Image-guided femtosecond laser-assisted cataract surgery in Peters anomaly type 2. J Cataract Refract Surg. 2015;41(11):2353–7. https://doi.org/10.1016/j.jcrs.2015.10.045. PMID: 26703482.
37. Srinivasan S, Ting DS, Snyder ME, Prasad S, Koch HR. Prosthetic iris devices. Can J Ophthalmol. 2014;49(1):6–17.
38. Mostafa YS, Osman AA, Hassanein DH, Zeid AM, Sherif AM. Iris reconstruction using artificial iris prosthesis for management of aniridia. Eur J Ophthalmol. 2018;28(1):103–7.

Cataract Associated with ROP and Other Retinal Pathologies

16

Abhidnya Surve, Chirakshi Dhull, and Sudarshan Kumar Khokhar

16.1 Introduction

Preterm babies with retinopathy of prematurity (ROP) can have poor visual prognosis if not treated early. Presence of cataract in these individuals may further delay proper screening and adequate treatment. Cataract can also develop post-treatment for ROP, making follow-up assessment of disease activity difficult. Amblyopia is another important component to be addressed in these small individuals. This chapter highlights the different aspects of cataract in a ROP case including the causes, pathophysiology, types, and management. The preoperative workup, intraoperative challenges and postoperative care required in such babies is discussed.

Supplementary Information The online version of this chapter (https://doi.org/10.1007/978-981-16-0212-2_16) contains supplementary material, which is available to authorized users.

A. Surve
R P Center, AIIMS, New Delhi, India

C. Dhull
Eye Q Hospital, Rohtak, Haryana, India

S. K. Khokhar (✉)
Professor Ophthalmology, Dr. RP Centre for Ophthalmic Sciences, All India Institute of Medical Sciences, New Delhi, India

16.2 Epidemiology

Cataract is defined as any opacity in the lens and prevalence of 1.2–6 cases per 10,000 infants [1]. The normal development of fetus occurs up to 40 weeks gestational age (GA). Those babies born before 34 weeks gestational age, having birth weight less than 1750 g and those >34 weeks GA or >1750 g with high-risk factors are at risk for retinopathy of prematurity (ROP) and hence screened [2]. The incidence of ROP in these preterm babies has increased due to an increased survival rate of preterm and poor health care regulations regarding neonatal care and screening guidelines. These preterm low birth weight babies are also at risk to have cataract and an incidence of 0.97–1.9% is seen in these preterms [3, 4]. These lenticular opacities can lead to difficulty in assessment of the posterior segment status and management of same.

16.3 Type of Cataract

The different morphologies of cataract seen in preterm babies include [3, 5–9]:

1. Focal opacities either punctate or vacuolated—These are usually transient, visually insignificantly and resolve spontaneously. Seen in approximately 2.7% of low birth weight infants [10, 11](Fig. 16.1)

S. K. Khokhar, C. Dhull (eds.), *Essentials of Pediatric Cataract Surgery*,
https://doi.org/10.1007/978-981-16-0212-2_16

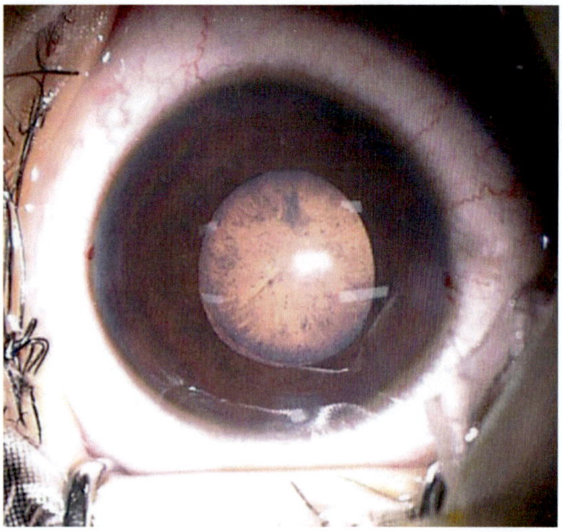

Fig. 16.1 Fifty-two weeks post-gestation age patient with cataract pulverulenta, Zone 2 spontaneously regressed ROP

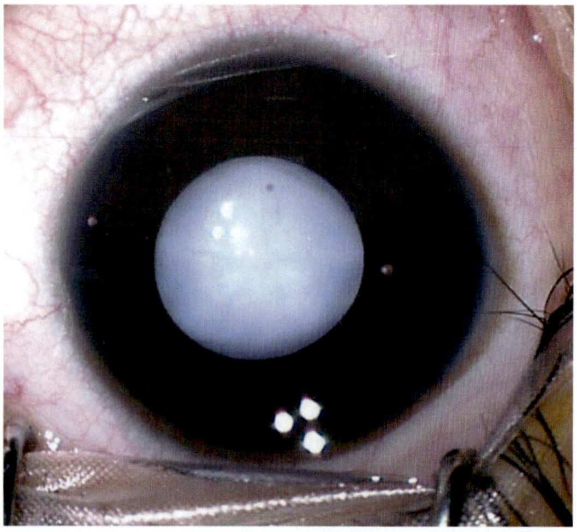

Fig. 16.2 Forty weeks post-gestation age patient with total cataract, 4 weeks following laser therapy for Zone 1 stage 3 ROP

2. Zonular cataract
3. Total cataract (Fig. 16.2)
4. Anterior or posterior subcapsular cataract
5. Complicated cataract—Seen as posterior subcapsular cataract with polychromatic luster or partially absorbed membranous cataract. Usually associated with retinal detachment.

16.4 Causes

Infantile cataract can develop due to intrauterine infections, drug-related, metabolic disorders, or inherited disorders. While many of these cases are bilateral, asymmetrical presentation is also commonly seen [1, 12]. In a premature child, cataract can form because of the systemic status, retinopathy of prematurity or due to treatment of same. Cataract development is seen at different duration ranging from 10 days to 13 months in laser-treated and 2 months to 5.6 years in post-vitrectomised eyes [3, 4, 13–15]. Pathophysiology of cataract in ROP can be divided according to the etiology:

1. Systemic factors
   The preterm babies are at risk of metabolic acidosis and sepsis during their NICU stay. These factors can lead to osmotic changes in the lens leading to development of cataract. The usual form seen is the bilateral clear vacuoles formation along the apices of posterior lens surface. These are transient and mostly clears over the course of several months but can progress to total opacification in some cases [1, 4, 10, 11].
2. Complicated cataract
   Complicated cataract is seen in those associated with retinal detachment, mostly in cases with advanced stage retinopathy [16]. It may present as posterior subcapsular cataract or partially absorbed membranous cataract.
3. Posttreatment
   Cataract in preterm child may or may not be associated with systemic treatment and ocular management [4, 8, 15]. The actual incidence of the same in retinopathy of prematurity may be less reported.

(a) Steroid-induced cataract: Though long-term steroids are known to cause cataract, there are no reports of steroid-induced cataract in preterm babies.

(b) Cryotherapy

Cryotherapy was previously used as a treatment for threshold ROP. It can cause more inflammation due to blood-retinal barrier breakdown. But cataract was not seen as a major complication in various studies [17–19].

(c) Laser

Laser is preferred over cryotherapy because of lesser complications of pain, adnexal edema, exudative retinal detachment, vitreoretinal traction, and vitreous hemorrhage. The incidence of cataract in laser-treated ROP ranges from 0.003 to 6% [4, 15, 20–23]. The type of laser used in treatment of ROP includes argon, diode and df-NdYAG laser. Argon laser had higher association with cataract among them [15, 24]. Prominent anterior vasculosa lentis, inadvertent burns placed on the iris or ciliary body and confluent laser therapy are the risk factors for cataract formation post-laser in a preterm baby. Following mechanisms play a role:

Thermal injury

The total amount of laser energy used depends on the type, power, duration of laser and number of laser spots. Lens protein and hemoglobin absorbs the energy of laser. This is especially important in case of persistent tunica vasculosa lentis (TVL), commonly present in preterm babies [20]. The incidence of cataract is lower in cases with diode laser energy as longer wavelength energy (810 nm) is lesser absorbed by hemoglobin as compared to argon laser [25]. However, some studies have found no correlation between development of cataract and energy of the laser used [4].

Tunica Vasculosa Lentis (TVL)

Premature infants have some amount of intact TVL. The hemoglobin absorbs laser energy at the lens surface leading to alteration in permeability of lens anterior capsule. This further affects the osmotic balance and leads to formation of cataract. In a very premature child, the disease may present in more aggressive form like aggressive posterior ROP (APROP) which has iris neovascularization with poor pupillary dilatation, hazy vitreous and severe plus disease. These cases require higher power, duration and more laser leading to higher energy being used, further increasing the risk. But studies have also shown similar incidence of cataract in ROP cases not having prominent TVL indicating other factors also do play a role [20, 21].

Anterior segment ischemia

The anterior segment of the eye is supplied by the anastomosis of anterior ciliary artery (ACA) and long posterior ciliary artery (LPCA). Damage to the LPCA can lead to anterior segment ischemia [26]. It can present as congestion, corneal edema, shallow anterior chamber, hyphema, cataract, posterior synechiae in the acute phase and hypotony, iris atrophy, ciliary body atrophy in the late phase. Some of these eyes do progress to phthisis bulbi [26, 27].

Uveal effusion

The higher amount of thermal energy and the immature blood-retinal barrier puts the baby at higher risk of uveal effusion. It can lead to anterior rotation of ciliary body and shallow anterior chamber which may cause corneo-lenticular apposition and cataract formation [25].

(d) Post-injection

In adults, cataract incidence varies in cases receiving intravitreal anti-VEGF [28, 29]. VEGF is an important molecule involved in the cascade of events in ROP. It is one of the factors involved in both angiogenesis and vasculogenesis phase. The use of intravitreal anti-VEGF in ROP allows for fast disease regression and improved vascular re-growth. This allows for a better field of vision but various regression patterns including vascular arrest along with high risk of recurrence is noted [23, 30, 31].

Cataract in anti-VEGF most commonly occurs due to the lens injury. In preterm babies, the lens is thicker as compared to other ocular structures and the pars plana is also not formed [32, 33]. Hence, if one is not familiar with the anatomy of these small eyes, there is a higher chance of mechanical lens injury. The injection in these children is usually given at 1.75 mm from the limbus with the needle tip directed posteriorly towards the optic disc. But, there have been reports of cataract formation in post-intravitreal anti-VEGF with no lens injury documented, which could be probably relate to the molecule itself (Figs. 16.3 and 16.4). Preexisting dehiscence of the posterior capsule has also been suspected [9]. Also until now, there is no level I evidence of the ocular, visual, systemic and neurodevelopmental safety profile of anti-VEGF in these babies.

(e) Post-surgery

Stage 4 or 5 ROP can be associated with cataract or the retina can be near the posterior capsule which may necessitate lensectomy along with vitrectomy to achieve optimal results. Cataract formation after lens sparing vitrectomy for ROP surgery can occur but is

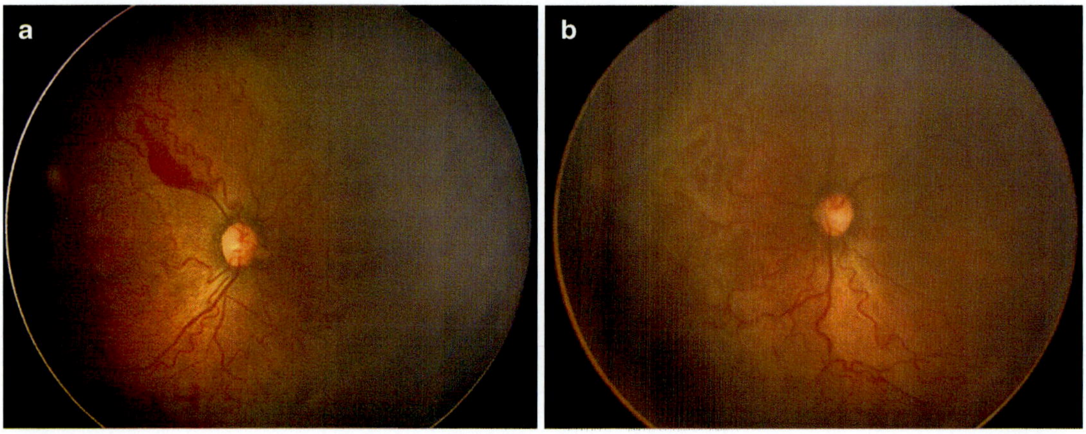

Fig. 16.3 Twenty-eight-week-old baby patient with bilateral Zone 1 APROP - Aggressive posterior retinopathy of prematurity OD&OS

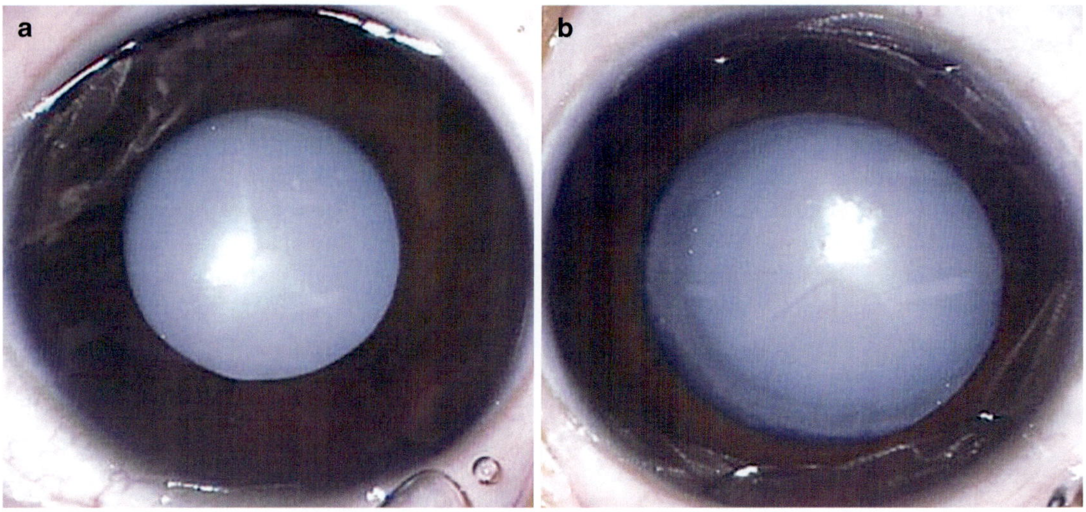

Fig. 16.4 Same patient as Fig. 16.3, developed bilateral total cataract OD&OS 6 weeks after anti-VEGF administration

less frequent as compared to pars plana vitrectomy in adults [3, 13, 14]. The lens retina approximation is one of the risk factors for cataract formation because of the probability of lens touch. The chemical changes also are known to occur with vitrectomy itself and depending on the type of tamponade agent used.

16.5 Management

Treatment of ROP is important and first priority as early intervention in these cases can prevent adverse outcomes. Obscuration of posterior segment visualization by cataract can preclude the screening and management of these cases. Hence, the need to manage cataract as soon as possible is essential to allow intervention for the posterior segment, monitor the disease and prevent amblyopia. As discussed, lensectomy might be required in addition to vitrectomy in some cases of stage 4 and stage 5 ROP, where the lens is cataractous or the retina is in close approximation with the lens. In cases where retina is hazily seen allowing staging of the disease but laser could not be performed, early cataract surgery is required for management of the posterior segment and prevent progression of ROP.

16.5.1 Preoperative Challenges

Pediatric cataract surgery is challenging in terms of smaller eye with lesser scleral rigidity, higher elasticity of anterior capsule, and steeper anterior curvature of lens. The anterior segment in a preterm child is further different from a normal child eye in terms of steeper cornea, shallow anterior chamber, more anteriorly inserted iris, thicker and more spherical lens [33, 34]. Further these parameters may vary with spontaneously regressed and laser-treated ROP. These differences not only pose intraoperative challenges but also affect the pattern of ocular growth [5, 33, 35–38]. This has a significant effect on the selection of appropriate intraocular lens power and the amount of under-correction required in these babies. Poor pupillary dilatation can further create problems during surgery.

Tropicamide (0.5%) and phenylephrine (2.5%) combination is used for dilatation in these preterm babies. As used for ROP screening, the drops should be instilled two times 10 min apart half an hour before the surgery. In cases with APROP, neovascularization of iris is often present. This causes non-dilation of the pupil, difficulty in visualization of lens status and posterior segment, and risk of bleeding. These cases are also at risk of having postoperative inflammation, posterior synechiae and visual axis opacification (VAO). Also, the posterior segment in these cases needs urgent treatment to avoid further complications leading to poor visual prognosis. Preoperative B-scan imaging is important to rule out the possibility of retinal detachment in cases where posterior segment is not visible. Preoperative ultrasound biomicroscopy (UBM) can help us to determine the area of the posterior synechiae, whether the posterior iris has adhered to anterior capsule, the status of the posterior capsule for presence of any preexisting posterior capsular defects and the sulcus to sulcus diameter (Fig. 16.2). The preoperative detection of preexisting posterior capsular defect can help one to anticipate complications and take necessary steps to prevent them. In APROP cases with severe neovascularization in absence of retinal detachment, intravitreal anti-VEGF before cataract surgery may help in the regression of the neovascularization. This decreases the risk of bleeding and allows dilatation of the pupil. All the challenges including posterior segment status, treatment required, amblyopia therapy, prognosis, need for postoperative care, refractive correction, and complications associated should be explained to the parents/caregivers.

16.5.2 Intraoperative Challenges

- Approach and dilatation
  The preferable approach in preterm babies is superior corneal incision as with other pediatric cases. The superior wound is covered with the upper eyelid and hence is at lesser risk of trauma and exposure, thereby decreasing the

risk of infection. Pupillary miosis and posterior synechiae can be present especially in cases with advanced ROP or APROP. The use of high-density viscocohesive like Healon-GV is preferred to maintain the anterior chamber and have minimum fluctuations in anterior chamber. The synechiae could be initially released to assess pupillary dilatation. In case of non-dilating pupil, various maneuvers like mechanical stretching, sphincterotomy, and use of mechanical devices like iris hooks can be tried. The use of other mechanical devices like the Malyugin ring in such small eyes is not preferable due to lesser space for maneuvering these devices.

- Anterior capsulorhexis and lens aspiration:
  The anterior capsule can be stained using 0.06% Trypan Blue dye to visualize it. Trypan blue dye is known to have biochemical effects on the lens capsule, decreasing its elasticity [39]. The anterior continuous capsulorhexis (ACC) can be started with the capsulotomy 26 Gauge needle and further performed using capsulorhexis forceps. The forceps allow for controlled maneuvering of the elastic capsule. But before starting the anterior chamber should be formed with high-density viscocohesive substance like Healon-GV which would allow minimum fluctuation in anterior chamber and flatten the anterior capsule in the center. Appropriate size of the ACC is approximately 5 mm. The use of Callisto guided marking system can help us in this aspect. The lens aspiration can be performed using bimanual technique which allows complete removal of the lens matter without undue stress on the bag. Any residual lens matter could lead to excess inflammation in these pediatric cases and hence preferably be avoided.
- Posterior capsulorhexis, vitrectomy and fundus examination
  A posterior continuous capsulorhexis (PCC) can be made after partially filling the posterior chamber with high-density viscocohesive. Complete fill should be avoided as these may lead to increased bowing of the posterior capsule causing increasing angulation of the instrument leading to difficult maneuvering. Also, there is an increase in the pressure on the posterior capsule especially at the posterior-most point creating a high risk of irregular extension. The PCC is performed with capsulorhexis forceps after initiation with a capsulotomy needle (Fig. 16.3a). This is followed by anterior vitrectomy (AV). The anterior vitrectomy as in other pediatric cataract cases should cover beyond the margin and 2 mm deeper from the posterior capsule. A complete anterior vitrectomy and PCC reduces the chances of postoperative posterior capsular opacification (PCO) significantly [40, 41]. However, caution must be exercised and overzealous anterior vitrectomy beyond the margins should be avoided as these cases may have peripheral vitreoretinal traction. The posterior segment can be visualized at this stage using endoilluminator and wide-angle retinal lens (Fig. 16.3). The anterior chamber should be formed with viscoelastic before inserting the endoilluminator. This allows us to assess the status of optic disc, posterior pole and also the periphery. Hence, zone of vascularization, presence of ROP, stage, and presence of plus disease can be determined. This visualization helps in further management of the posterior segment as postoperative examination with speculum and indentation may not be possible in the initial 2 weeks considering the wound stability.
- Intraocular lens (IOL)
  Another question arises if the IOL can be placed, and if yes, what power to be used? The intraocular lens can be placed if the size of corneal diameter >9 mm, the sulcus to sulcus diameter >8 mm, axial length >17 mm and if no additional ocular features precluding the use of IOL are present. The type of IOL depends on the availability of sulcus. In cases where the anterior and posterior capsulorhexis is intact and well sized, the IOL can be placed in the bag while in compromised capsulorhexis, a multipiece IOL can be placed in the sulcus (Fig. 16.3b). Optic capture involves fixing the lens optic behind the posterior capsule while the haptics remains in place allowing

better stabilization of the lens. In case of no capsular support, iris-fixated IOL or ACIOL can also be used. These ROP cases usually have myopia, thin sclera and retinal involvement. Hence, scleral fixated IOL are avoided. The IOL power in pediatric cases depends on the age of the patient at the time surgery, preoperative biometry and predicted postoperative change [12, 42]. Various formulae have been given over a period, but variance is seen more in children less than 2 years [42, 43]. Further, these preterm eyes will have more growth at a rapid rate initially as compared to normal eyes. The usual correlation between the axial length and refractive error is not seen in small preterm babies [13, 34]. Also, those treated with laser will have more axial length growth as compared to those treated with anti-VEGF or spontaneously regressed. These factors need to be taken into consideration as these cases may require more under-correction as compared to normal eyes.

- Technique—A single piece hydrophobic acrylate IOL can be placed in the bag using proper technique if the criteria for IOL placement are fulfilled. A 3.5 mm incision allows easy insertion of injector without any undue pressure on the wound, thereby maintaining the anterior chamber. The anterior chamber and the intraocular bag should be adequately filled with viscocohesive substance. While injecting the IOL, the leading haptic should be placed against the posterior surface of the anterior capsule to avoid any unnecessary strain on posterior capsule and dislocation of the IOL into the vitreous cavity. The trailing haptic can be released in the pupillary plane and then tucked in the bag using a Sinskey hook. The viscoelastic should be completely removed and wound sutured using 10-0 monofilament nylon suture. In cases where IOL cannot be placed, secondary IOL can be planned after 2 years of age.
- Intraoperative challenges in vitrectomized eyes:

  Further cataract surgery in a vitrectomized eye would be moreover challenging [44, 45]. The loss of posterior support can lead to hypotony, zonular instability, complicated capsulorhexis, and damage to the posterior capsule. Zonular instability along with the increased iris lens diaphragm mobility may lead to anterior chamber depth fluctuation. In cases with lens touch or preexisting defect which may be detected on the UBM, there is risk of posterior dislocation of the lens fragments. The sudden collapse of the anterior chamber should be avoided at any step in these cases. The irrigation parameters to be kept on the lower side and the overfilling of AC with viscoelastic to be avoided. Hydrodelineation should be done gently while hydrodissection and lens rotation should be completely avoided [46]. The lens aspiration should be performed trying to maintain the posterior cortex which should be aspirated at the end. In case of a posterior capsular opening, it's important not to panic and remove the instruments suddenly from the eye. The anterior chamber should be formed with a combination of Sodium hyaluronate 3.0%-Chondroitin sulfate 4.0% (Viscoat) before removing instruments. It coats the posterior capsular opening and prevents posterior dislocation of the lens matter. Lens matter in the anterior chamber can be removed using a vitreous cutter or wire vectis followed by complete anterior vitrectomy. Depending on the sulcus availability, a multipiece IOL can be placed. If the defect at the posterior capsule is small, it can be converted to PCC and a single piece IOL can be placed in the bag.

In cases with posteriorly dislocated lens fragments, depending on the amount, further approach can be decided. If the fragments size is small, it can be left as most of the time absorbs completely. Steroids may be required to avoid inflammation in these cases. If the fragments amount is large, a vitreoretinal surgeon may be called upon to remove it from the posterior segment. Simultaneous bilateral cataract surgery in one sitting is considered in small babies to avoid the risk of repeated anesthesia and the danger of developing amblyopia in case one eye is operated and the other could not be done due to systemic risk.

16.5.3 Postoperative

The postoperative complications of cataract surgery include inflammation, pupillary membrane formation, posterior synechiae, glaucoma, reproliferation of lens material, posterior capsule opacity, and retinal detachment. Postoperative treatment with topical cycloplegics and steroids is important. The severity of postoperative inflammation is higher in cases with iris neovascularization and those having posterior synechiae because of the iris manipulation and bleeding risk. Hence, topical steroids are required frequently and tapered slowly over a long period in these cases. This prevents the postoperative formation of posterior iris synechiae which may hamper visualization of the retina especially in the periphery and could lead to glaucoma.

Follow-up post cataract surgery should be synchronized with ROP monitoring and treatment to prevent unwanted outcomes. In children, refractive changes after cataract surgery are extensively studied and myopic shift is seen. This shift was more in younger children and aphakic eyes. Long-term refractive changes as previously described depends on various factors including gestational age, age of the child at the time of surgery, presence of ROP, type of treatment received and progression of myopia over a period [35–38, 42]. How much each of these factors contributes and affects the growth of the eyeball is unknown and still being studied. Hence, frequent refraction with appropriate correction glasses should be provided to avoid amblyopia. The glasses with appropriate fitting and counseling of the parents/caregivers to ensure use of glasses are needed.

Improvement in visual acuity and fixation is evident after cataract surgery in ROP cases but is limited because of the ocular morbidities (Table 16.1) [3, 6, 44, 47]. VAO is common after pediatric cataract surgery in children less than 1 year and depends whether PCCC and anterior vitrectomy is done or not [40, 48]. This can cause significant vision loss with risk of amblyopia. Hence, the importance of performing PCCC with anterior vitrectomy and to look for VAO in follow-up period [41]. To avoid VAO, PCCC should be done in all cases less than 6 years. Anterior vitrectomy to be done till 5 years of age. In older cases with mental retardation and those who cannot cooperate for slit lamp YAG capsulotomy, PCCC and anterior vitrectomy can be done [12]. Glaucoma is a common complication associated with both premature babies and pediatric cataract surgery [40, 49, 50]. The difference in the anterior segment of these individuals increases the risk of glaucoma [33]. Hence, the intraocular pressure and the optic disc cupping in these individuals should be monitored on follow-up. Retinal detachment (RD) is also one of the complications seen with pediatric cataract surgery and well documented after cataract surgery in adult ROP cases [6, 47, 51]. In preterm children with ROP, RD occurred in 3.5% of cases after cataract surgery [3]. It can occur in the preterm babies with progression of the ROP itself, and hence cannot be attributed to the cataract surgery alone. The ETROP study had 16% cases with RD after treatment by 9 months of the corrected age. Thus, the disease itself is at risk of progression even after treatment and good prognosis is obtained in stage 4 as compared to stage 5 ROP disease [13, 19]. Thus, these cases need a long-term follow-up for early detection of RD and intervention for the same.

Preterm children with cataract are at risk of vision loss because of various factors including retinal changes, glaucoma, and amblyopia. With an appropriate approach and combined effort of pediatrician, ophthalmologist, and anesthesiologist, early identification, prompt intervention, precise surgical techniques, proper counseling, and postoperative care including amblyopia management, these children can have good vision.

16.6 Cataract in Other Pediatric Retinal Disorders

Pediatric cases and adult cases differ in the type of retinal detachment along with cause and outcome of the same. The anatomical and functional outcomes are different from the adult cases [52]. The pediatric cases may be detected late as symp-

Table 16.1 Studies on cataract surgery in retinopathy of prematurity babies

Sr. No.	Author	Journal, year	No. of eyes	Previous retinal treatment (eyes)	Gestational age (wks)	Birth weight (g)	Age at surgery	Follow-up	PCIOL	Type of cataract (eyes)	Intraoperative complications	Postoperative complication (eyes)	Vision
1.	Yu et al.	J Cataract Refract Surg, 2004	8 eyes–ROP (stage 1-2, Stage 2-2, Stage 3-4)	Cryotherapy-3	26–36 (30)	800–2500 (1439)	0.2–5.5 y (1.5 y)	0.5–3.1 y (1.4 y)	Primary-1 Secondary-3	T-4 N-4		Pupillary membrane-1 Esotropia-1	Central steady reflex-5 Not centered reflex-1 BCVA >20/200-4
2.	Ezisi et al.	Br J Ophthalmol, 2017	28 eyes (stage 4–13)	Retinal surgery-19 Scleral buckle-1 Laser-3	–		0.2m–12 y (18.9 m)	1–132 m (2 y)	Primary-19	T-12 Z-5 N-4 PSC-5 ASC-1	PCR-2	VAO-4 Secondary glaucoma-2 IOL capture-1	BCVA >20/200-11 Myopic shift 2 y (pseudophakic-3.07D; aphakic-8.75D)
3.	Nguyen et al.	Open J of Ophth, 2017	19 eyes	Laser-13 Retinal surgery-5 Intravitreal injection-1	24.8	747 ± 233	Mean-6.7 y	1.5–16.8 y (10.1 y)	Primary-15 Secondary-2 Sulcus fixated-2	–	PCR-3 Pupillary miosis-3 Anterior capsular fibrosis-3 Posterior synechiae-3	VAO-10 Pupillary membrane-1 Acute angle closure glaucoma-1 Band-shaped keratopathy-3 Optic atrophy-6 Nystagmus-6 Strabismus-7	BCVA >20/200-11
4.	Quan et al.	Retina cases & brief report, 2015	3 eyes (stage 3-2, Stage 4-1)	Diode laser-3	22–26	–	–	11–13 y	Secondary-1	T-3		Anterior segment ischemia, cataract, phthisis bulbi	No PL to PL positive Refraction −5 to −17.5
5.	Krolicki TJ et al.	JAMA Ophthalmology, 1995	14 eyes (Regressed-10)	Retinal treatment-4 Cryotherapy-2	–	–	16–43 y (34.9 y)	4–269 m	Primary-8	N-9 PSC-4 ASC-1	PCR—2	VAO-6 Glaucoma-5	BCVA >20/200-5
6.	Farr et al.	Am J Ophthalmol, 2001	20 eyes	Retinal surgery-2 Cryotherapy-1	–	–	17–73 y (44.6 y)	6–103 m (32 m)	Primary-16 Scleral fixated-2	–	Zonular weakness-2	Retinal detachment-1 Glaucoma—8 eyes	BCVA >20/200-13

(continued)

Table 16.1 (continued)

Sr. No.	Author	Journal, year	No. of eyes	Previous retinal treatment (eyes)	Gestational age (wks)	Birth weight (g)	Age at surgery	Follow-up	PCIOL	Type of cataract (eyes)	Intraoperative complications	Postoperative complication (eyes)	Vision
7	Kaiser et al.	Am J Ophthalmol, 2008	66 eyes (18%-No peripheral changes, 38%-stage 1, 15%-stage 2, 21%-stage 3, 8%-stage 4)	–	24–30 (27)	679–1698 (1018)	7–66 y (40.31 y)	1 m–38.1 y (12 y)	–	–		Retinal tear or retinal detachment—15	BCVA > 20/200-39 BCVA < 4/200-13
8	Chandra et al.	Indian pediatics, 2016	2 eyes (APROP)	Laser-2	26	1200	36 wks	40 wks	Aphakic	T-2			Mild vitreous hemorrhage
9	Khokhar et al.	J Pediatr Ophthalmol Strabismus, 2019	2 eyes (APROP)	Intravitreal bevacizumab	28	1050	35 wks	–	Primary	T-2	–	–	–
10	Vanathi et al.	J Pediatr Ophthalmol Strabismus, 2019	3 eyes (stage 3-3)	Intravitreal anti-VEGF-3	28–30	980–1040	9 m–2 y (14 m)	3–6 m	Primary-3	Z-1 PSC-2	Peripheral dehiscence of posterior capsule-1		BCVA >20/200-1

wks weeks, *m* months, *y* years, *g* grams, *VEGF* vascular endothelial growth factor, *PCIOL* posterior capsular intraocular lens, *T* total, *N* nuclear, *Z* zonular, *PSC* posterior subcapsular, *ASC* anterior subcapsular, *VAO* visual axis opacification, *PCR* posterior capsular rupture, *BCVA* best corrected visual acuity, *PL* perception of light focused toms are usually ignored and difficulty in obtaining medical history [52]. The presence of cataract may further complicate the scenario. Posterior segment abnormalities can be associated with lens disorders like cataract or subluxated lens. The anatomical and functional success is poorer in pediatric cases with lens disorders as compared to those without lens involvement [53]. The various pediatric vitreoretinal disorders with cataract include incontinentia pigment, Coats disease, persistent hyperplastic primary vitreous (PHPV), familial exudative vitreoretinopathy (FEVR), and Stickler syndrome. Few of them are described here.

16.7 Coats Disease

Coats disease is seen in young males as a unilateral presentation characterized by telangiectatic vessels and exudation. Lenticular involvement seen in 8–28% of cases with Coats disease especially in the advanced stages includes total white cataract, posterior subcapsular cataract and less commonly as anterior subcapsular cataract [54–56]. The possible factors affecting the cataract formation in coats disease includes stage of the disease, extension of telangiectasia and exudation, presence of exudative retinal detachment, rubeosis iridis and neovascular glaucoma [56]. Presence of the exudative retinal detachment and advanced stage of the disease was one of the important factors in association with cataract formation and also a significant predictor for worse final visual outcome [56]. The cortical degeneration and the posterior migration of the lens epithelium was seen in enucleated eyes of cases with Coats disease and cataract [57]. The chronic exudation and inflammation do play a role in the cataract formation. The breakdown of the blood-retinal barrier and the oxidative stress are key factors. Though laser treatment is known to cause cataract in ROP, its role in coats disease with cataract have not been explored. Tunica vasculosa lentis which is a risk factor in ROP cases is not seen with coats disease. Hence, probably laser does not have any role in cataract formation. Cataract extraction does improve the fundus visualization but may not necessarily lead to improvement in vision.

16.8 Persistent Hyperplastic Primary Vitreous (PHPV)

PHPV is a congenital abnormality with failure of regression of the embryologic primary vitreous and hyaloid vasculature. Most cases are unilateral with microphthalmos, cataract, persistent hyaloid vasculature, and persistent tunica vasculosa lentis [58]. Advanced cases can have severe microphthalmos, foveal hypoplasia, retinal dysplasia or retinal detachment. PHPV is of three types—anterior, posterior, and combined. The posterior PHPV has poorer prognosis as compared to anterior PHPV [59, 60]. But untreated PHPV have high rate of progressing to phthisis bulbi, secondary glaucoma or painful blind eye requiring enucleation. The removal of the anterior traction relieves the pulling force on the ciliary body does decreasing the possibility of phthisis bulbi [59].The anatomical differences makes it difficult to perform cataract surgery and further implantation of an IOL is a challenge. In cases where corneal diameter is more than 10 mm and adequate capsular support is present, IOL implantation can be done. Being unilateral disease most of the time, amblyopia is another concern. The surgical outcomes are further compromised by high rate of intraoperative and post-operative complications like hyphemia, vitreous hemorrhage, recurrent VAO, glaucoma, strabismus and retinal detachment [59–61]. The presence of vascular membrane and stalk is a risk factor for bleeding. Diathermy or Fugo plasma blade can be used to cauterize the same [62].

16.9 Hereditary Syndromes

Cataract has been associated with various hereditary syndrome including Stickler syndrome, FEVR, retinitis pigmentosa, Usher syndrome, and others. In most of the diseases, it appears to be a secondary effect of the vitreoretinal degeneration and underlying effect rather than being a primary component of the genetic disorder. Further, the high risk of retinal detachment inherent to the pathology and to vitreal changes induced after the cataract surgery can significantly affect the visual outcome. Thus, follow-up examination of the fundus post cataract surgery is important at every visit to detect any posterior segment changes earlier.

Many studies have documented a higher association of same with retinitis pigmentosa [63]. The posterior subcapsular type is the most common type seen in retinitis pigmentosa and causes significant glare abnormalities especially in advanced cases with decrease in the visual fields (Fig. 16.5). But many of these present at a later stage of life. Cases with normal macular area may significantly benefit from the cataract surgery. Also some amount of zonular laxity is known to be associated with RP and these cases are hence prone to have subluxations or postoperative anterior capsular phimosis (Fig. 16.6) [64–66]. Hence, few considerations to be kept in mind while performing the surgery. The preoperative evaluation should include assessment of the visual fields if possible to explain the prognosis and benefits obtained by surgery. The ACC should be adequate and in case of any zonular laxity, CTR can be placed in the bag.

Lens involvement in Wagner disease is seen in adolescent age group and includes discrete anterior and posterior polar dot-like opacities, PSC, and nuclear sclerosis. They slowly progress to visual incapacitation at a later stage. The cataract surgery in these cases can cause vitreous changes and its related complications [67]. Stickler syndrome, also known as hereditary progressive arthro-ophthalmopathy, is a connective tissue disorder presenting with ocular, hearing abnormalities, midfacial underdevelopment, palatal abnormalities, mild spondyloepiphyseal dysplasia or precocious arthritis [68]. Ocular involvement can include myopia, glaucoma, strabismus, vitreoretinal degeneration, retinal detachment or cataract. Lens involvement is seen as wedge and fleck cataracts distinctively (Fig. 16.7) [69]. In a study of 70 members of 22 families, they found that the prevalence of cataract was 20% below the age of 10 years and increased to 83% in more than 50 years group [70]. FEVR is considered as one of the differential diagnosis of ROP. These cases develop cataract and retinal detachment as late complications. However, the pathogenesis of the cataract in same is unclear.

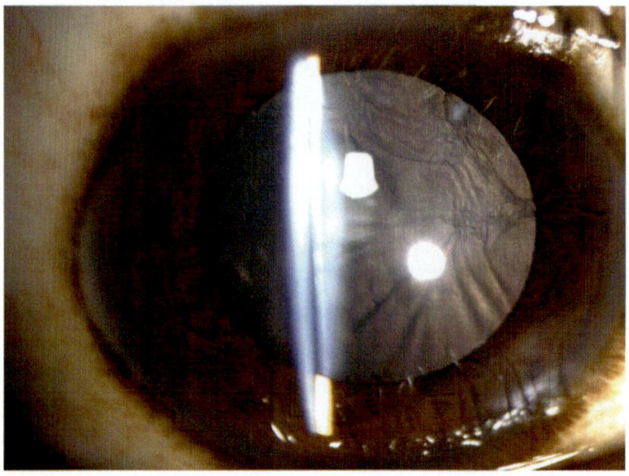

Fig. 16.5 Thirteen-year-old patient with retinitis pigmentosa with anterior and posterior subcapular cataract with folds in the capsule and mild fibrosis

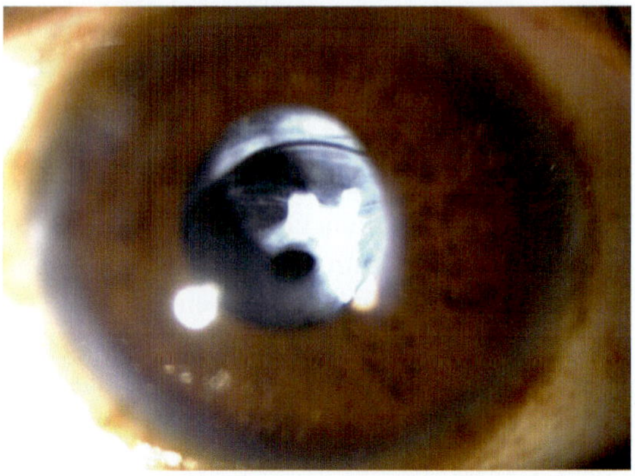

Fig. 16.6 Pseudophakia with severe anterior capsular phimosis 2 years after surgery in OS of the same patient as Fig. 16.5. Note no capsular tension ring put in OS

16.10 Ocular Trauma

Posterior segment can be involved in both the open and closed globe injuries and can be also associated with lens involvement. After the primary injury repair, one can assess the status of the posterior segment using ultrasonography in the setting of cataract. In presence of retinal

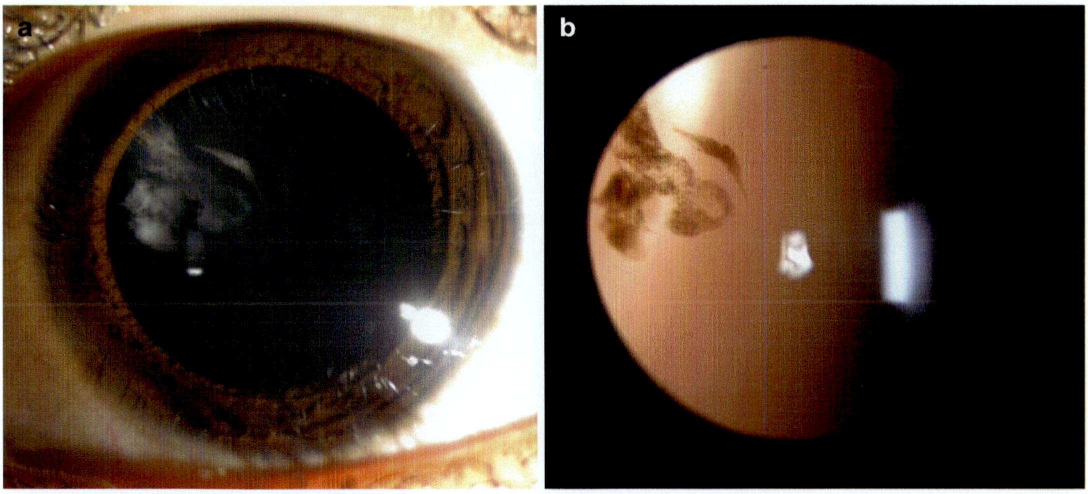

Fig. 16.7 Wedge-shaped cataract in 8-year-old boy with Stickler syndrome. (**a**) Diffuse illumination picture. (**b**) Retro-illumination picture

detachment or endophthalmitis, removal of lens by phacoemulsification or lens aspiration may be required for posterior segment management. The technique of lens aspiration further depends on the multiple factors like mode of injury, cornea status, cornea clarity, intactness of anterior and posterior capsule, or presence of hypotony. Thus stepwise method evaluating each step is required in cases with traumatic cataract and posterior segment abnormalities. Further secondary IOL implantation, wearing appropriate refractive error glasses and occlusion therapy after management for trauma related posterior segment injuries and cataract in children allows treatment of deprivation amblyopia and obtain good vision [71].

16.10.1 Ocular tumor

Retinoblastoma (RB) is the commonest intraocular malignancy of childhood. It is differential diagnosis for leukocoria. Ultrasonography is required to make a presumptive diagnosis of RB. USG showing mass lesion with calcification is highly suggestive (Fig. 16.8). Rather than the disease, cataract is most commonly a complication of radiation therapy received in the course of disease treatment [72]. Simultaneous occurrence of cataract with retinoblastoma is <1% [73, 74]. Surgical outcomes in radiation induced cataract depend on the primary location of regressed RB, with macular lesion showing worse prognosis than peripheral lesions.

Keypoints
- Cataract in ROP children can be because of the systemic status, retinal detachment, ROP itself or treatment of ROP.
- Early diagnosis and management of cataract is important to plan for posterior segment intervention.
- In case of severe neovascularization, anti-VEGF injection may be useful for stabilization of the disease till cataract is managed.
- Preoperative USG and UBM can help in determining preexisting retinal detachment and posterior capsular defect.
- A combined approach with postoperative care and counseling is important to maintain good vision in these preterm individuals. Long-term follow-up is necessary.
- Pediatric retinal disorders differ from adult disorder in term of cause and outcome.

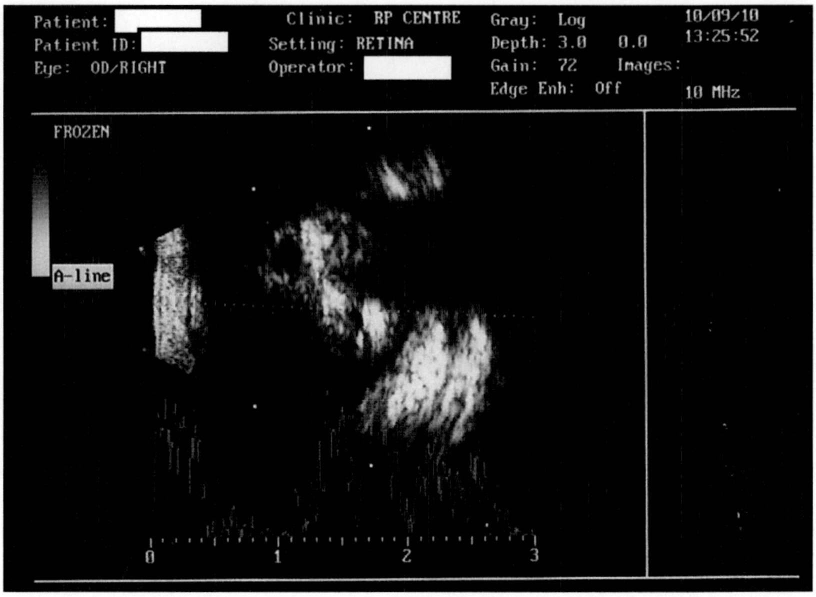

Fig. 16.8 USG showing mass lesion in the posterior segment with calcification suggestive of retinoblastoma

Presence of cataract further affects the prognosis.

- Regular follow-up with fundus examination is important after cataract surgery in pediatric cases with vitreoretinal abnormalities.

References

1. Lambert SR, Drack AV. Infantile cataracts. Surv Ophthalmol. 1996;40(6):427–58. https://doi.org/10.1016/S0039-6257(96)82011-X.
2. Vander JF, McNamara JA, Tasman W, Brown GC. Revised indications for early treatment of retinopathy of prematurity. Arch Ophthalmol. 2005;123(3):406–7; discussion 409–10. https://doi.org/10.1001/archopht.123.3.406-b.
3. Ezisi CN, Kekunnaya R, Jalali S, et al. Cataract surgery in children with retinopathy of prematurity (ROP): surgical outcomes. Br J Ophthalmol. 2017;101(8):1128–31. https://doi.org/10.1136/bjophthalmol-2016-309392.
4. Davitt BV, Christiansen SP, Hardy RJ, Tung B, Good WV, Early Treatment for Retinopathy of Prematurity Cooperative Group. Incidence of cataract development by 6 months' corrected age in the Early Treatment for Retinopathy of Prematurity study. J AAPOS. 2013;17(1):49–53. https://doi.org/10.1016/j.jaapos.2012.10.011.
5. Yu YS, Kim S-J, Chang BL. Cataract surgery in children with and without retinopathy of prematurity. J Cataract Refract Surg. 2004;30(1):89–94. https://doi.org/10.1016/S0886-3350(03)00059-2.
6. Krolicki TJ, Tasman W. Cataract extraction in adults with retinopathy of prematurity. Arch Ophthalmol. 1995;113(2):173–7. https://doi.org/10.1001/archopht.1995.01100020057028.
7. Vanathi M, Kumawat D, Singh R, Chandra P. Iatrogenic crystalline lens injury in pediatric eyes following intravitreal injection for retinopathy of prematurity. J Pediatr Ophthalmol Strabismus. 2019;56(3):162–7. https://doi.org/10.3928/01913913-20190211-02.
8. Chandra P, Khokhar S, Kumar A. Bilateral total cataract after laser treatment of aggressive posterior retinopathy of prematurity. Indian Pediatr. 2016;53(Suppl 2):S157–8.
9. Khokhar S, Chandra P, Gupta Y, Kumawat D, Dhull C. Bilateral total cataract after intravitreal bevacizumab injection in aggressive posterior retinopathy of prematurity. J Pediatr Ophthalmol Strabismus. 2019;56:e28–30. https://doi.org/10.3928/01913913-20190219-02.
10. Alden ER, Kalina RE, Hodson WA. Transient cataracts in low-birth-weight infants. J Pediatr. 1973;82(2):314–8. https://doi.org/10.1016/s0022-3476(73)80180-5.
11. Drack AV, Burke JP, Pulido JS, Keech RV. Transient punctate lenticular opacities as a complication of argon laser photoablation in an infant with retinopathy of prematurity. Am J Ophthalmol. 1992;113(5):583–4. https://doi.org/10.1016/s0002-9394(14)74733-6.
12. Khokhar SK, Pillay G, Dhull C, Agarwal E, Mahabir M, Aggarwal P. Pediatric cataract. Indian J Ophthalmol. 2017;65(12):1340–9. https://doi.org/10.4103/ijo.IJO_1023_17.
13. Choi J, Kim JH, Kim S-J, Yu YS. Long-term results of lens-sparing vitrectomy for stages 4B and 5 retinopathy of prematurity. Korean J Ophthalmol. 2011;25(5):305–10. https://doi.org/10.3341/kjo.2011.25.5.305.

14. Lakhanpal RR, Davis GH, Sun RL, Albini TA, Holz ER. Lens clarity after 3-port lens-sparing vitrectomy in stage 4A and 4B retinal detachments secondary to retinopathy of prematurity. Arch Ophthalmol. 2006;124(1):20–3. https://doi.org/10.1001/archopht.124.1.20.
15. Gold RS. Cataracts associated with treatment for retinopathy of prematurity. J Pediatr Ophthalmol Strabismus. 1997;34(2):123–4.
16. Knight-Nanan DM, Algawi K, Bowell R, O'Keefe M. Advanced cicatricial retinopathy of prematurity--outcome and complications. Br J Ophthalmol. 1996;80(4):343–5. https://doi.org/10.1136/bjo.80.4.343.
17. Trese MT, Shokoohi FK. Immediate complications of cryotherapy in children. Retina (Philadelphia, Pa). 1990;10(2):159.
18. Cryotherapy for Retinopathy of Prematurity Cooperative Group. Multicenter trial of cryotherapy for retinopathy of prematurity. Preliminary results. Arch Ophthalmol. 1988;106(4):471–9. https://doi.org/10.1001/archopht.1988.01060130517027.
19. Repka MX, Tung B, Good WV, et al. Outcome of eyes developing retinal detachment during the Early Treatment for Retinopathy of Prematurity Study (ETROP). Arch Ophthalmol. 2006;124(1):24–30. https://doi.org/10.1001/archopht.124.1.24.
20. Christiansen SP, Bradford JD. Cataract in infants treated with argon laser photocoagulation for threshold retinopathy of prematurity. Am J Ophthalmol. 1995;119(2):175–80. https://doi.org/10.1016/s0002-9394(14)73870-x.
21. O'Neil JW, Hutchinson AK, Saunders RA, Wilson ME. Acquired cataracts after argon laser photocoagulation for retinopathy of prematurity. J AAPOS. 1998;2(1):48–51. https://doi.org/10.1016/s1091-8531(98)90110-0.
22. Paysse EA, Miller A, Brady McCreery KM, Coats DK. Acquired cataracts after diode laser photocoagulation for threshold retinopathy of prematurity. Ophthalmology. 2002;109(9):1662–5. https://doi.org/10.1016/s0161-6420(02)01169-7.
23. Mintz-Hittner HA, Kennedy KA, Chuang AZ. BEAT-ROP Cooperative Group. Efficacy of intravitreal bevacizumab for stage 3+ retinopathy of prematurity. N Engl J Med. 2011;364(7):603–15. https://doi.org/10.1056/NEJMoa1007374.
24. Cuthbertson F, Newsom R. UK retinopathy of prematurity treatment survey. Eye (Lond). 2007;21(2):156–7. https://doi.org/10.1038/sj.eye.6702230.
25. Campolattaro BN, Lueder GT. Cataract in infants treated with argon laser photocoagulation for threshold retinopathy of prematurity. Am J Ophthalmol. 1995;120(2):264–6. https://doi.org/10.1016/s0002-9394(14)72627-3.
26. Kaiser RS, Trese MT. Iris atrophy, cataracts, and hypotony following peripheral ablation for threshold retinopathy of prematurity. Arch Ophthalmol. 2001;119(4):615–7.
27. Quan AV, Pineles SL, Tsui I, Velez FG. Phthisis bulbi following lensectomy in retinopathy of prematurity eyes previously treated with laser photocoagulation. Retin Cases Brief Rep. 2015;9(1):67–71. https://doi.org/10.1097/ICB.0000000000000086.
28. Fung AE, Rosenfeld PJ, Reichel E. The International Intravitreal Bevacizumab Safety Survey: using the internet to assess drug safety worldwide. Br J Ophthalmol. 2006;90(11):1344–9. https://doi.org/10.1136/bjo.2006.099598.
29. Meyer CH, Rodrigues EB, Michels S, et al. Incidence of damage to the crystalline lens during intravitreal injections. J Ocul Pharmacol Ther. 2010;26(5):491–5. https://doi.org/10.1089/jop.2010.0045.
30. Stahl A, Lepore D, Fielder A, et al. Ranibizumab versus laser therapy for the treatment of very low birthweight infants with retinopathy of prematurity (RAINBOW): an open-label randomised controlled trial. Lancet. 2019;394(10208):1551–9. https://doi.org/10.1016/S0140-6736(19)31344-3.
31. Chen TA, Shields RA, Bodnar ZH, Callaway NF, Schachar IH, Moshfeghi DM. A spectrum of regression following intravitreal bevacizumab in retinopathy of prematurity. Am J Ophthalmol. 2019;198:63–9. https://doi.org/10.1016/j.ajo.2018.09.039.
32. Hairston RJ, Maguire AM, Vitale S, Green WR. Morphometric analysis of pars plana development in humans. Retina (Philadelphia, Pa). 1997;17(2):135–8. https://doi.org/10.1097/00006982-199703000-00009.
33. Chang SHL, Lee Y-S, Wu S-C, et al. Anterior chamber angle and anterior segment structure of eyes in children with early stages of retinopathy of prematurity. Am J Ophthalmol. 2017;179:46–54. https://doi.org/10.1016/j.ajo.2017.04.010.
34. Fledelius HC. Pre-term delivery and the growth of the eye an oculometric study of eye size around term-time. Acta Ophthalmol. 1992;70(S204):10–5. https://doi.org/10.1111/j.1755-3768.1992.tb04915.x.
35. Laws DE, Haslett R, Ashby D, O'Brien C, Clark D. Axial length biometry in infants with retinopathy of prematurity. Eye. 1994;8(4):427–30. https://doi.org/10.1038/eye.1994.101.
36. Azad RV, Lakshminarayana P, Kumar H, Talwar D, Pal N, Chandra P. Ocular growth pattern in cryotherapy- and laser-treated infants with prethreshold retinopathy of prematurity. J Pediatr Ophthalmol Strabismus. 2005;42(3):149–54.
37. Axer-Siegel R, Bourla D, Kremer I, Weinberger D, Snir M. Effect of peripheral retinal ablation with cryotherapy versus diode laser photocoagulation on axial length in the growing rabbit eye. Br J Ophthalmol. 2006;90(4):491–5. https://doi.org/10.1136/bjo.2005.082768.
38. Cook A, White S, Batterbury M, Clark D. Ocular growth and refractive error development in premature infants with or without retinopathy of prematurity. Invest Ophthalmol Vis Sci. 2008;49(12):5199–207. https://doi.org/10.1167/iovs.06-0114.

39. Dick HB, Aliyeva SE, Hengerer F. Effect of trypan blue on the elasticity of the human anterior lens capsule. J Cataract Refract Surg. 2008;34(8):1367–73. https://doi.org/10.1016/j.jcrs.2008.03.041.
40. Astle WF, Alewenah O, Ingram AD, Paszuk A. Surgical outcomes of primary foldable intraocular lens implantation in children: understanding posterior opacification and the absence of glaucoma. J Cataract Refract Surg. 2009;35(7):1216–22. https://doi.org/10.1016/j.jcrs.2009.02.028.
41. Vasavada AR, Praveen MR, Tassignon M-J, et al. Posterior capsule management in congenital cataract surgery. J Cataract Refract Surg. 2011;37(1):173–93. https://doi.org/10.1016/j.jcrs.2010.10.036.
42. Khokhar SK, Tomar A, Pillay G, Agarwal E. Biometric changes in Indian pediatric cataract and postoperative refractive status. Indian J Ophthalmol. 2019;67(7):1068–72. https://doi.org/10.4103/ijo.IJO_1327_18.
43. McClatchey SK. Choosing IOL power in pediatric cataract surgery. Int Ophthalmol Clin. 2010;50(4):115–23. https://doi.org/10.1097/IIO.0b013e3181f0f2e0.
44. Nguyen H, Yen KG. Outcome of cataract surgery in patients treated for retinopathy of prematurity. Open J Ophthalmol. 2017;7(4):293–302. https://doi.org/10.4236/ojoph.2017.74038.
45. Cole CJ, Charteris DG. Cataract extraction after retinal detachment repair by vitrectomy: visual outcome and complications. Eye (Lond). 2009;23(6):1377–81. https://doi.org/10.1038/eye.2008.255.
46. Saeed MU, Prasad S. Management of cataract caused by inadvertent capsule penetration during intravitreal injection of ranibizumab. J Cataract Refract Surg. 2009;35(11):1857–9. https://doi.org/10.1016/j.jcrs.2009.05.050.
47. Farr AK, Stark WJ, Haller JA. Cataract surgery by phacoemulsification in adults with retinopathy of prematurity. Am J Ophthalmol. 2001;132(3):306–10. https://doi.org/10.1016/s0002-9394(01)01006-6.
48. O'Keefe M, Fenton S, Lanigan B. Visual outcomes and complications of posterior chamber intraocular lens implantation in the first year of life. J Cataract Refract Surg. 2001;27(12):2006–11. https://doi.org/10.1016/s0886-3350(01)00973-7.
49. Bremer DL, Rogers DL, Good WV, Tung B, Hardy RJ, Fellows R. Glaucoma in the Early Treatment for Retinopathy of Prematurity (ETROP) study. J AAPOS. 2012;16(5):449–52. https://doi.org/10.1016/j.jaapos.2012.06.011.
50. Chandra P, Tewari R, Salunkhe N, Kumawat D, Chaurasia AK, Gupta V. Short-term incidence and management of glaucoma after successful surgery for stage 4 retinopathy of prematurity. Indian J Ophthalmol. 2019;67(6):917. https://doi.org/10.4103/ijo.IJO_33_18.
51. Kaiser RS, Fenton GL, Tasman W, Trese MT. Adult retinopathy of prematurity: retinal complications from cataract surgery. Am J Ophthalmol. 2008;145(4):729–735.e1. https://doi.org/10.1016/j.ajo.2007.11.007.
52. Rumelt S, Sarrazin L, Averbukh E, Halpert M, Hemo I. Paediatric vs adult retinal detachment. Eye (Lond). 2007;21(12):1473–8. https://doi.org/10.1038/sj.eye.6702511.
53. Wang NK, Chen TL, Lai CC, et al. Clinical characteristics and surgical outcomes of pediatric retinal detachments with lens disorders. J Pediatr Ophthalmol Strabismus. 2009;46(3):160–7. https://doi.org/10.3928/01913913-20090505-07.
54. Shields JA, Shields CL, Honavar SG, Demirci H. Clinical variations and complications of Coats disease in 150 cases: the 2000 Sanford Gifford Memorial Lecture. Am J Ophthalmol. 2001;131(5):561–71. https://doi.org/10.1016/S0002-9394(00)00883-7.
55. Shields JA, Shields CL, Honavar SG, Demirci H, Cater J. Classification and management of Coats disease: the 2000 Proctor Lecture. Am J Ophthalmol. 2001;131(5):572–83. https://doi.org/10.1016/S0002-9394(01)00896-0.
56. Daruich A, Matet A, Munier FL. Cataract development in children with Coats disease: risk factors and outcome. J AAPOS. 2018;22(1):44–9. https://doi.org/10.1016/j.jaapos.2017.09.009.
57. Chang MM, McLean IW, Merritt JC. Coats' disease: a study of 62 histologically confirmed cases. J Pediatr Ophthalmol Strabismus. 1984;21(5):163–8.
58. Goldberg MF. Persistent fetal vasculature (PFV): an integrated interpretation of signs and symptoms associated with persistent hyperplastic primary vitreous (PHPV). LIV Edward Jackson Memorial Lecture. Am J Ophthalmol. 1997;124(5):587–626.
59. Pollard ZF. Persistent hyperplastic primary vitreous: diagnosis, treatment and results. Trans Am Ophthalmol Soc. 1997;95:487–549.
60. Jinagal J, Gupta PC, Ram J, et al. Outcomes of cataract surgery in children with persistent hyperplastic primary vitreous. Eur J Ophthalmol. 2018;28(2):193–7. https://doi.org/10.5301/ejo.5001017.
61. Johnson CP, Keech RV. Prevalence of glaucoma after surgery for PHPV and infantile cataracts. J Pediatr Ophthalmol Strabismus. 1996;33(1):14–7. https://doi.org/10.3928/0191-3913-19960101-05.
62. Sinha R, Bali SJ, Kumar C, et al. Results of cataract surgery and plasma ablation posterior capsulotomy in anterior persistent hyperplastic primary vitreous. Middle East Afr J Ophthalmol. 2013;20(3):217–20. https://doi.org/10.4103/0974-9233.114794.
63. Heckenlively J. The frequency of posterior subcapsular cataract in the hereditary retinal degenerations. Am J Ophthalmol. 1982;93(6):733–8. https://doi.org/10.1016/0002-9394(82)90469-X.
64. Dikopf MS, Chow CC, Mieler WF, Tu EY. Cataract extraction outcomes and the prevalence of zonular insufficiency in retinitis pigmentosa. Am J Ophthalmol. 2013;156(1):82–88.e2. https://doi.org/10.1016/j.ajo.2013.02.002.
65. Gocho K, Kameya S, Akeo K, et al. High-resolution imaging of patients with Bietti crystalline dystrophy with CYP4V2 mutation. Lai TY, ed. J

Ophthalmol. 2014;2014:283603. https://doi.org/10.1155/2014/283603.
66. Jackson H, Garway-Heath D, Rosen P, Bird AC, Tuft SJ. Outcome of cataract surgery in patients with retinitis pigmentosa. Br J Ophthalmol. 2001;85(8):936–8. https://doi.org/10.1136/bjo.85.8.936.
67. Manning LM. Wagner's hereditary vitreoretinal degeneration. Aust J Opthalmol. 1980;8(1):29–33. https://doi.org/10.1111/j.1442-9071.1980.tb00885.x.
68. Robin NH, Moran RT, Ala-Kokko L. Stickler syndrome. In: Adam MP, Ardinger HH, Pagon RA, et al., editors. GeneReviews®. Seattle: University of Washington; 1993. http://www.ncbi.nlm.nih.gov/books/NBK1302/. Accessed June 2, 2020.
69. Seery CM, Pruett RC, Liberfarb RM, Cohen BZ. Distinctive cataract in the Stickler syndrome. Am J Ophthalmol. 1990;110(2):143–8. https://doi.org/10.1016/S0002-9394(14)76982-X.
70. Liberfarb RM, Hirose T, Holmes LB. The Wagner-Stickler syndrome: a study of 22 families. J Pediatr. 1981;99(3):394–9. https://doi.org/10.1016/s0022-3476(81)80324-1.
71. Bai H, Meng X, Wang D, Han J. Treatment for amblyopia after surgery for cataract and vitreoretina in pediatric ocular trauma. Eye Sci. 2013;28(2):68–72.
72. Brooks HL Jr, Meyer D, Shields JA, Balas AG, Nelson LB, Fontanesi J. Removal of radiation-induced cataracts in patients treated for retinoblastoma. Arch Ophthalmol. 1990;108:1701–8.
73. Brown GC, Shields JA, Oglesby RB. Anterior polar cataracts associated with bilateral retinoblastoma. Am J Ophthalmol. 1979;87:276.
74. Balasubramanya R, Pushker N, Bajaj MS, Ghose S, Kashyap S, Rani A. Atypical presentations of retinoblastoma. J Pediatr Ophthalmol Strabismus. 2004;41:18–24.

Management of Subluxated Lens and Spherophakia

17

Sagnik Sen, Chirakshi Dhull,
Sudarshan Kumar Khokhar, and Kamal Kishore

17.1 Management of Subluxated Lenses and Spherophakia

Chirakshi Dhull and Sudarshan Kumar Khokhar

17.1.1 Introduction

17.1.1.1 Ectopia Lentis

Subluxation or dislocation of lens or ectopia lentis is defined as the shift of the lens from its original location, i.e., the patellar fossa either partially or completely, anteriorly into the anterior chamber or posteriorly towards the vitreous cavity (Fig. 17.1). Subluxation of lens may occur post-trauma or due to predisposing hereditary conditions like Marfan syndrome or Homocystinuria. Spontaneous dislocation may be a common cause of lens dislocation. Post-traumatic dislocation may also happen due to the zonules being weak. However, significant closed globe injury can also cause dislocation of a healthy lens due to zonular injury.

17.1.1.2 Spherophakia

Spherophakia is a very rare ocular disease in which the crystalline lens is spherical instead of its oval shape (Fig. 17.2) and may occur either as an isolated condition or may be a part of hereditary diseases like Marfan syndrome, Weil-Marchesani syndrome, etc. and may or may not be associated with lens subluxation [1]. Most patients have high myopia which can be corrected by spectacles or contact lenses. Movement of the lens into the anterior chamber may intermittently cause acute glaucoma attacks and may be associated with retinal detachment due to repeated vitreous traction and break formation.

Subluxated lens management has evolved over the last half a decade with advancement in surgical instruments and improvement in surgeon experience in handling complicated scenarios. While partial subluxation or anterior dislocation of lenses can be adequately handled by anterior segment surgeons, posterior subluxation or dislocation into the vitreous cavity may require a collaborative effort of both anterior and posterior segment surgeons. After the primary removal of the dislocated lens, the next important management step is refractive rehabilitation by placement

Supplementary Information The online version of this chapter (https://doi.org/10.1007/978-981-16-0212-2_17) contains supplementary material, which is available to authorized users.

S. Sen
Aravind Eye Hospital, Madurai, India

C. Dhull (✉)
Eye Q Hospital, Rohtak, Haryana, India

S. K. Khokhar
Professor Ophthalmology, Dr. RP Centre for Ophthalmic Sciences, All India Institute of Medical Sciences, New Delhi, India

K. Kishore
Illinois Retina and Eye Associates, Peoria, IL, USA

S. K. Khokhar, C. Dhull (eds.), *Essentials of Pediatric Cataract Surgery*,
https://doi.org/10.1007/978-981-16-0212-2_17

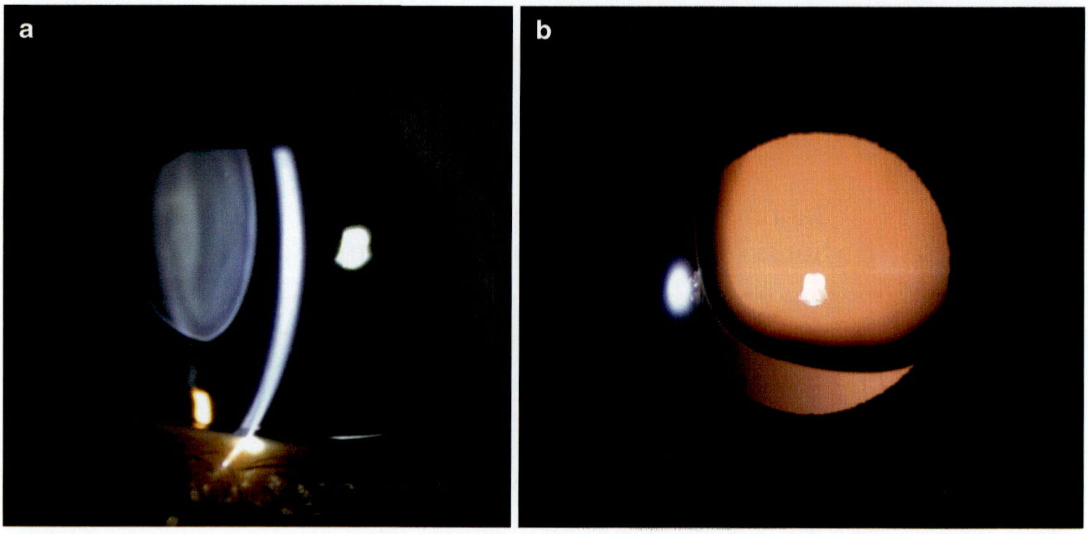

Fig. 17.1 Lenticular subluxation. (**a**) Slit-examination, (**b**) retroillumination picture of supero-temporally subluxated clear lens

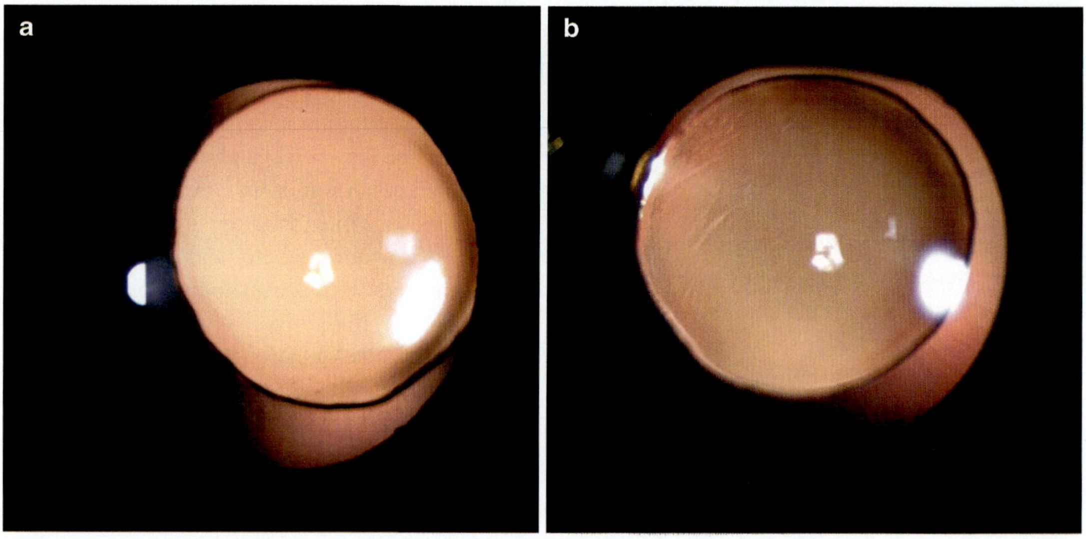

Fig. 17.2 Microspherophakia. (**a**, **b**) Retro illumination picture of right and left eye respectively showing small clear lens, with margins of the lens seen 360° along with stretched zonules

of an intraocular lens, which again depends on the availability of capsular support. Depending on whether adequate capsular support is present, the cases may be handled by anterior segment or posterior segment surgeons. In this chapter, we would be dealing with the various challenging scenarios which might be faced by ophthalmologists during management of such difficult cases.

17.1.2 Clinical History and Examination

All patients must undergo a complete ophthalmological history taking and examination to arrive at a proper etiological diagnosis regarding the subluxation. History should be elicited regarding duration of symptoms, pattern of progression of vision loss, direct trauma to the eye (closed globe or open globe), previous ocular surgery, family history of similar ocular illness or any surgery because of them, and history of using thick glasses.

17.1.2.1 Ectopia Lentis

A detailed systemic evaluation should also be carried out to look at body deformities and heart ailments. It is of prime concern that one rules out systemic diseases causing the subluxation. Most common diseases associated are Marfan syndrome, Homocystinuria, Weil-Marchesani syndrome and Hyperlysinemia. Table 17.1 lists some of the pointers towards diagnosis of systemic cases. Etiology of ectopia lens may be classified based on the following categories:

1. **Genetic without systemic manifestations**
    - Simple ectopia lentis
    - Ectopia lentis et pupillae
    - Ectopia lentis with spherophakia
2. **With systemic manifestations**
    - Marfan syndrome (Modified Ghent's diagnostic criteria in Table 17.2) (Fig. 17.3)
    - Weil-Marchesani syndrome (Diagnostic criteria in Table 17.3) (Fig. 17.4)

Table 17.1 Comparison of clinical features of some systemic causes of lens subluxation [1, 2]

	Marfan syndrome	Homocystinuria	Weil-Marchesani
Inheritance	Autosomal dominant	Autosomal recessive	Autosomal recessive
Skeletal	Arachnodactyly Laxity of joints Deformity of sternum	Occasional arachnodactyly Osteoporosis	Stocky build Short digits Tight joints Brachycephaly
Vascular	Dilatation of aorta root	Dilatation and thrombosis of medium-sized vessels	None
Mental retardation	Absent	Often present	Absent
Gait	Normal	Charlie Chaplin gait	Normal
Lens	Subluxation is stable, zonular fibers are strong and stretched	Subluxation is progressive, zonular fibers are weak and unstable	Spherophakia commonly associated and pathognomonic

Table 17.2 Modified Ghent's criteria for Marfan syndrome

Isolated patient

1. Aortic root dilatation (z >= 2) And Ectopia lentis
2. Aortic root dilatation (z >= 2) And FBN1 mutation
3. Aortic root dilatation (z >= 2) And Systemic score >= 7 points
4. Ectopia lentis And FBN1 mutation

Positive family history

1. Ectopia lentis
2. Systemic score >= 7
3. Aortic root dilatation (z >= 2)

Systemic signs

Wrist AND Thumb sign [3]
Wrist OR Thumb sign [1]
Pectus carinatum [2]
Pectus excavatum or chest asymmetry [1]
Hindfoot deformity [2]
Plain flat foot [1]
Spontaneous pneumothorax [2]
Dural ectasia [2]
Protrucio acetabulae [2]
Scoliosis or thoracolumbar kyphosis [1]
Reduced elbow extension [1]
3/5 facial features [1]
Skin striae [1]
Severe myopia [1]
Mitral valve prolapse [1]
Reduced upper segment/ lower segment ratio [1]

Diagnostic scenarios

I Aortic involvement AND Ectopia lentis
II Aortic involvement AND FBN1 mutation
III Aortic involvement AND Systemic involvement
IV Aortic involvement AND Family history
V Ectopia lentis AND FBN1 mutation
VI Ectopia lentis AND Family history
VII Systemic involvement AND Family history

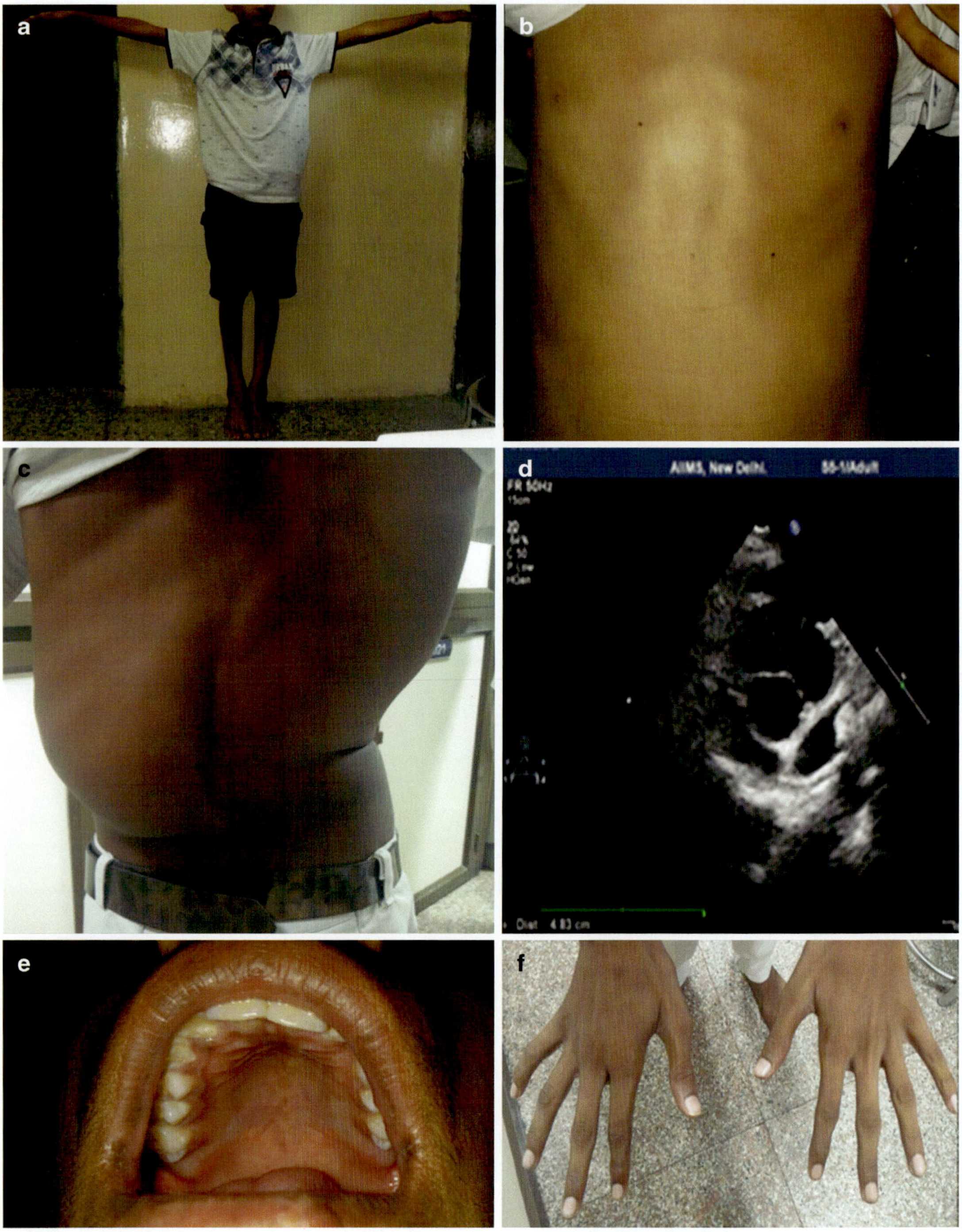

Fig. 17.3 Marfan's syndrome. (**a**) Increased arm span, increased upper segment to lower segment ratio. (**b**) Pectus carinatum. (**c**) Kyphoscoliosis. (**d**) Echocardiogram with aortic root regurgitation. (**e**) High arched palate. (**f**) Positive thumb sign. (**g**) Positive wrist sign

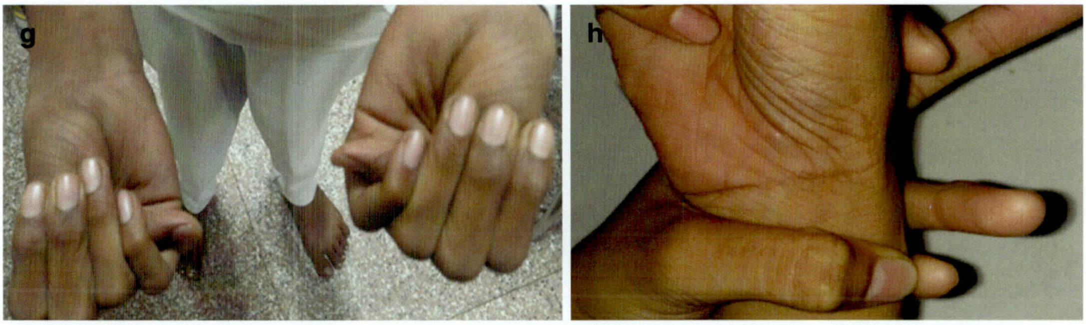

Fig. 17.3 (continued)

Table 17.3 Diagnostic criteria for Weil-Marchesani syndrome

Body abnormalities	Eye abnormalities	Airway abnormalities	Cardiac abnormalities
Brachymorphy Brachycephaly Brachydactyly Short stubby hand	Ectopia lentis Spherophakia High myopia Secondary glaucoma	Maxillary hypoplasia Narrow palate Stiff joints Limited neck movement Malaligned teeth	Prolonged QTc interval Mitral valve prolapse Mitral regurgitation Aortic stenosis Pulmonary stenosis Pulmonary hypertension

- Hyperlysinemia
- Sulfite oxidase deficiency

3. **Primary ocular causes**
   - Pseudoexfoliation syndrome
   - Trauma
   - Myopia
   - Glaucoma/buphthalmos
   - Aniridia
   - Retinitis pigmentosa

17.1.2.2 Spherophakia

Systemic associations have been found with Homocysteinemia, Weil-Marchesani syndrome, Marfan's syndrome, Alport's syndrome, Hyperlysinemia, congenital rubella syndrome, megalocornea-spherophakia-secondary glaucoma, arrhythmogenic right ventricular dysplasia type 1, spinocerebellar ataxia, etc. Prevalence of spherophakia is unclear because of the rare occurrence of the disease. Spherophakia has been seen to commonly occur in patients of Weil-Marchesani syndrome (WMS) and the prevalence of WMS has been estimated at 1:100000. Data from India has shown that 1.2% of children presenting with lens abnormalities have spherophakia [3].

17.1.3 Preoperative Investigations

- **Systemic**: Blood investigations for Homocysteinemia, urine for Homocystinuria, cardiac electrophysiology and electrocardiography, coagulation parameters, chest X-ray (Table 17.4)
- **Ocular**:
  - **Slit lamp biomicroscopy** to document type of subluxation (anterior or posterior), degrees of subluxation with status of equatorial zonules (stretched, broken), fundus examination to rule out posterior segment pathologies like pathological myopia, retinal peripheral degeneration (breaks/ lattices), assess whether the subluxated lens is crystalline or cataractous (along with grade of cataract), presence of vitreous in anterior chamber, undilated and dilated refraction to assess the best corrected visual acuity (to rule out amblyopia)
  - **Gonioscopic evaluation** to look at angles and to rule out pseudoexfoliative material

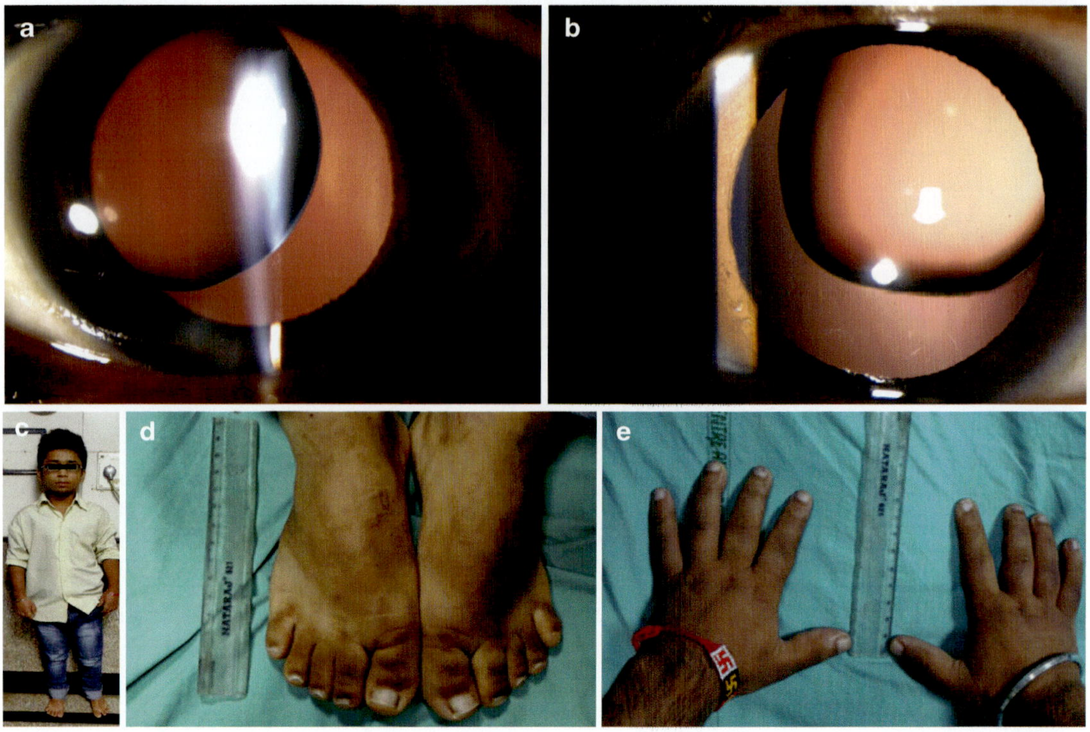

Fig. 17.4 Sixteen-year-old boy with Weil-Marchesani syndrome with spherophakia. (**a**, **b**) Retro illumination picture of right and left eye respectively showing spherophakia with supero-temporal subluxation and broken zonules. (**c**) Notice short stature of the patient. (**d**) Small feet with short toes. (**e**) Short, stubby fingers are seen

Table 17.4 Systemic investigations in hereditary diseases

Systemic disease	Investigations
Marfan syndrome	Cardiac electrophysiology and electrocardiography, chest X-ray, skeletal X-ray
Homocystinuria	Coagulation parameters, urine and serum for homocysteine levels
Weil-marchesani syndrome	Cardiac electrophysiology and electrocardiography, skeletal X-ray
Sulfite oxidase deficiency	Musculoskeletal evaluation

- **Ocular ultrasound** to assess the axial length of the eyeball, as syndromes like Marfan syndrome may be associated with myopia
- **Ocular ultrasound biomicroscopy** and **Anterior segment optical coherence tomography** may be used to assess the zonular status if pupil(s) cannot be dilated due to any reason. Ultrasound biomicroscopy produces two-dimensional cross-sectional images of the anterior segment showing morphology of the anterior chamber angle, iris, ciliary body, zonules, and lens. High resolution optical coherence tomography of the anterior segment gives a cross-sectional image of the lenticular anatomy and is useful to determine the shape of the lens and the orientation of the iris-lens diaphragm to identify pupillary block (Fig. 17.5).

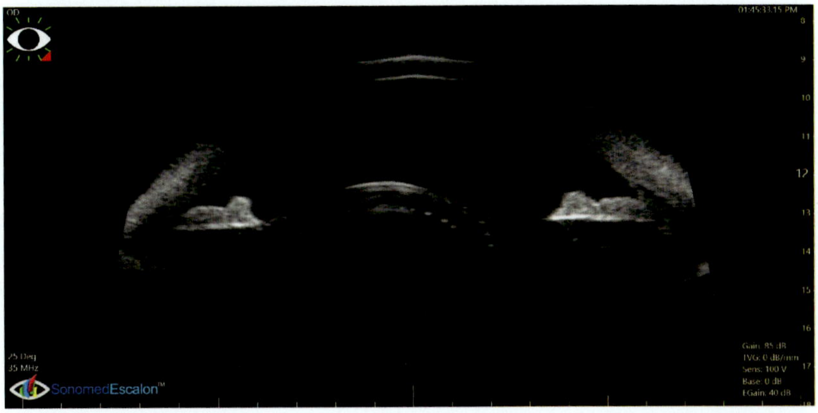

Fig. 17.5 Ultrasound biomicroscopy of subluxated lens showing no tilt, stretched zonules and minimal opacification of lens

– **Biometry** using either immersion ultrasound biometry or IOL Master Optical biometry is used to determine axial length, keratometry and intraocular lens power using SRK-T, Hoffer-Q or Holladay I formulae.

17.1.4 Management Approaches to Lens Subluxation

Not all cases of ectopia need immediate surgical intervention. The various different clinical scenarios of subluxation which need intervention can be summarized as follows:

- High lenticular myopia and myopic astigmatism which can cause amblyopia in children
- Progressive subluxation in children
- Lens dislocation anteriorly
  - Dislocation of crystalline lens into the anterior chamber
  - Dislocation of soft cataractous lens into the anterior chamber
- Lens dislocation posteriorly
  - Dislocation of crystalline lens into vitreous
  - Dislocation of soft cataractous lens into vitreous
- Lens dislocation associated with perforating ocular injuries
- Glaucoma—pupillary block, anterior subluxation into anterior chamber causing inverse glaucoma, mechanical angle closure due to secondary angle closure
- Lens-induced uveitis
- Retinal detachment due to chronic traction

17.1.4.1 Conservative Management

Eyes which do not need immediate surgery must undergo a dilated refraction and wear refractive correction, especially so in children to prevent amblyopia. Several spherophakia eyes have very high lenticular myopia, which need just a full refractive correction. However, such patients may opt in for lens management because of cosmetic reasons.

17.1.4.2 Lens Management

Surgical management of ectopia lentis is a daunting task. Cases presenting with severe forms of subluxation of more than 270°, progressive causes of subluxation such as Marfan's syndrome and anterior dislocation of lens in spherophakia are among some of the most complicated cases. Depending on the location of the dislocated lens, capsular bag status, amount of subluxation, various different techniques have been described over the years. Earliest methods of lens removal consisted of ICCE through a 6 mm incision at the corneoscleral limbus. However, this technique led to vitreous traction due to loss of posterior chamber leading to anterior movement of vitreous resulting in a higher risk of retinal detachment [4]. Hence modern procedures have focused on minimum size of entry into the anterior chamber, with removal of the lens and/ or the capsular bag causing minimum disturbance to the vitreous phase or if at all perform a dry anterior vitrectomy. Posterior dislocation however requires a complete vitrectomy by a vitreoretinal surgeon.

1. **Subluxation of clear lens**
   - **Intralenticular lens aspiration**
   – **Conventional technique** using bimanual irrigation-aspiration probe followed by vitrector [5]

     In this technique, after completion of aspiration of lens material using a bimanual irrigation-aspiration cannula, a vitrectomy cutter is used to remove the capsular bag

     Modified technique using vitrector only (Fig. 17.6) [6]

     In this technique, both the lens and the capsular bag are removed with the help of the vitrectomy cutter, and no change of instruments is needed.

- **Pars plana lensectomy**

  In eyes having posterior dislocation of entire lens or >270° subluxation, it may be preferable to involve a vitreoretinal surgeon to handle the case. Standard 3-port pars plana vitrectomy along with a lensectomy can be performed with or without the implantation of an intraocular lens. Anterior segment surgeons may attempt removing the lens through the anterior route also based on clinical judgment. Limited anterior vitrectomy without the insertion of a posterior infusion line can minimize vitreous traction. However, some surgeons believe unnecessary vitreous traction may

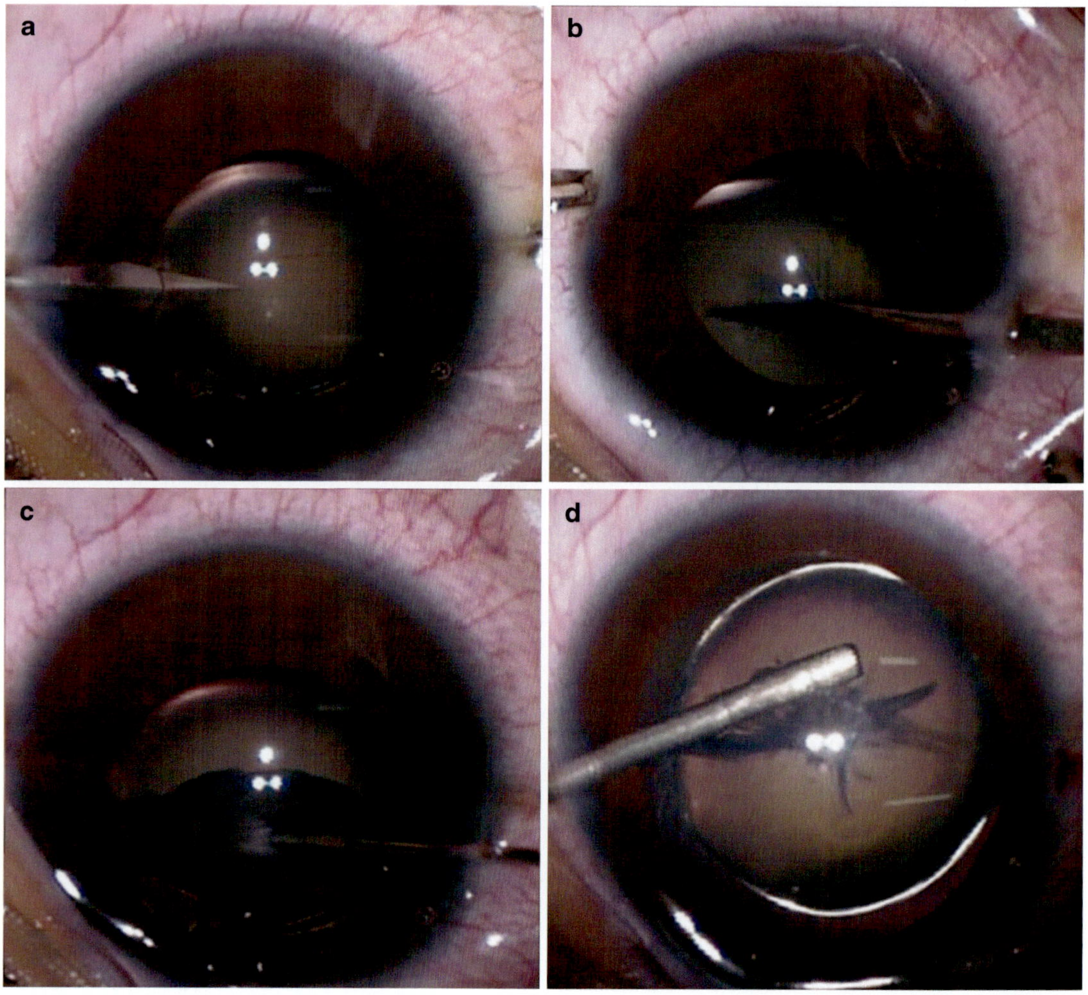

Fig. 17.6 Lensectomy with ACIOL (**a–c**) two MVR entry with entry in the lens. (**d**) Irrigation port of vitrectomy cutter inside lens. (**e**) Lensectomy with cutter. (**f**) Capsular bag removed with cutter. (**g**) AC formed with air. (**h**) ACIOL placed under air. (Source S Khokhar et al.)

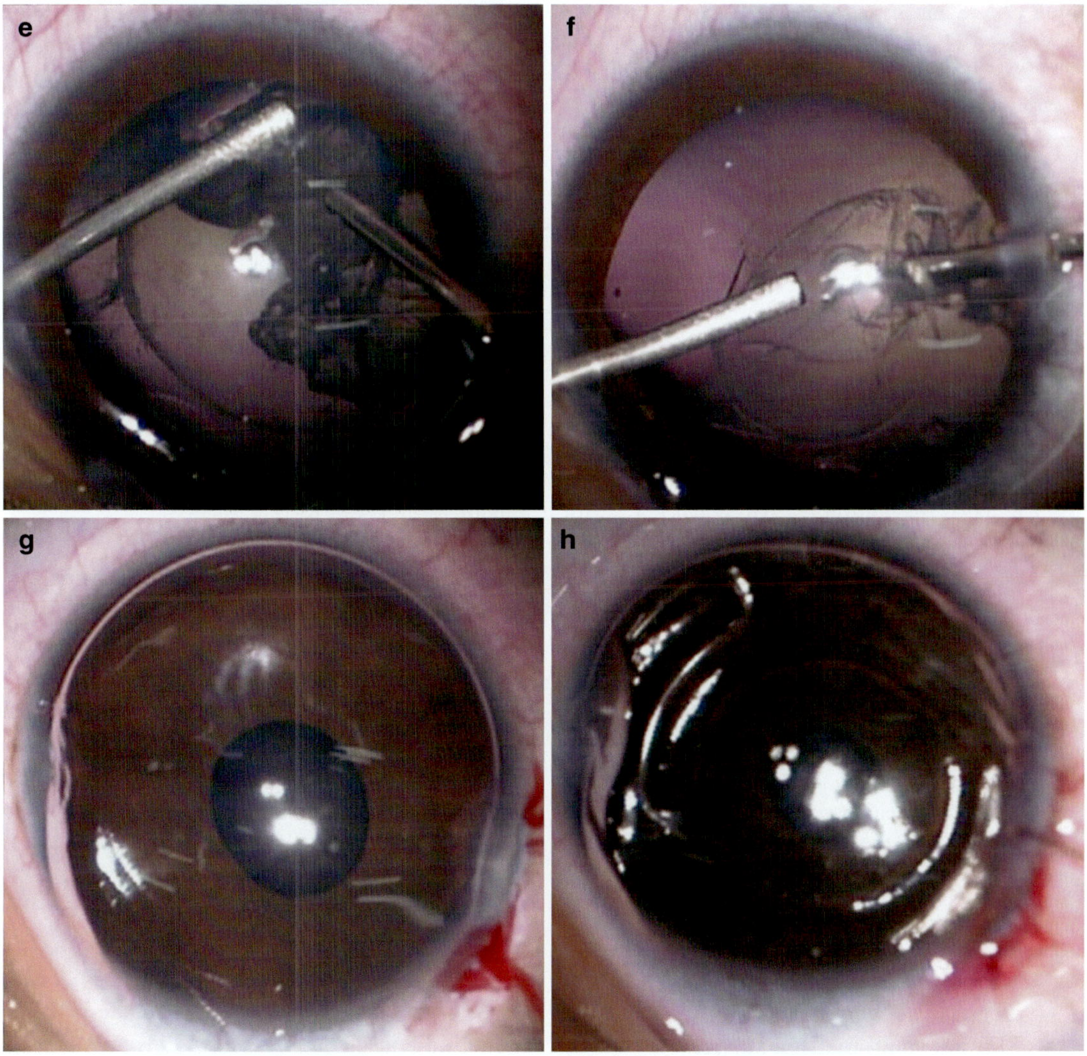

Fig. 17.6 (continued)

predispose the eyes to future retinal complications [7–11].

2. **Subluxation of cataractous lenses**
   - **Phacoaspiration/ Lens aspiration with assistive devices**

     A careful capsulorhexis is warranted keeping in mind the location of the zonular laxity. However, after aspiration of the lens matter, a surgeon may need some surgical assistive devices like the capsular tension ring (CTR), capsular tension segment (CTS), Cionniring,etc.Thesepolymethylmethacrylate rings may be inserted into the capsular bag any time, before phacoemulsification, during or after the aspiration of cortex is done [12–14]. Capsular supportive devices enhance the safety and efficacy during phacoemulsification and IOL implantation, and can maintain the circular contour of the capsular bag. They also avoid the collapsing of the capsular bag after lens aspiration and provide additional support to the bag by pushing it towards its original position in the patellar fossa. This in turn helps prevent IOL decentration or bag contraction. During phacoaspiration, a careful hydrodissection should be done to reduce stress on the zonules by sudden surge of intracapsular pressure. Minimum manipulation of the nucleus should be attempted during aspiration and if possible, performing aspiration

Table 17.5 Summary of surgical procedure according to the degree of zonular dehiscence in cases of traumatic/ non-progressive subluxated lenses

Degree of zonular dehicense	Preferred procedure
Up to 4 clock hours	CTR with IOL
>3–6 clock hours	Modified CTR with single loop
>6–9 clock hours	Modified CTR with double loop with IOL
9 or more clock hours	ICCE with SFIOL/ACIOL

after prolapsing the lens matter in the anterior chamber may also be beneficial. Cortical matter may be removed by viscodissection and reduced traction on the bag equator. Careful phacoaspiration in experienced hands may give very good outcomes in such cases [15, 16]. The degree of zonular dehiscence/ laxity and the choice of surgical procedure may be summarized as in Table 17.5. These surgical decisions are taken for cases with traumatic dislocation or hereditary non-progressive ectopia lentis. For progressive ectopia lentis mostly lens with bag is removed and a scleral-fixated intraocular lens may be preferred. The age of the patient may also be an indicator as to which surgery might be attempted, keeping in mind the future potential of a bag and lens drop into vitreous cavity in future in cases of progressive subluxation and broken zonules.

- **Manual small incision surgery**

  Manual small incision cataract surgery (SICS) may be attempted to remove subluxated lenses in resource limited settings with similar visual outcomes to phacoemulsification. However, authors have reported lesser bag retention, and more complications with SICS than phaco (higher chance of increasing the zonular dehiscence and escaped capsulorhexis), especially in eyes with >180° subluxation and presence of lens coloboma [17, 18].
- **Pars plana lensectomy**

  During pars plana lensectomy to remove cataractous subluxated lens, after removal of core vitreous, perfluorocarbon liquid may be injected to lift the nucleus away from the macula for protection from vitrector or fragmatome [19]. Now, the surgeon needs to assess the grade of cataract and decide whether the vitrectomy cutter would be adequate for efficiency of removal of the lens or a fragmatome needs to be inserted through a separate sclerotomy [20].

17.1.4.3 Role of Ocular Viscoelastic Devices

Viscodispersive agents like Viscoat may be used to fill the area of zonular dehiscence to compartmentalize the anterior chamber from the posterior chamber, preventing the vitreous from entering the anterior chamber and the drop of lens material posteriorly.

17.1.4.4 Choice of Intraocular Lenses for Refractive Rehabilitation

The options for intraocular lens implantation after lensectomy include, angle-supported anterior chamber IOLs (ACIOL), iris-enclavated IOLs, posterior chamber IOLs (PCIOL) and scleral-fixated IOL (SFIOL) [21–23]. The choice of the IOL depends on the availability of capsular support and surgeon experience and expertise.

Anterior Chamber Intraocular Lens

Angle-supported ACIOLs have been reported to have complications like corneal endothelial cell loss, peripheral anterior synechiae (PAS) formation and glaucoma due to chronic anterior chamber irritation [24]. Some of these complications have been listed in Table 17.6. Iris-enclavated lenses avoid the angle related complications and may be placed anterior or posterior to the iris [25, 26]. However, iris-claw

Table 17.6 Complications arising from ACIOLs and SFIOLs

ACIOL	SFIOL
Endothelial decompensation	Chance of decentration
Glaucoma	Concern regarding haptic extrusion
Pigment dispersion	Scleral flap necrosis
Movement if unstable	If sutured, long-term suture breakage
De-enclavation accidentally	Retinal detachment

lenses may not be available in every setup, and ACIOLs have been previously shown to be an effective choice of IOL in pediatric ectopia patients [27].

Steps of angle-supported ACIOL surgery

- Lens aspiration
- Bag removal by vitrectomy cutter ± Core vitrectomy (retina specialist)
- Check anterior chamber for remnant of vitreous strands
- Use vitrector to make a surgical iridetomy
- Put pilocarpine into the anterior chamber and inject air bubble
- Increase the size of the corneal entry wound with MVR blade
- Insert ACIOL (Kelman multiflex) under air
- Suture corneal wound

The technique of iris-claw fixation is discussed in subsequent subsection.

Posterior Chamber Intraocular Lens

In eyes with lesser degree of zonular dehiscence, placing a PCIOL in the bag may be considered [15]. In this regard, a "dual-support technique" of insertion of a capsular tension segment (CTS) with tension ring (CTR) along with a PCIOL in case of spherophakia has been described to stabilize the bag-IOL complex and prevent it from dropping into the vitreous cavity (Fig. 17.7) [16]. Such patients tend to perform well in terms of IOL stability and tilt in the long term (Fig. 17.8).

Scleral-Fixated Intraocular Lens

Another effective method of IOL implantation, especially in eyes without any capsular support, is scleral fixation of intraocular lens (SFIOL), which may be sutured or sutureless. Scleral-fixated IOLs are rid of the angle related problems and various techniques of scleral fixation have been described. However, several complications have been reported with sutured SFIOLs, like suture breakage, decentration of IOL, exposure of haptic by conjunctival erosion, retinal detachment, suprachoroidal hemorrhage, and endophthalmitis (Table 17.3) [28, 29]. Scharioth et al. have described a sutureless technique of haptic burial, using two diametrically opposite scleral tunnels with a 24-gauge cannula, which gets rid of several disadvantages of the sutured technique, like instability of globe and anterior chamber, especially while passing scleral sutures, leading to corneal endothelial damage and improper placement of scleral sutures [30, 31]. SFIOLs have been described safely for both ectopia lentis and spherophakia eyes [32, 33].

Steps of SFIOL surgery

- Two partial thickness scleral tunnels are made at diametrically opposite points using MVR blade, 1.5 mm from the limbus (Gabor's flapless technique) or two flaps 1.5 × 1.5 mm in size are lifted at diametrically opposite points, with partial thickness tunnels, using a crescent blade (flap technique)
- Standard 3-port pars plana vitrectomy is performed with lensectomy
- Two sclerotomies are made near the tunnels
- Multi-piece monofocal IOL is injected into the anterior chamber
- Leading haptic of the IOL is taken out of one sclerotomy using intravitreal forceps or by using docking technique with a 24-gauge needle
- Tailing haptic is taken out of the other sclerotomy and the haptics are tucked into the scleral tunnels
- In cases of flaps, the flap is closed either with the help of sutures or glue and centration of the IOL is checked.

The technique of Gore-tex-fixated SFIOL is discussed in the subsequent subsection.

IOL choice has to be made on a case-to-case basis. ACIOLs should be avoided in eyes at risk of glaucoma or having any corneal pathology. In eyes with conjunctival or scleral thinning, SFIOLs should be avoided due to risk of exposure by erosion [34].

17.1.4.5 Glaucoma Management

Glaucoma may be seen in these eyes and may have different presentations. Pupillary block may occur due to anterior subluxation of the lens, leading to spontaneous shift of iris-lens diaphragm anteriorly. Sometimes, and more so in cases of spherophakia, where the lens is globular, the anterior subluxation may cause secondary angle closure glaucoma due to shallow anterior chamber. The spherophakic lens may also wander into the anterior chamber and cause "inverse glaucoma," where pupillary miosis traps the lens in the anterior chamber, causing mechanical angle closure. Lens-induced uveitis may also cause chronic glaucoma due to trapping of inflammatory cells in the angle.

Pupillary block glaucoma cases are treated with topical and/or systemic medications and laser or surgical peripheral iridotomy. Some surgeons have suggested trabeculectomy for control of intraocular pressure. Simple lens extraction may also control intraocular pressure to some extent, however, a future trabeculectomy may be required eventually. Inverse glaucoma cases are treated with immediate lens extraction.

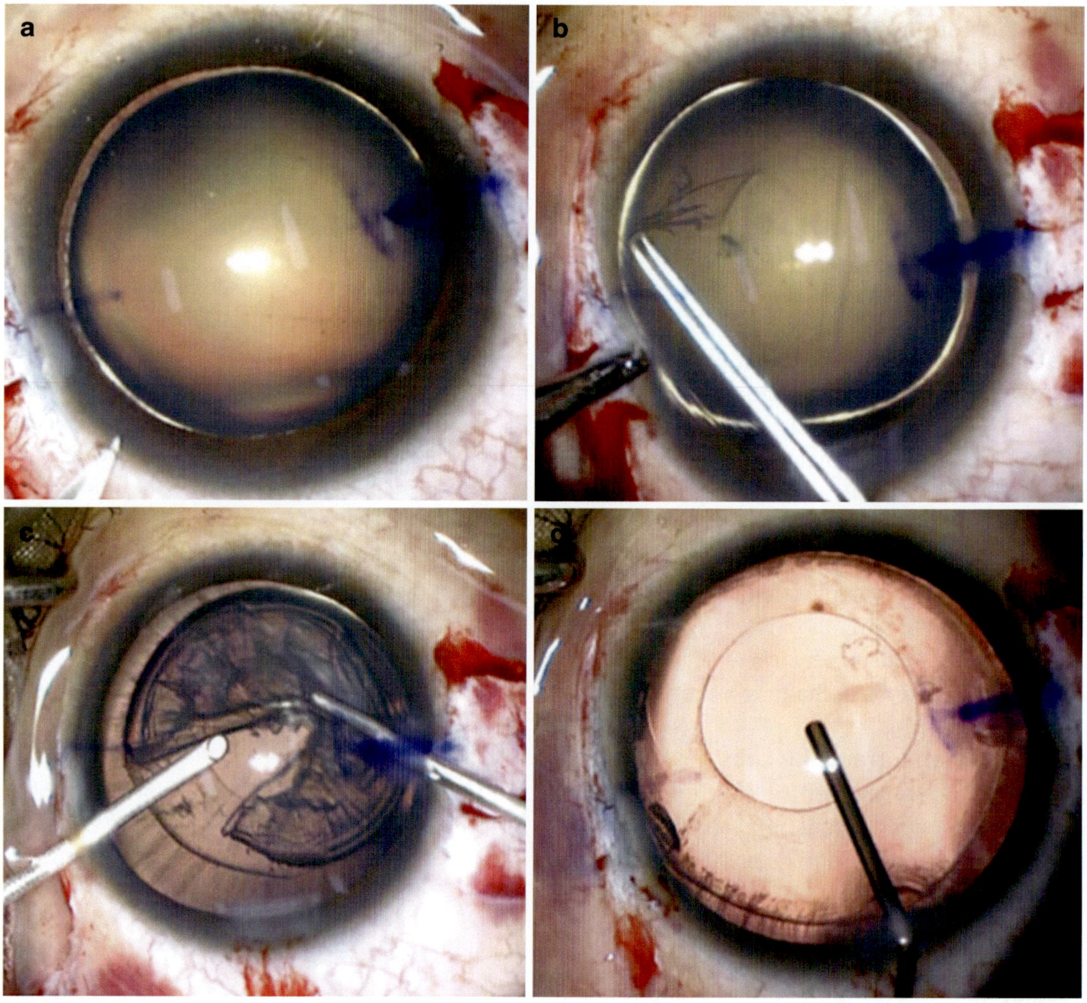

Fig. 17.7 Dual fixation technique (**a**) Spherophakia with two scleral tunnel 180° across. (**b**) Anterior capsulorhexis completed using Utrata forceps. (**c**) Lensectomy performed inside the bag. (**d**) Intact bag after completion on lensectomy. (**e**) 9-0 prolene being used to fix Cionni ring with sclera. (**f**) Cionni ring in the bag. (**g**) CTS in the bag (opposite side). (**h**) Final position after placing IOL with superior and inferior fixation

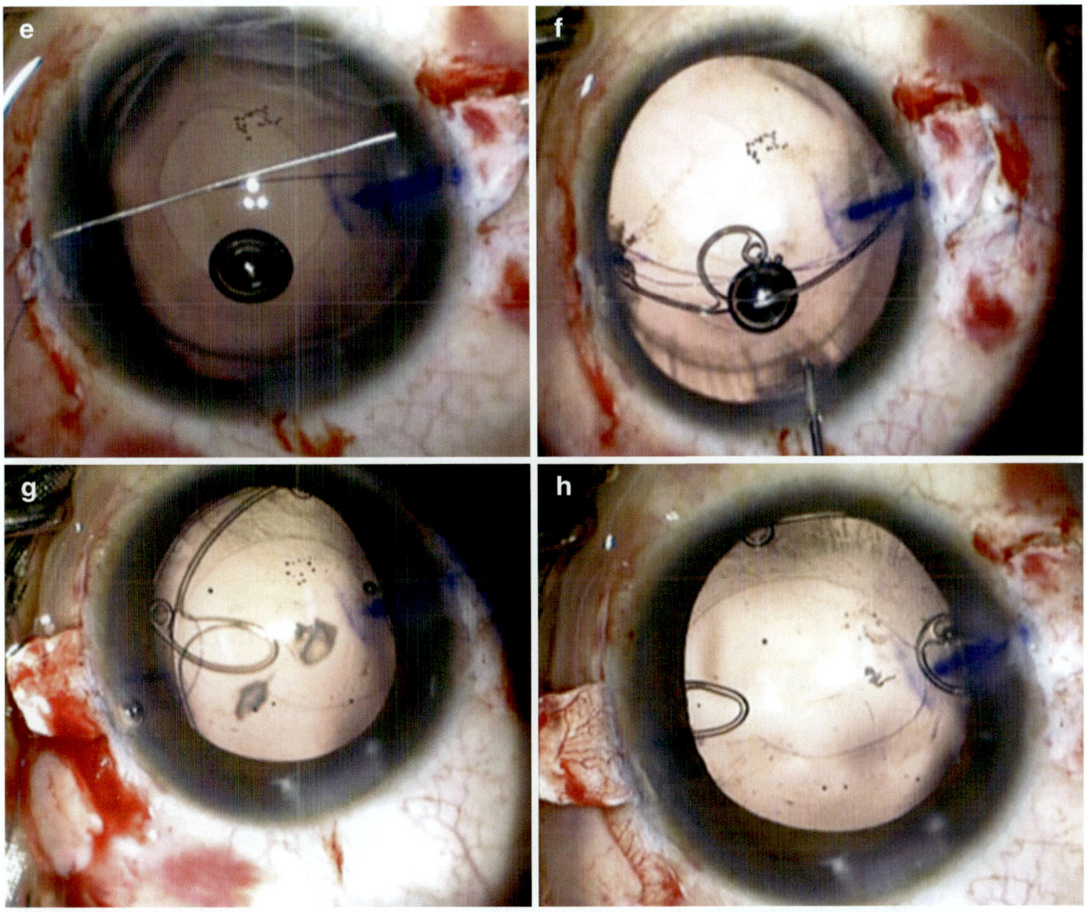

Fig. 17.7 (continued)

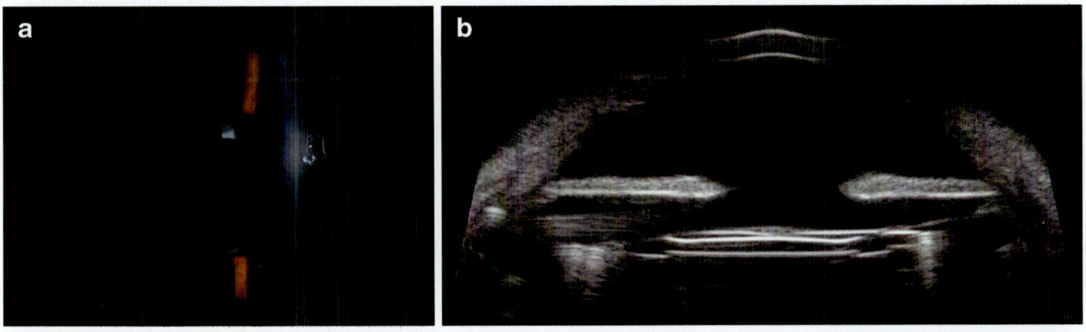

Fig. 17.8 Postoperative picture of the same patients after 3 years. (**a**) Slit examination showing fibrosis of anterior capsule and IOL in bag with no clinical tilt. (**b**) UBM of the patient showing IOL in bag with good centration and no tilt. Note the reverberations from both the edges of the IOL-bag complex caused by loop of cionni ring and CTS

Summary of glaucoma management:

- Medical management with beta blockers and miotics
- Peripheral iridotomy (relieves pupillary block)
- Lensectomy (relieves pupillary block and inverse glaucoma)
- Trabeculectomy (in recalcitrant cases)

17.1.5 Visual Rehabilitation

A major limitation to the treatment of ectopia lentis is the very high chance of amblyopia in these eyes. These eyes may already be amblyopic due to lenticular myopia (spherophakia) or uncorrected aphakia due to shifting of lens from the visual axis. A lot of cases of ectopia lentis and spherophakia may just need refractive error correction, with good improvement and maintenance of visual acuity for prolonged periods of time without any complication. Surgery is to be performed for those selected cases which do not have a chance of improvement with refractive correction or are at risk of losing vision from lens drop or glaucoma. Bilateral surgery is to be preferred in children with progressive ectopia lentis, since unilateral surgery may lead to anisometropia which has a strong amblyogenic potential. However, in cases of traumatic subluxation, unilateral surgery is unavoidable and post-surgical management of amblyopia should be given prime importance.

17.1.6 Long-Term Complications

- Amblyopia
- Glaucoma (primary or secondary)
- Lens with bag drop into the vitreous
- Retinal break development due to prolonged vitreous traction
- Retinal detachment
- Prolonged inflammation and band shaped keratopathy

17.1.7 Conclusion

Management of subluxation of lens in pediatric age group is a complex issue, with a lot of confusion in management related to severity of disease, age of patient, associated complications, and the best method of surgery and following refractive rehabilitation. In this chapter we have summarized the various approaches to surgery and the importance of a holistic management of subluxation and spherophakia eyes.

17.2 Gore-Tex Sutured One-Piece PMMA IOL

Kamal Kishore

17.2.1 General Considerations

In the absence of adequate capsular or zonular support, a scleral-sutured posterior chamber IOL is an acceptable option [35]. Ab externo technique, originally described by Lewis in 1991 is more precise and predictable compared to blind ab-interno passage of sutures and is currently the favored method for suture fixation of IOL [36]. In recent years, there is also a trend towards more posterior scleral penetration site to 2.5–3 mm from the posterior or surgical limbus to reduce the risk of optic capture, rubbing of the iris by IOL, and intraocular hemorrhage [37]. Traditionally, 10-0 polypropylene (Prolene®, Ethicon) has been employed for this purpose, but there are reports of late suture breakage of Prolene leading to dislocation of IOL, particularly in younger patients [38, 39].

Expanded polytetrafluoroethylne (ePTFE, Gore-Tex®, W.L. Gore and Associates, Newark, DE) suture is widely used for a variety of cardiac and vascular procedures due to its strength, lack of inflammation and nonabsorbable properties, but is currently off-label for ophthalmic use. Compared to other nonabsorbable materials, Gore-Tex® is soft, pliable, strong and has minimal memory allowing for easier handling and reduced risk of twisting, knotting, and breakage. The thinnest available suture size CV-8 which is approximately USP size 7-0 is a monofilament suture designed for arteriovenous fistulas and distal femoro-popliteal vascular procedures [40], and was first used off-label for scleral fixation of a posterior chamber IOL in 2012 [41]. There have been several publications of Gore-Tex fixation of a posterior chamber IOL [42–45]. The 3/8th circle 9 mm needle supplied with Gore-Tex CV-8 suture is not suitable for suture passage through the sclera for IOL fixation and needs to be cut off. Therefore, techniques involving Gore-Tex for scleral fixation of an IOL involve creation of sclerotomies in ab externo manner with a suitable instrument, such as an MVR blade [41, 43], 15° blade [46], or MIVS trocars—25 or 23 g [42, 47], followed by suture retrieval through the sclerotomy by handoff with a pair of instruments. As CV-8 Gore-Tex is thicker in diameter compared to 9-0 or 10-0 Prolene, and the suture has to be handed off to and retrieved with an instrument for passage through the sclera, relatively larger sclerotomies need to be made, usually 3–5 mm apart on each side. Therefore, unlike techniques involving Prolene, scleral flaps are not made for Gore-tex fixation. Instead, the knots are rotated into the suture track and a segment of Gore-Tex is left behind in the subconjunctival space after covering it with both Tenon's capsule and conjunctiva where it is well tolerated without any tissue reaction or inflammation.

17.2.2 Choice of IOL

The initial publications by Slade (2012), Snyder (2014) and Khan MA (2014) used a one-piece PMMA lens with eyelets on both haptics (Model CZ70BD, Alcon, Fort Worth, TX) [41, 42, 46]. This lens has an optic diameter of 7 mm and overall diameter of 12.5 mm with thin, smooth, 5° posteriorly slanted haptics and has been used extensively for suture fixation to the sclera for more than a quarter century with an excellent track record. However, it requires a relatively large 7.5 mm incision. Akreos AO 60 (Bausch and Lomb, Bridgewater, NJ), a foldable planar lens, became very popular in subsequent years due to eyelets in its four haptics ensuring a true four-point fixation [43]. However, it is made of soft hydrophilic acrylic material with a theoretical risk of cheese wiring later in life. In addition, reports of opacification of this lens from intraocular air, gas or silicone oil are a serious concern [48–50]. The overall diameter of Akreos AO60 lens is only 10.7 mm, rather short for ciliary sulcus. A foldable one-piece hydrophobic acrylic lens with an eyelet at each optic haptic junction (enVista MX60, Bausch and Lomb, Bridgewater, NJ) has been used for this purpose [47]. However, this lens has thick square haptics, not suitable for sulcus placement, and there is a recent report of eyelet fracture leading to lens dislocation following Gore-Tex fixation of enVista lens [51].

Therefore, my personal preference for scleral suturing of an IOL is for Alcon CZ70BD lens.

17.2.3 IOL Power

If sclerotomies are made 2 mm from the limbus, the lens power should be reduced by 1 diopter from "in the bag" calculation. However, if sclerotomies are placed 3 mm behind the limbus, the same power as determined for capsular bag fixation can be used [52].

17.2.4 Surgical Technique

A toric IOL marker is used to mark the cornea at 3 and 9 O'clock positions. Conjunctival peritomy is performed to provide exposure in superior 270° with relaxing incision at each end located at least one clock hour away from proposed sclerotomy sites. Hemostasis is achieved with an eraser tip ophthalmic cautery. Four marks are placed on the sclera, two on either side, 2.5 mm posterior to limbus, 4 mm apart and straddling the horizontal meridian. A 7.5 mm long scleral incision is made with a diamond blade set at 350 μm. A crescent blade or equivalent is used to create a tunnel at the base of this incision into clear cornea without entering the anterior chamber. Four 25-g valved cannulas are placed with MIVS trocars making straight entry perpendicular to the globe. A thorough vitrectomy is performed, with particular attention to the areas of previously placed cannulas. Peripheral retina is inspected, and all retinal pathologies are treated with laser. A thorough vitrectomy may reduce the risk of late retinal detachment [53].

Thereafter, a paracentesis is made with a 15° blade in inferotemporal quadrant and infusion is shifted to the anterior chamber. The superior incision is opened with a 2.75 mm keratome. The sclerotomies into which the knot will be rotated are enlarged slightly with 25 g trocar, or a 23-g MVR blade. The Gore-Tex CV-8 suture is cut in half after cutting and discarding its needles. One end of each half is introduced into the anterior chamber and retrieved through inferior sclerotomies on each side with a pair of bent 25-g vitreoretinal endgrasping forceps. The other end of both sutures is threaded through the eyelet of CZ70BD lens. After that the free end is introduced into the anterior chamber and is retrieved by transferring to the 25-g endgrasping forceps introduced through the superior sclerotomy on each side. The IOL is displaced to one side as needed for this step. Care should be taken to maintain correct orientation of sutures. A drop of OVD is placed over the lens optic and the leading haptic is introduced into the anterior chamber. An assistant removes the slack from the suture as the IOL is advanced. The leading haptic is placed behind the iris followed by the trailing haptics. The sutures are pulled on both sides. The lens should center automatically. The iris is stroked a little to ensure that the pupil is round and there is no iris root tuck. The suture is gently tied on one side with a double throw and a slip knot taking care to avoid overtightening. Knot is made permanent on the other side using 2-1-1-1 throws. The knot on the first side is also made permanent. Knots are rotated into opposite sclerotomies (one superior and one inferior). Suture is trimmed about 1 mm from the knot and ends buried into the wound. Sclerotomies are checked for wound leak and if present, closed with 7-0 vicryl suture. Usually it is not necessary.

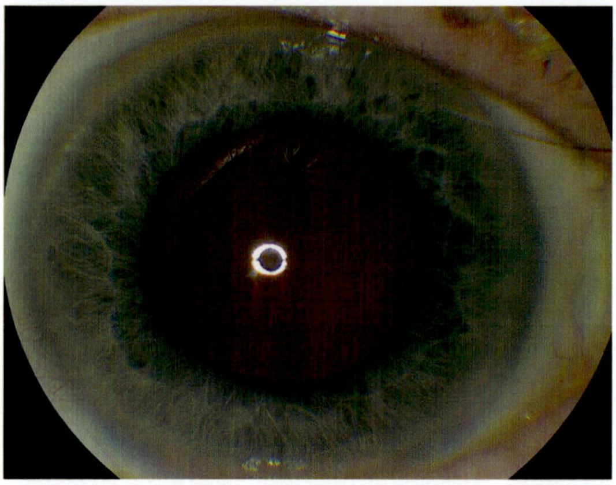

Fig. 17.9 Well-centered Gore-Tex sutured IOL

Superior incision is closed with interrupted or continuous 10-0 nylon suture. The conjunctiva is closed with multiple 7-0 vicryl sutures making sure that Gore-Tex is well covered (Fig. 17.9).

17.2.5 Dos

1. Have a vigilant assistant.
2. Maintain globe stability, avoid wound leak and hypotony.
3. Good vitrectomy especially in the regions of sclerotomies.
4. Inspect peripheral retina and treat retinal pathologies as needed.
5. Use valved cannulas for sclerotomies to minimize wound leak. I prefer 25-g as those almost never need sutured but need to be enlarged a little bit for rotating the knot. 23-g sclerotomies have also been described.
6. Anterior chamber maintainer. No need to fill the AC with an OVD.
7. Pass distal suture end first.
8. Bend 25-g end grasping forceps over a 20 mL syringe to make suture grasping easier, particularly on the nasal side.
9. Take the slack from Gore-Tex as the leading haptic is inserted into the anterior chamber and behind the iris to prevent suture entan-

glement, or the optic passing through redundant suture loop.

10. Minimize intraoperative hypotony. Consider closing the wound with one suture after the IOL has been inserted prior to tying Gore-tex and rotating the knots.
11. Use slip knot to secure first haptic before tying the knot on the other side
12. Stroke the iris with a spatula to make sure there is no tuck of the iris root. Acetylcholine (Miochol) or carachol (Miostat) can also be injected.
13. Rotate knots towards opposite sides (one superior and other inferior).
14. Rotate the knots before trimming the suture.
15. Ensure good coverage of Gore-Tex with both Tenon's and conjunctiva.

17.2.6 Don't

1. Apply excessive cautery. It causes necrosis and poor healing.
2. Use this technique in eyes with unhealthy conjunctiva from previous eye surgery, particularly scleral buckle surgery. Neither conjunctiva nor Tenon's grows over Gore-Tex and a conjunctival defect or suture exposure by conjunctival retraction is very difficult to manage later on.
3. Tie suture until both haptics have been delivered behind the iris. It is very easy to torque the lens.
4. Don't tie sutures too tight which can torque or tilt the lens.
5. Leave knot under the conjunctiva.

Financial Disclosures or Conflict of Interest None

References

1. Nelson LB, Maumenee IH. Ectopia lentis. Surv Ophthalmol. 1982;27:143–60.
2. Easty DL, Sparrow JM. Oxford textbook of ophthalmology, vol. I. Oxford: Oxford University Press; 1999. p. 708.
3. Khokhar S, Agarwal T, Kumar G, Kushmesh R, Tejwani LK. Lenticular abnormalities in children. J Pediatr Ophthalmol Strabismus. 2012;49:32–7.
4. Naeser K, Baggesen K, Knudsen EB. Retinal detachment following intracapsular cataract extraction. A 10-year follow-up study. Acta Ophthalmol Scand. 1998;76(6):727–30.
5. Sinha R, Sharma N, Vajpayee RB. Intralenticular bimanual irrigation: aspiration for subluxated lens in Marfan's syndrome. J Cataract Refract Surg. 2005;31(7):1283–6.
6. Khokhar S, Aron N, Yadav N, Pillay G, Agarwal E. Modified technique of endocapsular lens aspiration for severely subluxated lenses. Eye (Lond). 2018;32(1):128–135. https://doi.org/10.1038/eye.2017.160. Epub 2017 Aug 11. PMID: 28799565; PMCID: PMC5770709.
7. Shortt AJ, Lanigan B, O'Keefe M. Pars plana lensectomy for the management of ectopia lentis in children. J Pediatr Ophthalmol Strabismus. 2004;41:289–94.
8. Miraldi Utz V, Coussa RG, Traboulsi EI. Surgical management of lens subluxation in Marfan syndrome. J AAPOS. 2014;18:140–6.
9. Wu-Chen WY, Letson RD, Summers CG. Functional and structural outcomes following lensectomy for ectopia lentis. J AAPOS. 2005;9:353–7.
10. Hubbard AD, Charteris DG, Cooling RJ. Vitreolensectomy in Marfan's syndrome. Eye. 1998;12(Pt 3a):412–6.
11. Dehgan MH, Soleimanizad R, Ahmadieh H, Azarmina M, Sohelian M, Moradian S, et al. Outcomes of lensectomy in hereditary lens subluxation. Iran J Ophthalmic Res. 2006;1:92–5.
12. Hara T, Hara T, Yamada Y. 'Equator ring' for maintenance of the completely circular contour of the capsular bag equator after cataract removal. Ophthalmic Surg. 1991;22:358–9.
13. Cionni RJ, Osher RH. Management of zonular dialysis with endocapsular ring. J Cataract Refract Surg. 1995;21:245–9.
14. Osher R. New approach: synthetic zonules. Video J Cat Refract Surg. 1997:13.
15. Khokhar S, Pangtey MS, Sony P, Panda A. Phacoemulsification in a case of spherophakia. J Cataract Refract Surg. 2003;29:845–7.
16. Khokhar S, Gupta S, Kumar G, Rowe N. Capsular tension segment in a case of spherophakia. Cont Lens Anterior Eye. 2012;35:230–2.
17. Goel R, Kamal S, Kumar S, et al. Feasibility and complications between phacoemulsification and manual small incision surgery in subluxated cataract. J Ophthalmol. 2012;2012:205139.
18. Goel R, Kamal S, Khurana B, Kumar S, Malik KP, Bodh SA, Singh M. Manual small incision cataract surgery for subluxated cataract with lens coloboma. Cont Lens Anterior Eye. 2012;35(2):89–91. https://doi.org/10.1016/j.clae.2011.12.001. Epub 2011 Dec 30. PMID: 22209392.
19. Nagpal M, Jain P. Dropped lens fragment, dislocated intraocular lens. Dev Ophthalmol. 2014;54:234–42.

20. Chiang A, Garg SJ, Alshareef RA, et al. Removal of posterior segment retained lens material using the OZil phacoemulsification handpiece versus fragmatome during pars plana vitrectomy. Retina. 2012;32:2119–26.
21. Morrison D, Sternberg P, Donahue S. Anterior chamber intraocular lens (ACIOL) placement after pars plana lensectomy in pediatric Marfan syndrome. J AAPOS. 2005;9(3):240–2.
22. Kumar M, Arora R, Sanga L, Sota LD. Scleral-fixated intraocular lens implantation in unilateral aphakic children. Ophthalmology. 1999;106(11):2184–9.
23. Asadi R, Kheirkhah A. Long-term results of scleral fixation of posterior chamber intraocular lenses in children. Ophthalmology. 2008;115(1):67–72.
24. McAllister AS, Hirst LW. Visual outcomes and complications of scleral-fixated posterior chamber intraocular lenses. J Cataract Refract Surg. 2011;37:1263–9.
25. Lifshitz T, Levy J, Klemperer I. Artisan aphakic intraocular lens in children with subluxated crystalline lenses. J Cataract Refract Surg. 2004;30(9):1977–81.
26. Dureau P, De Laage de Meux P, Edelson C, Caputo G. Iris fixation of foldable intraocular lenses for ectopia lentis in children. J Cataract Refract Surg. 2006;32:1109–14.
27. Khokhar S, Pillay G, Sen S, et al. Clinical spectrum and surgical outcomes in spherophakia: a prospective interventional study. Eye. 2018;32(3):527–36.
28. Schechter RJ. Suture-wick endophthalmitis with sutured posterior chamber intraocular lenses. J Cataract Refract Surg. 1990;16:755–6.
29. Heilskov T, Joondeph BC, Olsen KR, Blankenship GW. Late endophthalmitis after transscleral fixation of a posterior chamber intraocular lens. Arch Ophthalmol. 1989;107:1427.
30. Gabor SG, Pavlidis MM. Sutureless intrascleral posterior chamber intraocular lens fixation. J Cataract Refract Surg. 2007;33:1851–4.
31. Scharioth GB, Prasad S, Georgalas I, Tataru C, Pavlidis M. Intermediate results of sutureless intrascleral posterior chamber intraocular lens fixation. J Cataract Refract Surg. 2010;36:254–9.
32. Subbiah S, Thomas PA, Jesudasan CAN. Scleral-fixated intraocular lens implantation in microspherophakia. Indian J Ophthalmol. 2014;62:596–600.
33. Kannan NB, Kohli P, Pangtey BPS, Ramasamy K. Evaluation of sutureless, glueless, flapless, intrascleral fixated posterior chamber intraocular lens in children with ectopia lentis. J Ophthalmol. 2018; https://doi.org/10.1155/2018/3212740.
34. Kalevar A, Dollin M, Gupta RR. Opacification of scleral-sutured Akreos AO60 intraocular lens after vitrectomy with gas tamponade: case series. Retina Cases Brief Rep 2017.
35. Wagoner MD, Cox TA, Ariyasu RG, et al. Intraocular lens implantation in the absence of capsular support: a report by the american academy of ophthalmology. Ophthalmology. 2003;110(4):840–59.
36. Lewis JS. Ab externo sulcus fixation. Ophthalmic Surg. 1991;22(11):692–5.
37. Ma DJ, Choi HJ, Kim MK, et al. Clinical comparison of ciliary sulcus and pars plana locations for posterior chamber intraocular lens transscleral fixation. J Cataract Refract Surg. 2011;37(8):1439–46.
38. Price MO, Price FW Jr, Werner L, et al. Late dislocation of scleral-sutured posterior chamber intraocular lenses. J Cataract Refract Surg. 2005;31(7):1320–6.
39. Vote BJ, Tranos P, Bunce C, et al. Long-term outcome of combined pars plana vitrectomy and scleral fixated sutured posterior chamber intraocular lens implantation. Am J Ophthalmol. 2006;141(2):308–12.
40. https://www.goremedical.com/resource/AM3020-EN3. Accessed 3 July 2020.
41. Slade DS, Hater MA, Cionni RJ, et al. Ab externo scleral fixation of intraocular lens. J Cataract Refract Surg. 2012;38(8):1316–21.
42. Khan MA, Gerstenblith AT, Dollin ML, et al. Scleral fixation of posterior chamber intraocular lenses using gore-tex suture with concurrent 23-gauge pars plana vitrectomy. Retina. 2014;34(7):1477–80.
43. Terveen DC, Fram NR, Ayres B, et al. Small-incision 4-point scleral suture fixation of a foldable hydrophilic acrylic intraocular lens in the absence of capsule support. J Cataract Refract Surg. 2016;42(2):211–6.
44. Khan MA, Gupta OP, Pendi K, et al. Pars plana vitrectomy with anterior chamber versus gore-tex sutured posterior chamber intraocular lens placement: long-term outcomes. Retina. 2019;39(5):860–6.
45. Su D, Stephens JD, Obeid A, et al. Refractive outcomes after pars plana vitrectomy and scleral fixated intraocular lens with gore-tex suture. Ophthalmol Retina. 2019;3(7):548–52.
46. Snyder ME, Perez MA. Tiltless and centration adjustable scleral-sutured posterior chamber intraocular lens. J Cataract Refract Surg. 2014;40(10):1579–83.
47. Su D, Borkar D, Gupta O. Scleral fixation of posterior chamber hydrophobic acrylic intraocular lenses using gore-tex suture. Retina. 2019;39(Suppl 1):S30–2.
48. Kalevar A, Dollin M, Gupta RR. Opacification of scleral-sutured akreos Ao60 intraocular lens after vitrectomy with gas tamponade: case series. Retin Cases Brief Rep. 2020;14(2):174–7.
49. Cao D, Zhang H, Yang C, et al. Akreos adapt AO intraocular lens opacification after vitrectomy in a diabetic patient: a case report and review of the literature. BMC Ophthalmol. 2016;16:82.
50. Rubin U, Baker CF. Akreos lens opacification under silicone oil. Can J Ophthalmol. 2018;53(5):e188–90.
51. Gupta RR, Seamone ME, Pollmann A. Dislocation of a scleral-fixated, hydrophobic, single-piece acrylic intraocular lens secondary to eyelet fracture from Gore-Tex suture. JVRD. 2019;3:395–8.
52. Botsford BW, Williams AM, Conner IP, et al. Scleral fixation of intraocular lenses with gore-tex suture: refractive outcomes and comparison of lens power formulas. Ophthalmol Retina. 2019;3(6):468–72.
53. Davies EC, Pineda R II. Complications of scleral-fixated intraocular lenses. Semin Ophthalmol. 2018;33(1):23–8.

Index

S. K. Khokhar, C. Dhull (eds.), *Essentials of Pediatric Cataract Surgery*,
https://doi.org/10.1007/978-981-16-0212-2

R